CORNEA
HANDBOOK

CORNEA HANDBOOK

WILLIAM B. TRATTLER, MD

Center for Excellence in Eye Care
Assistant Professor of Ophthalmology
University of Miami's Bascom Palmer Eye Institute
Miami, Florida

PARAG A. MAJMUDAR, MD

Mid West Eye Professionals
Palos Surgie Center
Palos Heights, IL

JODI I. LUCHS, MD, FACS

Assistant Clinical Professor of Ophthalmology and Visual Sciences
Albert Einstein College of Medicine
Bronx, NY
Director of the Department of Refractive Surgery
Long Island Jewish/North Shore University Health System
Wantagh, NY

TRACY S. SWARTZ, OD, MS

Center Director, VisionAmerica
Huntsville, AL

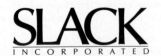

SLACK
INCORPORATED

ISBN: 978-1-55642-842-5

Published by: SLACK Incorporated
                  6900 Grove Road
                  Thorofare, NJ 08086 USA
                  Telephone: 856-848-1000
                  Fax: 856-853-5991
                  www.slackbooks.com

Contact SLACK Incorporated for more information about other books in this field or about the availability of our books from distributors outside the United States.

Library of Congress Cataloging-in-Publication Data

Cornea handbook / [edited by] William B. Trattler ... [et al.].
       p.   ; cm.
    Includes bibliographical references and index.
    ISBN 978-1-55642-842-5
  1. Cornea--Diseases--Handbooks, manuals, etc. I. Trattler, William B.
    [DNLM: 1. Corneal Diseases--Handbooks. 2. Cornea--surgery--Handbooks. WW 39 C813 2010]
    RE336.C633 2010
    617.7'19--dc22

                                                    2009041572

Last digit is print number: 10   9   8   7   6   5   4   3   2   1

DEDICATIONS

The *Cornea Handbook* shows how friends working together can make a wonderful contribution to the ophthalmic literature. I want to thank each of the chapter authors for their hard work and dedication. I would, of course, also like to thank Tracy Swartz, whose fantastic organizational skills, keen eyes, and editing abilities helped keep this project relatively on time.

I would like to thank my mentors, including Jim McCulley, MD; Wayne Bowman, MD; Steven Orlin, MD; Michael Sulewski, MD; and Nick Volpe, MD; who provided me with a solid background for advancing my understanding of corneal diseases and conditions. I would also like to thank my colleagues and staff at the Center For Excellence In Eye Care in Miami, who I have been fortunate to work with over the past 11 years. In particular, I have been lucky to practice with my father, Henry, whose love for his patients and profession showed me that we can make a positive impact on our patients' lives by understanding and treating their eye conditions.

Of course, it has been with the loving support of my wife, Jill, and my children Ali, Jeremy, and Josh that has allowed me to accomplish so much, including this book on the fundamentals of corneal diseases and conditions. Although still many years away, I am hoping my love for helping patients will pass on to my kids so that one day we may also practice together.

William B. Trattler, MD

To my wonderful wife, Brooke, without whose constant love, support, and patience I could not have completed his project,

To my children, Ethan, Evan, and Elana for constantly reminding me of the meaning of life,

To my brothers, Gregg and Scott, for their support and encouragement, and

To my father, Saul, for showing me the way.

Jodi I. Luchs, MD

To my 4 mentors, Drs. Verinder S. Nirankari and Kenneth M. Goins, who instilled in me a love for the cornea, and Drs. Richard F. Dennis and Randy J. Epstein, with whom I have had the privilege of practicing for the past 12 years.

To my father, who always encouraged me to write as a means of self-growth and continued learning.

To my wife, Dr. Sonali P. Majmudar, and my daughters Shivani and Ishani, for their unconditional love and support.

Parag A. Majmudar, MD

To Daniel, my husband, for allowing me to pursue this project, and to Jackson, Jessica, and Mackenzie, for their unconditional love and their constant reminder of my need to play.

To Doug Horner, for his support and guidance; to Michael Duplessie, for sharing his expertise; and to Ming Wang, for opening doors that lead to this project.

Tracy S. Swartz, OD, MS

CONTENTS

Dedications .... *v*

About the Editors .... *ix*

Contributing Authors .... *xi*

Preface .... *xv*

Chapter 1.   Anatomy and Physiology of the Cornea 1
             Tal Raviv, MD, FACS

Chapter 2.   Bacterial Corneal Infections 13
             David Varssano, MD

Chapter 3.   Nonbacterial Corneal Ulcers..23
             David M. Sachs, MD; Henry D. Perry, MD; and Eric D. Donnenfeld, MD

Chapter 4.   Corneal Inflammatory Disorders..37
             João Malta, MD; Fatima K. Ahmad, MD; Shahzad I. Mian, MD;
             and Alan Sugar, MD

Chapter 5.   Ocular Surface Disorders 61
             Ahmad Kheirkhah, MD; V.-K. Raju, MD, FRCS, FACS;
             and Scheffer C. G. Tseng, MD, PhD

Chapter 6.   Corneal Dystrophies...75
             Sean Pieramici, MD; Natalie Afshari, MD; and Jodi I. Luchs, MD, FACS

Chapter 7.   Corneal Ectatic Disorders...109
             J. Bradley Randleman, MD and Michelle B. Crosby, MD, PhD

Chapter 8.   Systemic and Immunologic Conditions of the Cornea.................123
             Howard A. Lane, MD, FACS and Jodi I. Luchs, MD, FACS

Chapter 9.   Metabolic and Congenital Disorders..141
             Tracy S. Swartz, OD, MS; Michael D. Duplessie, MD;
             and Jodi I. Luchs, MD, FACS

Chapter 10.   Anterior Segment Neoplasia 163
             David A. Hollander, MD, MBA

Chapter 11.   Corneal Trauma and Burns..191
             Pedram Hamrah, MD and Richard A. Eiferman, MD, FACS

Chapter 12.   Dry Eye..201
             Sanjay N. Rao, MD

Chapter 13.   Diagnostic Instrumentation 225
             Emil William Chynn, MD, MBA and Conswalla Shavers, MD

Chapter 14.   Corneal Surgery..249
             Yassine J. Daoud, MD and Terry Kim, MD

Chapter 15. Refractive Surgery 269
        Jerome Charles Ramos-Esteban, MD; Sonya Bamba, MD;
        and Ronald R. Krueger, MD

Index.. *295*

ABOUT THE EDITORS

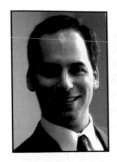

William B. Trattler, MD, is currently practicing at the Center for Excellence in Eye Care specializing in refractive, corneal, and cataract eye surgery and is a volunteer assistant professor of ophthalmology at the University of Miami's Bascom Palmer Eye Institute.

After graduating from Dartmouth College, he attended medical school at the University of Miami School of Medicine and completed his ophthalmology residency at the University of Pennsylvania, Scheie Eye Institute. He spent an additional year for subspecialty training in cornea and refractive surgery at the University of Texas Southwestern Medical Center in Dallas. During his corneal fellowship, he performed research on dry eye and blepharitis. Dr. Trattler has continued his involvement in research and has participated in numerous phase 3 and phase 4 studies in areas ranging from cataract and refractive surgery to dry eye and blepharitis.

Dr. Trattler has authored many books, articles, and textbook chapters including *Microbiology Made Ridiculously Simple*, a textbook he helped coauthor that is used by medical, nursing, and veterinary students throughout the world. In 2002, Dr. Trattler received the Outstanding Young Ophthalmologist Leadership Award from the Florida Society of Ophthalmology. In 2006, he was named one of the top 50 Cataract & Refractive Surgery Opinion Leaders, as voted on by readers of *Cataract & Refractive Surgery Today*.

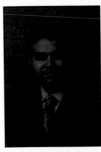

Parag A. Majmudar, MD, is a fellowship-trained corneal and refractive surgery specialist. Raised primarily in New Jersey, Dr. Majmudar graduated with a bachelor of arts degree from Lehigh University in Bethlehem, PA, as part of an accelerated honors program in medical education. While at Lehigh University, Dr. Majmudar was elected as a member of the Phi Beta Kappa National Honor Society. After receiving his degree at the Medical College of Pennsylvania in Philadelphia, where he was elected to the prestigious Alpha Omega Alpha Honor Society, Dr. Majmudar completed his ophthalmology residency at the University of Chicago. During his residency, he was elected chief resident by his teachers and peers.

He followed his residency with a subspecialty fellowship in cornea, external diseases, and refractive surgery at Rush University Medical Center in Chicago and joined Chicago Cornea Consultants, where he has been practicing since 1998. He has also maintained an academic affiliation at Rush Medical College, where he has attained the rank of associate professor of ophthalmology, and is active in the clinical and surgical education of the residents at Rush University Medical Center. He was also the codirector of the Rush University Corneal fellowship program.

Dr. Majmudar is a highly regarded international lecturer and instructor on the subjects of corneal and refractive surgery. He is also an active participant in clinical research activities. Dr. Majmudar is an active member of the American Society of Cataract and Refractive Surgery as well as the American Academy of Ophthalmology, and he recently received the Academy's Achievement Award.

He is an International Council Representative from the United States for the International Society of Refractive Surgery.

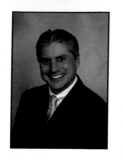

Jodi I. Luchs, MD, FACS graduated from the University of Pennsylvania in 1987 and received his MD in 1991 from the Albert Einstein College of Medicine in New York. He completed an internship at the Mount Sinai Medical Center and his ophthalmology residency at Long Island Jewish Medical Center. He was a fellow in cornea/external disease at Wills Eye Hospital. Following his training, Dr. Luchs joined South Shore Eye Care in 1996.

Dr. Luchs is the Director of the Department of Refractive Surgery for the Long Island Jewish/North Shore University Health System, where he continues to be a member of the Cornea Service. He is also an assistant clinical professor of ophthalmology and visual sciences at the Albert Einstein College of Medicine. He has numerous publications on cornea, external diseases, and refractive surgery to his credit, including one textbook, and has lectured nationally and internationally. Dr. Luchs is board certified by the American Board of Ophthalmology and a fellow of the American Academy of Ophthalmology, the American College of Surgeons, and the Nassau Academy of Medicine. He is also a member of the American Society of Cataract and Refractive Surgery as well as the International Society of Refractive Surgery.

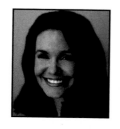

Tracy Schroeder Swartz, OD, MS, FAAO, currently serves as the Center Director of VisionAmerica in Huntsville, AL, where she practices consultative optometry, specializing in ocular surface disease and dry eye. Originally from Wisconsin, Dr. Swartz attended Indiana University School of Optometry, graduating in 1994.

After completing her doctorate, she pursued a master's degree in physiological optics, specializing in pediatrics. She served as faculty at the IU School of Optometry for 4 years and earned the Indiana chapter of the American Academy of Optometry Gordon Heath Fellowship, 1996.

After completion of her master's, she relocated to metro DC, where she specialized in refractive and corneal surgery. She later joined Wang Vision Institute in Nashville, Tenn. Here she served as Director of Clinical Operations, Residency Director for the Optometric Residency Program, and adjunct faculty to Indiana University School of Optometry. While there, she edited two textbooks with Ming Wang, MD, PhD: *Corneal Topography in the Wavefront Era* (SLACK Incorporated, Thorofare, NJ, 2006) and *Irregular Astigmatism: Diagnosis and Treatment* (SLACK Incorporated, Thorofare, NJ, 2007), as well as authoring numerous book chapters on refractive surgery, topography, aberrometry, and anterior segment disease. She served as coeditor for the literature review column for *Cataract and Refractive Surgery Today* from 2003 to 2008, and currently serves on the editorial board of *Optometry Times*. She is adjunct faculty for the School of Optometry at the University of Waterloo, and is on the board of the Optometric Council of Refractive Technology.

CONTRIBUTING AUTHORS

Fatima K. Ahmad, MD (Chapter 4)
Wills Eye Institute
Philadelphia, PA

Natalie Afshari, MD (Chapter 6)
Duke University Eye Center
Durham, NC

Sonya Bamba, MD (Chapter 15)
Louisiana State University
Department of Ophthalmology
New Orleans, LA
Formerly of the Cleveland Clinic
Cole Eye Institute
Cleveland, OH

Emil William Chynn, MD, MBA (Chapter 13)
Park Avenue Laser Vision
New York, NY

Michelle B. Crosby, MD, PhD (Chapter 7)
San Francisco, CA

Yassine J. Daoud, MD (Chapter 14)
Wilmer Eye Institute
Baltimore, MD

Eric D. Donnenfeld, MD (Chapter 3)
Ophthalmic Consultants of Long Island
Rockville Centre, NY
Clinical Professor of Ophthalmology
New York University
New York, NY
Trustee, Dartmouth Medical School
Hanover, NH

Michael D. Duplessie, MD (Chapter 9)
Bethesda, MD

Richard A. Eiferman, MD, FACS (Chapter 11)
Clinical Professor of Ophthalmology,
University of Louisville
Louisville, KY

Jerome Charles Ramos-Esteban, MD (Chapter 15)
Cleveland Clinic
Cole Eye Institute
Cleveland, OH

Pedram Hamrah, MD (Chapter 11)
Instructor, Department of
Ophthalmology
Director, Ocular Surface Imaging
Center
Attending Physician, Cornea and
Refractive Surgery
Massachusetts Eye & Ear Infirmary
Harvard Medical School
Boston, MA

David A. Hollander, MD, MBA (Chapter 10)
Assistant Clinical Professor of
Ophthalmology
Jules Stein Eye Institute
David Geffen School of Medicine at
UCLA
Greater Los Angeles VA Medical
Center
Los Angeles, CA

Ahmad Kheirkhah, MD (Chapter 5)
Ocular Surface Center
Miami, FL

Terry Kim, MD (Chapter 14)
Associate Professor of Ophthalmology
Cornea and Refractive Surgery
Duke University Eye Center
Durham, NC

Ronald R. Krueger, MD (Chapter 15)
Medical Director of Refractive Surgery
Cole Eye Institute
Professor of Ophthalmology
Cleveland Clinic
Lerner College of Medicine
Cleveland, OH

Howard A. Lane, MD, FACS (Chapter 8)
Cornea Service, Department of
Ophthalmology
North Shore University/Long Island
Jewish Health System
Manhasset, NY
Partner, South Shore Eye Care, LLP
Wantagh, NY and Massapequa, NY

João Malta, MD (Chapter 4)
W.K. Kellogg Eye Center, Department
of Ophthalmology and Visual
Sciences, University of Michigan
Ann Arbor, MI
Department of Ophthalmology,
Division of Cornea and External
Disease
Santa Casa de São Paulo,
São Paulo, Brazil

Shahzad I. Mian, MD (Chapter 4)
W.K. Kellogg Eye Center, Department
of Ophthalmology and Visual Sciences
University of Michigan
Ann Arbor, MI

Henry D. Perry, MD (Chapter 3)
Senior Founding Partner,
Ophthalmic Consultants of Long Island
Rockville Centre, NY
Medical Director,
Lions Eye Bank for Long Island
Manhasset, NY
Chief Cornea Service,
Nassau University Medical Center
East Meadow, NY

Sean Pieramici, MD (Chapter 6)
Milauskas Eye Institute
Rancho Mirage, CA

V.-K. Raju, MD, FRCS, FACS (Chapter 5)
Clinical Professor, Department of
Ophthalmology
West Virginia University
Medical Director, Eye Foundation of
America
Morgantown, WV

J. Bradley Randleman, MD (Chapter 7)
Associate Professor, Ophthalmology
Emory University School of Medicine
Emory Eye Center and Emory Vision
Atlanta, GA

Sanjay N. Rao, MD (Chapter 12)
Director, Cornea and Refractive
Surgery
Lakeside Eye Clinic, Inc.
Chicago, IL

Tal Raviv, MD, FACS (Chapter 1)
Assistant Professor of Ophthalmology
New York Medical College
Valhalla, NY
Adjunct Surgeon, Cornea Service and
Cataract Surgery Attending,
New York Eye and Ear Infirmary
Founding Partner, New York Laser Eye,
LLP
Private Practice
New York, NY

David M. Sachs, MD (Chapter 3)
Ophthalmic Consultants of Long
Island
Nassau University Medical Center
East Meadow, NY

Conswalla Shavers, MD (Chapter 13)
Bear, DE

Alan Sugar, MD (Chapter 4)
Professor of Ophthalmology &
Visual Sciences
W.K. Kellogg Eye Center,
University of Michigan Medical School
Ann Arbor, MI

Scheffer C. G. Tseng, MD, PhD, (Chapter 5)
Director, Ocular Surface Center
Medical Director, Ocular Surface
Research & Education Foundation
Director, Research & Development
Department
TissueTech, Inc.
Miami, FL

David Varssano, MD (Chapter 2)
Department of Ophthalmology
Tel Aviv Medical Center
Tel Aviv, Israel

PREFACE

Cornea Handbook was designed to provide our readers with a handy reference of up-to-date core information on important topics in cornea, external diseases, as well as corneal and refractive surgery. While there is a tendency when writing a textbook of this kind to become encyclopedic and include as much technical information as possible, it was our goal to include only the most clinically relevant information in an easily readable format. Accordingly, while this is not a comprehensive textbook encompassing all of cornea, external disease, and refractive surgery, it is a comprehensive collection of the essential conditions, their pathophysiology, clinical findings and treatments, as well as just the right amount of background information to provide an understanding of the condition. In this way, we hope to provide our readers with easy access to the important clinical points that will enhance their ophthalmic practice.

We have enlisted the expertise of well-recognized experts in cornea, external disease, and refractive surgery as contributing authors for each of the chapters in this text in order to bring the most up-to-date information to our readers. In addition, we have included a large number of color photographs throughout the text in order highlight the clinical findings in many important conditions.

While this textbook is organized in a similar fashion to a comprehensive anterior segment textbook—beginning with anatomy and physiology and concluding with anterior segment and refractive surgery—each chapter can be read individually. This text is suitable both for those beginning residency as well as clinicians already in practice.

Finally, we would like to acknowledge that none of us would have been able to complete this project without the tremendous support of our families at home. We are continually grateful for all of their love and encouragement, without which we would not have been able to deliver a product of this caliber. We hope that you enjoy reading and learning from it as much as we enjoyed putting it all together.

William B. Trattler, MD
Parag A. Majmudar, MD
Jodi I. Luchs, MD
Tracy S. Swartz, OD, MS

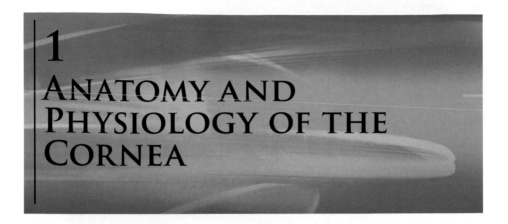

1
ANATOMY AND PHYSIOLOGY OF THE CORNEA

Tal Raviv, MD, FACS

The human cornea is a unique anatomical structure whose combination of form and function serves two critical roles: providing the primary refractive surface of the eye and protecting the intraocular contents from the environment and pathogens.

The cornea is an avascular tissue primarily composed of connective tissue stroma. Together with the contiguous limbus and sclera, it forms the outer shell of the eyeball. The mechanical strength of the stroma is provided by fibrous collagen, whose precise architecture in the cornea is critical for tissue transparency.

Maintenance of corneal shape and transparency are critical for refraction. Many components and processes work together to accomplish this, including properly functioning epithelium and endothelium, regulation of stromal hydration, and healthy interaction between structural components such as collagen and proteoglycans. Any disturbance to these processes through disease, trauma, or surgery may lead to corneal opacity, edema, and, ultimately, loss of transparency.

This chapter will review the fundamental structural and physiological processes of the cornea in order to provide a basis for the normal corneal condition as well as its pathophysiology.

GROSS ANATOMY

The cornea measures 11 to 12 mm horizontally and 9 to 11 mm vertically. It is approximately 0.5 mm thick centrally and up to 0.7 mm thick peripherally.[1] The refractive power of the cornea comes from the central 3 mm of the cornea where the surface is almost spherical, averages between 40 to 44 diopters, and comprises about two thirds of the eye's total refractive power.

The cornea is composed of an outer stratified squamous nonkeratinized epithelium, an acellular Bowman's layer, an inner connective tissue stroma with its resident keratocytes, Descemet's membrane, and a cuboidal monolayered endothelium (Figure 1-1). Devoid of vascularization, the cornea is bathed in tears anteriorly and aqueous humor posteriorly.

Trattler WB, Majmudar PA, Luchs JI, Swartz TS, eds.
Cornea Handbook (pp. 1-12)
© 2010 SLACK Incorporated

Figure 1-1. Corneal anatomy. Epithelium (A) composed of basal cells (E), wing cells (D), and squamous cells (C); Bowman's membrane (B); stroma (F); Descemet's membrane (G); and endothelium (H). (Image courtesy of Heidelberg Engineering, Gerhart, Germany.)

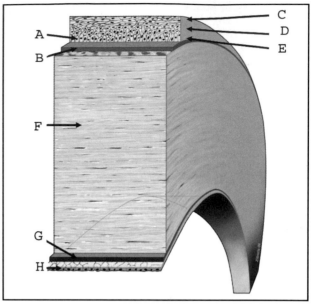

The cornea also receives support from the surrounding limbus and conjunctiva, as well as the adnexa, including the eyelids and associated glands. In harmony, these components ensure a smooth functioning ocular surface.

CORNEAL EPITHELIUM

The corneal epithelium has certain functions typical of other bodily epithelia, namely, as a diffusion barrier to water and solutes and a mechanical barrier to microorganisms (Figure 1-2). But unlike other epithelia of its type, it is specialized to function over an avascular stroma. Furthermore, it is unique in creating a smooth, transparent optical surface critical for refracting light. It also is one of the most densely innervated parts of the body, which is believed to help with a rapid wound-healing response.

The nonkeratinized, stratified squamous corneal epithelium has 5 to 7 layers of cells and is 50 to 52 µm thick (10% of the corneal thickness). In the healthy cornea, the thickness is uniform throughout. However, in response to stromal thinning conditions, such as following herpes simplex virus (HSV) keratitis or excimer laser ablation, the epithelium has tremendous ability to thicken by hyperplasia, thereby maintaining the smoothness of the surface.[2]

Epithelial cells can be morphologically divided into 3 groups: an inner single layer of columnar basal cells (Figure 1-3); 1 to 3 layers of wing cells (Figure 1-4); and 2 to 4 outer, flattened squamous cells (Figure 1-5). Only the basal cells are mitotically active, with each daughter cell differentiating and moving apically to become a wing cell and then a squamous surface cell before sloughing off into the tear film. This process normally takes about 7 to 14 days.[3]

The epithelial cells tightly adhere to each other and to their basement membrane through intercellular specialized junctional complexes. These include tight junctions, desmosomes or hemidesmosomes, and gap junctions. Associated with these adhesion complexes is the intracellular cytoskeleton composed of 3 types

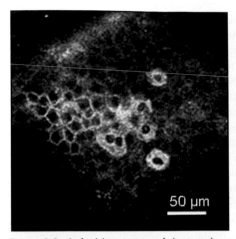

Figure 1-2. Confocal laser imaging of the corneal surface. (Image courtesy of Heidelberg Engineering, Gerhart, Germany.)

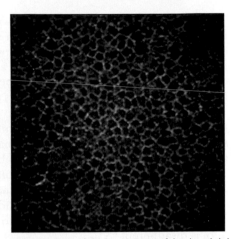

Figure 1-3. Confocal laser imaging of basal epithelial cells. (Image courtesy of Heidelberg Engineering, Gerhart, Germany.)

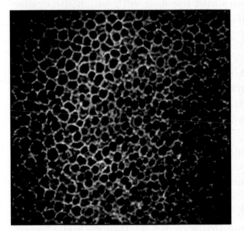

Figure 1-4. Confocal laser imaging of intermediate wing cells. (Image courtesy of Heidelberg Engineering, Gerhart, Germany.)

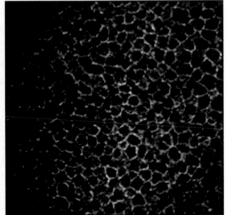

Figure 1-5. Confocal laser imaging of surface epithelium. (Image courtesy of Heidelberg Engineering, Gerhart, Germany.)

of protein filaments: intermediate filaments (composed of keratins), actin filaments, and microtubules. These elements contribute to the shape and motility of the epithelial cells.

Basal Cells

Basal cells are comprised of a single layer of columnar cells that adhere to their basement membrane. Like epithelia in other parts of the body, the basal cells secrete most of the components of their basement membrane. Its major components are type IV collagen and laminin. The basement membrane serves to maintain the polarity of the epithelial cells, provide a matrix for epithelial migration and structure (ie, during wound healing), and separate the epithelium from the stroma.

The basal cells give rise to daughter wing cells through mitosis and are in turn replenished by centripetal movement of stem cells in the basal layer of the limbal epithelium. The basal cells are differentiated from the limbal stem cells by the expression of a major keratin pair K12 and K3, believed to be important in handling trauma. A mutation in these corneal keratins leads to Meesmann's corneal dystrophy, with resultant epithelial cysts and fragility.[4]

Basal cells adhere to the basement membrane and the underlying stroma through anchoring complexes containing hemidesmosomes. The hemidesmosomes from the cytoplasmic side of the basal cell membrane connect to anchoring filaments that cross the basement membrane to coalesce with anchoring fibrils. The fibrils are composed of type VII collagen and terminate in the anterior 1 to 2 μm of stroma in structures called *anchoring plaques*.[5] These anchoring complexes are critical to epithelial stromal adhesion. In epidermolysis bullosa acquisita, a blistering disease with autoimmunity to type VII collagen, all stratified epithelium is disadherent.[6]

Altered epithelial basement membrane interactions are also found in the diabetic cornea. Studies have shown a lower density of desmosomes[7] and shorter anchoring fibrils[8] in diabetics. This is the basis for the increased preponderance of recurrent erosion syndrome in diabetics and the ease with which the epithelium is disrupted in diabetic patients during vitrectomy.

Wing Cells

These 1 to 3 layers of polygonal cells represent an intermediate state of differentiation between basal cells to superficial cells. The cells are characterized by abundant intracellular keratin tonofilaments. The cell membranes of adjacent wing cells and basal cells interdigitate and are connected by numerous desmosomes and gap junctions.

Desmosomes (maculae adherents) tightly connect cells, allowing minimal fluid to pass through. So firm are these connections that frequently epithelium sloughs off as a sheet in conditions such as bullous keratopathy or recurrent corneal erosions.

Gap junctions are channels formed between 2 cells' apposing plasma membranes. They allow for intercellular communication and are thought to be important for cell differentiation and migration. These junctions also act to electrically couple the cells so they operate as a syncytium to affect transepithelial ion transport.[9]

Squamous Cells

As the cells move apically from the basal and wing layer, they become terminally differentiated into 2 to 3 layers of flat squamous surface cells. These cells are characterized by a smaller size and fewer organelles than the other epithelial cells. As the outermost corneal layer, squamous cells have a specialized apical surface geared to maintaining the precorneal tear film and mucous layer. This tear-cornea interface represents the primary refracting surface of the eye and requires an extraordinarily smooth corneal surface.

Surface ridge-like folds in the apical membrane, called *microplicae*, and small fingerlike projections termed *microvilli*, serve to increase the surface area of each cell and thereby allow for better oxygen uptake and tear film adhesion.

The apical membrane also contains numerous glycoprotein and glycolipid molecules, collectively termed the *glycocalyx*. By virtue of the numerous oligosaccharide side chains in the glycocalyx, the membrane is conferred hydrophilic properties, which allows for intimate interaction with the mucinous layer of the tear film and maximum tear stability.

The squamous cells are tightly connected through numerous zonula occludens, or tight junctions. These junctions comprise an important intercellular barrier impenetrable to microorganisms and virtually impermeable to fluid, electrolytes, or other macromolecules. This prevents net flow of tear fluid into the stroma and forces material to flow through cells where it can be controlled. Because necessary nutrients are also excluded, these must be obtained through the aqueous.

STROMA

The stroma comprises about 90% of the corneal thickness and includes both Bowman's layer and the lamellar stroma. It is unique among the body's connective tissues because it is highly organized and transparent. In addition to its function in transmitting light, its tensile strength and contiguity with the sclera ensure a rigid framework for maintaining intraocular pressure (IOP), corneal curvature, and thus optical alignment.[10]

Bowman's Layer

This acellular region of densely woven collagen fibrils is considered to be the anterior portion of the stroma. Its collagen fibers differ from those of the corneal stroma in that they are randomly organized and of smaller diameter.[11]

The function of Bowman's is unknown. It may be responsible for maintaining epithelial uniformity, keeping optical stability, or for physically separating the active microenvironment of the epithelial cells from the keratocytes. Another theory is that Bowman's is a remnant derived from epithelia–stromal interactions during embryologic development.[12] Bowman's layer does not regenerate after injury.

Many mammals' corneas have no Bowman's layer yet maintain their corneal stability. Furthermore, the lack of any significant complications in the millions of people who are devoid of Bowman's layer following photorefractive keratectomy implies that it serves a less than critical role.

Stromal Components

Structurally, the stroma is composed almost entirely of extracellular matrix (ECM) components—predominantly collagen fibrils running parallel to the corneal surface separated by their associated proteoglycans (Figures 1-6 and 1-7). These matrix components are secreted and maintained by stromal fibroblasts, termed *keratocytes*, which reside between the lamellae. The cells comprise only about 10% of the stromal volume.[13]

Stromal keratocytes are long and flat, with many filopodial processes that interconnect to other keratocytes by gap junctions. The keratocytes form a syncytium and can coordinate healing activities and differentiation after injury. They are believed to be in a quiescent state in the normal cornea but can be activated after trauma or infection[14] and induced to synthesize ECM-degrading enzymes such as

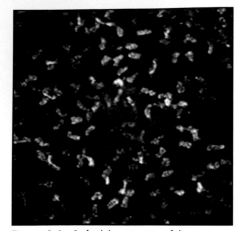

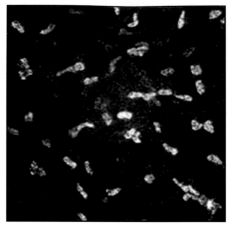

Figure 1-6. Confocal laser imaging of keratocytes in anterior stroma. (Image courtesy of Heidelberg Engineering, Gerhart, Germany.)

Figure 1-7. Confocal laser imaging of keratocytes in posterior stroma. (Image courtesy of Heidelberg Engineering, Gerhart, Germany.)

matrix metalloproteinases. The cells can also differentiate into myofibroblasts, as may occur following surface excimer ablation, creating the clinical appearance of subepithelial reticular haze.[15]

The stromal ECM's transparency is believed to be due to the uniquely regular alignment of its collagen fibrils. Interfiber distance is highly uniform (41.4 nm),[16] as is the consistent diameter of the corneal collagen (22.5 to 35 nm),[17] much smaller and more homogeneous than in other tissues. The regulation of this is believed to be related to the types and quantity of collagen present as well as its interaction with the major corneal proteoglycans, keratan sulfate and chondroitin/dermatan sulfate.

Of the 21 types of collagen found in the human body, the cornea has at least 11. The most predominant are the fibrillar collagens type I and type V. Type V collagen usually comprises 5% of other body connective tissue but makes up 15% to 20% of corneal collagen. Its interaction with type I collagen has been shown to limit the fibril diameter by 50%.[18]

The proteoglycans consist of a core protein and an associated glycosaminoglycan (GAG) side chain. The corneal proteoglycans were initially identified and named by their GAG carbohydrate side chains (also known as mucopolysaccharides) and more recently by their core proteins. The stromal GAGs are comprised of 65% keratan sulfate and 30% chondroitin/dermatan sulfate. Chondroitin/dermatan sulfate's primary core proteins are decorin and biglycan. The primary core proteins in keratan sulfate are lumican, keratocan, mimecan/osteoglycan, and fibromodulin.[19] Only keratocan is unique to the cornea.[20]

The proteoglycans serve to maintain the ordered spacing of the collagen fibrils and to modulate fibrillogenesis by limiting fibril size. A mutation in keratocan has been shown to cause cornea plana,[21] a condition of marked corneal flatness. Furthermore, the polyanionic GAG side chains are able to bind water molecules and account for the stroma's water-holding capacity. Thus, proteoglycans' central role in collagen fibrillogenesis and hydration is critical in maintaining corneal transparency.

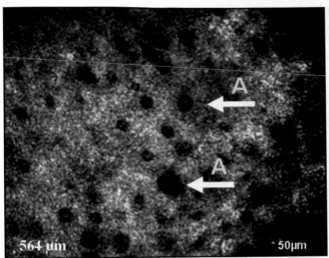

Figure 1-8. Confocal laser imaging of excrescences of Descemet's membrane in Fuchs' dystrophy.

Descemet's Membrane

The corneal endothelium rests on, and is separated from, the posterior stroma by its basement membrane, termed *Descemet's membrane*. This acellular layer, composed primarily of collagen type IV,[22] laminin, and fibronectin, is secreted by the endothelial cells and progressively thickens with age. In the adult eye it can reach up to 10 to 15 μm thick, making it one of the thickest basement membranes in the body.[23]

The collagen fibers in the stroma are not continuous with those in Descemet's as they are with Bowman's layer. This is evident in cataract surgery by the ease with which Descemet's can be detached by shearing force and is taken advantage of for lamellar surgeries such as deep anterior lamellar keratoplasty (DALK) and Descemet's stripping endothelial keratoplasty (DSEK). Furthermore, Descemet's is quite resistant to enzymatic proteolysis following corneal ulceration or other melting corneal disease and can remain intact as a bulging descemetocele.

In Fuchs' dystrophy, abnormal endothelial secretion leads to a thickened Descemet's with posterior excrescences known as *guttae* (Figure 1-8). By protruding into the endothelium, these focal thickenings are associated with thinning and enlargement of the overlying cells.

ENDOTHELIUM

The corneal endothelium is comprised of a single row of cells that form the cornea's posterior interface with the aqueous humor (Figure 1-9). The monolayer is composed of a regularly sized mosaic of polygonal cells (mostly hexagonal) whose principal role is regulating the water content of the corneal stroma.

Corneal endothelial cells do not substantially replicate in humans and therefore slowly decrease in density at a rate of 0.6% per year in the healthy cornea.[24] In adults the average cell density ranges from 2500 to 3000 cells/mm². As endothelial cells are lost, either by age, disease, or trauma, adjacent cells increase in size and spread to cover the defective area. Over time, this process leads to variability in the mean cell area (*polymegathism*) as well as a decrease in the number of regularly

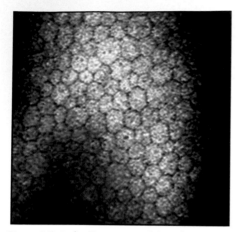

Figure 1-9. Confocal laser imaging of the endothelium in a healthy cornea. (Image courtesy of Heidelberg Engineering, Gerhart, Germany.)

shaped hexagonal cells (*pleomorphism*). Quantifying these characteristics clinically by specular microscopy can help assess endothelial health.

Structurally, endothelial cells have numerous organelles such as mitochondria, smooth and rough endoplasmic reticulums, and Golgi apparatus, indicative of the significant metabolic and secretory function of these cells. The apical surface is lined with microvilli and larger folds that increase the absorptive surface area with the aqueous.

The endothelial cells attach to each other through various interdigitations and junctional complexes in their lateral membranes but more of the macula occludens type than zonula occludens. By not completely encircling the cells,[25] as they do in the epithelium, these tight junctions form a more porous barrier to the aqueous humor. Also in the basolateral membrane reside the numerous ionic pumps responsible for corneal deturgescence. All of these structures are critical in the endothelium's dual role as nutrition gateway and hydration regulator.

CORNEAL NUTRITION

The high metabolic activities of the endothelium and epithelium require a constant supply of glucose and oxygen, in addition to other nutrients. Due to its avascular nature, the cornea relies on the tear film and aqueous for its nutritional needs.

With a restrictive epithelial barrier, the cornea obtains its supply of glucose, amino acids, vitamins, and other nutrients from the aqueous humor. The cornea is very sensitive to the aqueous's ionic concentration, osmolalities, and pH. In the early days of phacoemulsification, one of the reasons for the significant corneal edema was "incomplete" intraocular irrigating solutions, which lacked critical ions, proper buffering, antioxidants, or a sugar source.

Oxygen, conversely, is mostly supplied by diffusion from the atmosphere via the tear film. Any limitation between the air and the tear film, such as a contact lens, can disrupt the corneal oxygen supply with resultant hypoxia and edema.[26] During sleep, oxygen is delivered by the highly vascularized palpebral conjunctiva, albeit at a lower level (PO_2 of 8% versus 21% with the eyelid open[27]). As most clinicians can attest, the not infrequent combination of contact lens and overnight wear is an ideal setup for corneal edema and infectious keratitis.

REGULATION OF STROMAL HYDRATION AND TRANSPARENCY

Ideally, the human cornea maintains a 78% hydration level[28]; any major deviation can lead to corneal opacity. This constant is maintained primarily by the membrane properties of the endothelium and epithelium and the fluid flow characteristics of the stroma.

The cornea has an inherent tendency to imbibe water and swell. Stromal proteoglycans associated with collagen bind water and create a strong inward pressure gradient called the *swelling pressure*. The epithelium and endothelium, via a combination of barrier functions and active ion transport, act together to counteract this swelling pressure and prevent net fluid flow into the cornea.

Epithelial Regulation

The stratified epithelium, with its hydrophobic apical cell membrane and band-like tight junctions, acts principally as an impervious barrier to fluid flow from the tear film. The clinical application of fluorescein, an anionic molecule, illustrates this barrier function of intact epithelium. Visualization of fluorescein penetration into the stroma due to any host of pathologic conditions provides a measure of the barrier function.[29] In addition to its barrier function, the epithelium also maintains active transport systems, but they account for a very small part of active corneal hydration homeostasis.[30]

Evaporation can play a role in epithelial hydration. In the open eye, evaporation leads to a slightly hypertonic tear film, which can draw fluid from the cornea. This may account for the 5% increase in corneal thickness during sleep. In the borderline cornea, evaporation can be a factor in maintaining epithelial dehydration, as is seen in the diurnal variation of vision in early Fuchs' patients.

Endothelial Regulation

The endothelium is the prime structure in corneal hydration regulation—mostly through its ionic pumps but also with its barrier function. Though endothelial cells have a relatively "leaky" barrier, which allows for paracellular percolation of nutrient rich fluid, they are still 10 times more resistant to fluid flow than the stroma itself.[31]

The cells' ionic metabolic pumps, such as Na^+/K^+-ATPase and others, use energy-dependent active transport to secrete solute (such as bicarbonate[32] and sodium ions) into the aqueous humor. Water then passively follows the local osmotic gradient with net flow from stroma to aqueous. An osmotic gradient of only 2 to 3 mOsm needs to be maintained to preserve a balance.[33] Other recent experiments add to this transcellular transport theory and point to a role of paracellular fluid transport driven by electroosmotic coupling.[34]

Equilibrium between the active metabolic "pump" and the passive "leak" of solute and fluid across the semipermeable endothelium must be maintained to keep the stroma relatively dehydrated and transparent.

Corneal Edema

If the epithelium and endothelium are stripped from a cornea in vitro, the stroma will imbibe water and swell to about twice its normal size. Likewise, any disturbance, whether via trauma or disease, in the cornea's protective membranes often leads to corneal edema.

Endothelial dysfunction can occur acutely in surgical trauma or chronically in diseases such as Fuchs' dystrophy. In acute settings, initial corneal edema can be cleared as the endothelial function is restored. In chronic settings, as the

Figure 1-10. Bullous keratopathy. (Courtesy of Tracy S. Swartz, OD, MS.)

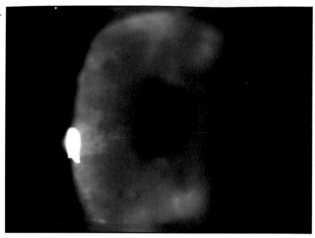

endothelial cells decrease in number and fall below a critical threshold, despite increased production of pump sites per cell, stromal dehydration can no longer be maintained and the cornea gradually swells.

Extra intrastromal fluid stretches and disorganizes the cornea's regular collagen alignment, decreasing transparency and causing opacity. Because the cornea can only expand posteriorly in size, swelling leads to folds in Descemet's membrane, clinically visible as striae.

In addition to stromal edema, epithelial edema can result from endothelial dysfunction as well as elevated IOP. In these scenarios, forward movement of stromal fluid and aqueous becomes trapped by the otherwise healthy epithelium. Fluid accumulates extracellularly in potential spaces between the basal epithelial cells and is clinically visible as microcystic edema. With prolonged edema, larger bullae develop as seen in bullous keratopathy (Figure 1-10).

Different IOP and endothelial function combinations can lead to edema. High IOP and normal endothelium as in acute angle closure glaucoma, or even normal IOP in Fuchs', are both sufficient. However, some IOP is necessary as the driving force for epithelial edema because it is not seen in phthisis, no matter how sick the endothelium or thick the stroma.[35]

A different type of reversible epithelial edema occurs with abusive contact lens wear. This is believed to be due to hypoxia or lactate buildup causing osmolar changes and intracellular (rather than extracellular) fluid buildup.[36]

CONCLUSION

The cornea's unique anatomic structure along with its specific physiologic functions allows it to excel as the transparent protective refractive surface of the eye. In the upcoming chapters, different pathologies and pathophysiologies of the cornea will be examined; most will have a deleterious effect on the cornea's hydration management, structural integrity, or ultimately its transparency. Our medical and surgical treatments to restore corneal transparency and, more recently, to refractively enhance the cornea will be explored.

Financial disclosure: Dr. Raviv is a speaker for Alcon, ISTA Pharmaceuticals, and Bausch & Lomb.

REFERENCES

1. Mishima S. Corneal thickness. *Surv Ophthalmol.* 1968;13(2):57-96.

2. Hanna KD, Pouliquen Y, Waring GO III. Corneal stromal wound healing in rabbits after 193-nm excimer laser surface ablation. *Arch Ophthalmol.* 1989;107:895-901.

3. Hanna C, Bicknell DS, O'Brien JE. Cell turnover in the adult human eye. *Arch Ophthalmol.* 1961;65:695-698.

4. Irvine AD, Corden LD, Swensson O, et al. Mutations in cornea-specific keratin K3 or K12 genes cause Meesmann's corneal dystrophy. *Nat Genet.* 1997;16:184-187.

5. Gipson IK, Spurr-Michaud S, Tisdale A, Keough M. Reassembly of the anchoring structures of the corneal epithelium during wound repair in the rabbit. *Invest Ophthalmol Vis Sci.* 1989; 30:425-434.

6. Woodley DT, Sarret Y, Briggaman RA. Autoimmunity to type VII collagen. *Semin Dermatol.* 1991;10:232-239.

7. Azar DT, Spurr-Michaud SJ, Tisdale AS, Gipson IK. Altered epithelial-basement membrane interactions in diabetic corneas. *Arch Ophthalmol.* 1992;110:537-540.

8. Azar DT, Spurr-Michaud SJ, Tisdale AS, Gipson IK. Decreased penetration of anchoring fibrils into the diabetic stroma. A morphometric analysis. *Arch Ophthalmol.* 1989;107:1520-1523.

9. Laux-Fenton WT, Donaldson PJ, Kistler J, Green CR. Connexin expression patterns in the rat cornea: molecular evidence for communication compartments. *Cornea.* 2003;22:457-464.

10. Gipson IK, Joyce NC, Zieske JD. The anatomy and cell biology of the human cornea, limbus, conjunctiva, and adnexa. In: Foster CS, Azar DT, Dohlman CH, eds. *Smolin and Thoft's The Cornea: Scientific Foundations and Clinical Practice.* Philadelphia, PA: Lippincott Williams & Wilkins; 2005:1-35.

11. Nishida T. Cornea. In: Krachmer J, Mannis M, Holland E, eds. *Cornea.* Philadelphia, PA: Elsevier Mosby; 2005:3-26.

12. Wilson SE, Hong JW. Bowman's layer structure and function: critical or dispensable to corneal function? A hypothesis. *Cornea.* 2000;19:417-420.

13. Edelhauser HF, Ubels JL. The cornea and the sclera. In: Kaufman PL, Alm A, eds. *Adler's Physiology of the Eye.* St. Louis, MO: Elsevier Mosby; 2003:47-114.

14. Li Q, Fukuda K, Lu Y, et al. Enhancement by neutrophils of collagen degradation by corneal fibroblasts. *J Leukoc Biol.* 2003;74:412-419.

15. Netto MV, Mohan RR, Sinha S, Sharma A, Dupps W, Wilson SE. Stromal haze, myofibroblasts, and surface irregularity after PRK. *Exp Eye Res.* 2006;82:788-797.

16. Hamada R, Pouliquen Y, Giraud JP, et al. Quantitative analysis on the ultrastructure of human fetal cornea. In Yamada E, Mishima S, eds. *The Structure of the Eye III.* Tokyo: Jpn J Ophthalmol; 1976:49-62.

17. Komai Y, Ushiki T. The three-dimensional organization of collagen fibrils in the human cornea and sclera, *Invest Ophthalmol Vis Sci.* 1991;32:2244-2258.

18. Birk DE. Type V collagen: heterotypic type I/V collagen interactions in the regulation of fibril assembly. *Micron.* 2001;32:223-237.

19. Tanihara H, Inatani M, Koga T, Yano T, Kimura A. Proteoglycans in the eye. *Cornea.* 2002; 21(suppl):62-69.

20. Corpuz LM, Funderburgh JL, Funderburgh ML, Bottomley GS, Prakash S, Conrad GW. Molecular cloning and tissue distribution of keratocan. Bovine corneal keratan sulfate proteoglycan 37A. *J Biol Chem.* 1996;271:9759-9763.

21. Pellegata NS, Dieguez-Lucenta JL, Joensuu T, et al. Mutations in KERA, encoding keratocan, cause cornea plana. *Nat Genet.* 2000;25:91.

22. Fitch JM, Birk DE, Linsenmayer C, Linsenmayer TF. The spatial organization of Descemet's membrane-associated type IV collagen in the avian cornea. *J Cell Biol.* 1990;110:1457-1468.

23. Gipson IK, Joyce NC. Anatomy and cell biology of the cornea, superficial limbus, and conjunctiva. In: Albert DM, Jakobiec FA, eds. *Principles and Practice of Ophthalmology.* Philadelphia, PA: W.B. Saunders; 2000:612-629.

24. Bourne WM, Nelson LR, Hodge DO. Central corneal endothelial cell changes over a ten-year period. *Invest Ophthalmol Vis Sci.* 1997;38:779-782.

25. McLaughlin BJ, Caldwell RB, Sasaki Y, Wood TO. Freeze-fracture quantitative comparison of rabbit corneal epithelial and endothelial membranes. *Curr Eye Res.* 1985;4:951-961.

26. Holden BA, Sweeney DF, Vannas A, et al. Effects of long-term extended contact lens wear on the human cornea. *Invest Ophthalmol Vis Sci.* 1985;26:1489-1501.

27. Efron N, Carney LG. Oxygen levels beneath the closed eyelid. *Invest Ophthalmol Vis Sci.* 1979;18:93-95.

28. Edelhauser HF. The balance between corneal transparency and edema. *Invest Ophthalmol Vis Sci.* 2006;47:1755-1767.

29. Yokoi N, Kinoshita S. Clinical evaluation of corneal epithelial barrier function with the slit-lamp fluorophotometer. *Cornea.* 1995;14:485-489.

30. Klyce SD. Transport of Na, Cl, and water by the rabbit corneal epithelium at resting potential. *Am J Physiol.* 1975;228:1446.

31. Arffa RC. *Grayson's Diseases of the Cornea.* St. Louis, MO: Mosby; 1997.

32. Hodson S, Miller F. The bicarbonate ion pump in the endothelium which regulates the hydration of rabbit cornea. *J Physiol.* 1976;263:563-577.

33. Klyce SD. Corneal physiology. In: Foster CS, Azar DT, Dohlman CH, eds. *Smolin and Thoft's The Cornea Scientific Foundations and Clinical Practice.* Philadelphia, PA: Lippincott Williams & Wilkins; 2005:37-58.

34. Diecke FP, Ma L, Iserovich P, Fischbarg J. Corneal endothelium transports fluid in the absence of net solute transport. *Biochim Biophys Acta.* 2007;1768:2043-2048.

35. Dohlman CH, Klyce SD. Corneal edema. In: Albert DM, Jakobiec FA, eds. *Principles and Practice of Ophthalmology.* Philadelphia, PA: W.B. Saunders; 2000:646-657.

36. Klyce SD. Stromal lactate accumulation can account for corneal oedema osmotically following epithelial hypoxia in the rabbit. *J Physiol.* 1981;321:49-64.

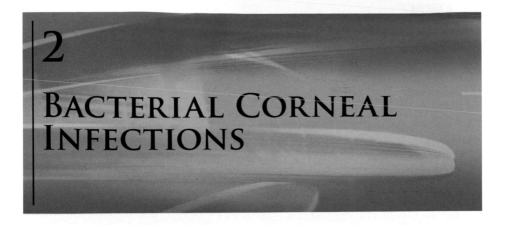

2

BACTERIAL CORNEAL INFECTIONS

David Varssano, MD

Corneal infections can be caused by viruses, fungi, parasites, and bacteria. These are collectively termed *microbial keratitis*. Bacterial corneal infections comprise a high percentage of all microbial infections and are a common but treatable cause of blindness worldwide.

The cornea is a thin, delicate structure, critical to the visual function. Even mild damage to the cornea near the visual axis is enough to permanently reduce visual acuity. Bacterial corneal infections involving the center of the cornea are a threat to vision, potentially causing significant damage within days. Management of such infections requires treatments that are effective and work rapidly to reduce the risk of vision loss.

The incidence of infectious corneal ulcers was reported to be 11.0 per 100 000 people per year in the United States in the 1980s,[1] a sharp rise from 2.5 per 100 000 people per year in the 1950s in the same location. In Scotland, the overall annual incidence of culture-proven microbial keratitis was a much lower 2.6 per 100 000 people,[2] although the estimate of the incidence of presumed microbial keratitis was 3.6 per 100 000. The incidence of infectious corneal ulcers in developing countries is much higher, reported to be 799 per 100 000 people a year in Nepal.[3] In southern India, the annual incidence of corneal ulceration was 113 per 100 000 people.[4] The much higher incidence in developing countries earned the label *silent epidemic*.[5,6]

MICROBIAL CAUSES

Almost any bacterial species can cause corneal infection and ulceration. The lid margin and the conjunctiva are populated by multiple species of bacteria.[7] However, there are natural barriers to infection that prevent the ability of these bacteria to initiate clinical infection in the cornea. These barriers include the antibacterial properties of the tear film due to the presence of proteins such as lysozyme, lactoferrin, and secretory IgA. An additional protection is the flow of tears across the ocular surface, which, combined with the shearing action of blinking, wash bacteria off the surface of the cornea and help to prevent bacterial

Trattler WB, Majmudar PA, Luchs JI, Swartz TS, eds.
Cornea Handbook (pp. 13-22)
© 2010 SLACK Incorporated

Table 2-1

RISK FACTORS FOR CORNEAL INFECTIONS

1. Contact lens wear
   - Especially when worn overnight
   - Soft contact lenses > rigid gas-permeable contact lenses
   - When contacts cleaned with homemade solutions
2. Surgical trauma
   - Surgical wound inoculation
   - Postoperative epithelial defect*
   - Suture-related infections
3. Nonsurgical trauma
   - Corneal abrasion
   - Corneal foreign body
   - Toxic medications
4. Dellen
5. Corneal injury caused by lid dysfunction
6. Trichiasis
7. Lagophthalmos (mechanical or neurologic)
8. Altered mental status (neurologic disease, substance abuse)
9. Corneal, conjunctival, or lacrimal dysfunction
10. Bullous keratopathy
11. Neurotrophic cornea
12. Ocular cicatricial pemphigoid
13. Stevens-Johnson syndrome
14. Graft-versus-host disease
15. Dysfunctional tear syndrome: dry eye, meibomian gland

*See Figure 2-1.

adherence. However, perhaps the most important barrier to the development of corneal infection is the presence of an intact, healthy corneal epithelium.

The most common species causing infection are *Staphylococcus*, followed by *Streptococcus, Pseudomonas, Enterobacteriaceae, Moraxella* species, and *Klebsiella pneumoniae*.[8-10] In the pediatric age group, the common pathogens are *Pseudomonas* and *Staphylococcus*.[11] In contact lens users, the bacterial pathogens are almost equally divided between gram-positive and gram-negative bacteria, although the most common species isolated is *Pseudomonas aeruginosa*.[12] Interestingly, the most common pathogen in bullous keratopathy-related corneal ulcers is *Streptococcus*.[13]

RISK FACTORS

Any factor that alters the health or integrity of the corneal epithelium and tear film is a potential risk factor (Table 2-1).[10] Contact lens wear is commonly associated with bacterial corneal infections. However, even proper lens care hygiene does not

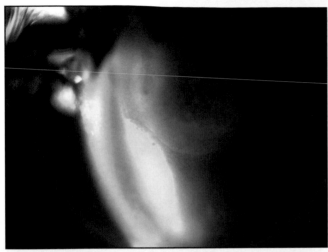

Figure 2-1. Bacterial keratitis in a patient 3 days following photorefractive keratectomy (PRK). The patient presented with severe pain and sudden loss of vision to count fingers at 2 feet. (Courtesy of Tracy S. Swartz, OD, MS.)

eliminate the risk of infection.[14] Approximately 30% of patients with contact lens-related corneal ulcers were compliant with the guidelines for contact lens wear.

PATHOGENESIS

Most bacteria are unable to penetrate the intact corneal epithelium. Exceptions include *Neisseria gonorrhea* (Figure 2-1), *Neisseria meningitides*, *Corynebacterium diphtheriae*, *Shigella*, and *Listeria*.[15] Bacterial colonization is initiated by adhesion of bacterial surface proteins (called *adhesins*) to receptors on the host cell surface. Other virulence factors include pili and flagella and extracellular products, such as alkaline protease, elastase, exoenzyme S, exotoxin A, endotoxin, slime polysaccharide, phospholipase C, and leukocidin.[15] After adhesion to the damaged or healthy epithelium, the bacteria proceed to invade the underlying stroma. This task is facilitated by bacterial proteinases that destroy the epithelial basement membrane and the extracellular matrix.[15] Exotoxins, released by the live bacteria, and endotoxins, released after microbial death, create damage and initiate inflammatory reactions through various pathways.

CLINICAL FEATURES

The clinical features of bacterial keratitis are not pathognomonic for any specific infectious agent. There are no biomicroscopic findings to identify a specific organism. The clinical presentation results from multiple variables: the virulence of the infecting organism(s), the method of inoculation, time since inoculation, previous status of the cornea, prior and concomitant antimicrobial and corticosteroid therapy, and other host factors[16] (Figure 2-2). Pain is the most common symptom of a bacterial corneal infection. Movement of the eyelids against an ulcer intensifies the pain.

Visual acuity is usually reduced, more when the involved area is in the visual pathway. Photophobia, blepharospasm, and tearing are other common symptoms. Purulent discharge is more likely to be present in advanced corneal ulcers. Other findings may include conjunctival hyperemia, chemosis, nonspecific papillary reaction, and lower and upper lid edema.

Figure 2-2. Hyperacute conjuncti-vitis. (Courtesy of Eric D. Donnenfeld, MD.)

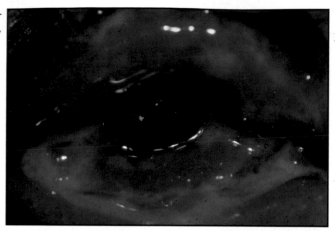

Figure 2-3. Severe conjunctival injection, pain, eroded epithelium, and underlying infiltrate suggest a bacterial ulcer. (Courtesy of Tracy S. Swartz, OD, MS.)

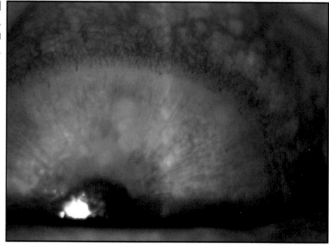

The most distinctive sign of bacterial corneal infection is a corneal ulcer: eroded epithelium, accompanied by an underlying stromal infiltrate (Figure 2-3). The ulcer is most often focal but can also be diffuse or multifocal. Multifocality of the corneal ulcers may be suggestive of polymicrobial or fungal infection.[17] When viewing the adjacent cornea with a thin slit and high magnification, one can observe a less consolidated cellular reaction in the stroma, termed *brawny edema*, extending along and between stromal lamellae. This cellular reaction tends to remain for days and weeks after the acute inflammation but disappears without scarring.

Anterior chamber reaction is another sign of bacterial keratitis. It ranges from mild through moderate to severe cell and flare. The nonsoluble content in the anterior chamber fluid (mainly proteins and inflammatory cells) reduce the aqueous clarity, and can be observed when using a 1 mm x 1 mm oblique slit.

As the nonsoluble content accumulates, some of it creates a gravitational sediment, hypopyon, in the lower iridocorneal angle. The hypopyon is generally sterile when Descemet's membrane is intact[15] (Figure 2-4). The magnitude of the hypopion can be documented by its height in millimeters from the limbus.

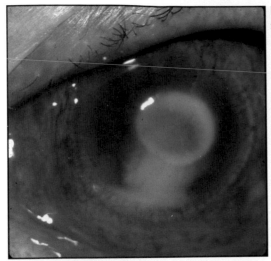

Figure 2-4. Anterior chamber response, when severe, results in a hypopion. (Courtesy of Eric D. Donnenfeld, MD.)

Treatment with antibiotics changes the clinical features, usually reducing the severity of signs and symptoms and altering the biomicroscopic appearance of the infected cornea. Corticosteroid treatment also reduces the signs and symptoms, sometimes producing short-term improvement for the first few days of treatment, but retards host defense mechanisms and enhances the danger of new opportunistic infections.[15]

The examination of the eye with suspected bacterial keratitis should include exact measurement of the findings. A detailed clinical drawing or photos are helpful for visit-to-visit comparison. The size of the epithelial defect and the size of the stromal infiltrate can be measured using the slit beam of the biomicroscope. The measurements are performed in 2 perpendicular meridians and repeated for comparison on subsequent examinations. A similar measurement can be performed on the height of the hypopyon, if present. The depth of the stromal infiltrate can be estimated, and any corneal thinning can be described as a percentage of the thickness of a healthy cornea (eg, "thin to 40% of normal").

With a severe stromal melt, all stromal lamellae can be lost, leaving only Descemet's membrane, which tends to bow outward due to the IOP. This situation is called a *descemetocele* (Figure 2-5). Minimal trauma can result in a perforation (Figure 2-6).

DIAGNOSIS

The initial diagnosis of a bacterial keratitis is based on its biomicroscopic appearance, such as the presence of an epithelial defect over a stromal infiltrate (Figure 2-7). The underlying microbial agent will only be learned following laboratory investigation, such as Gram stain or culture. However, in many cases, a presumed bacterial keratitis responds promptly to antibiotic therapy, yet has negative cultures.

Laboratory Investigation

Culturing of the infective agent by sampling the surface of the ulcer is the gold standard for diagnosis. This method is employed for some cases of microbial

Figure 2-5. Descemetocele occur with severe stromal melts and place the patient at high risk for perforation. (Courtesy of Tracy S. Swartz, OD, MS.)

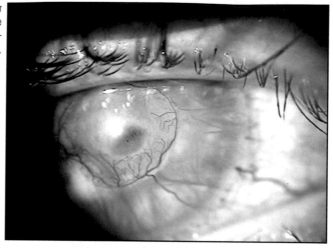

Figure 2-6. Corneal gluing may be required when bacterial keratitis results in perforation. (Courtesy of Eric D. Donnenfeld, MD.)

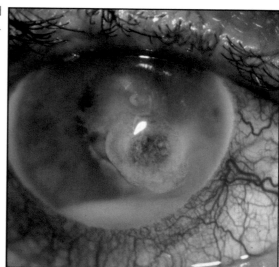

Figure 2-7. Ulcer with underlying infiltrate. (Courtesy of Eric D. Donnenfeld, MD.)

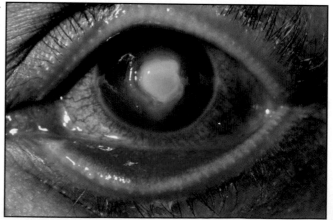

infections, whereas empiric treatment is employed for others. Sampling for stain-ing and culture is most revealing when performed before antibiotic treatment is initiated. However, positive bacterial cultures can be achieved even after antibi-otic treatment has been started. Patients on antibiotic treatment were only slightly more likely to be culture negative but significantly more likely to have a delay in pathogen recovery.[18] Although topical anesthetics are typically necessary for patients to tolerate culturing of the ocular surface, these anesthetics may contain benzalkonium chloride/EDTA, which can inhibit bacterial growth.[19] Material from the scraping should be inoculated directly onto the culture media. A plati-num spatula with a rounded flexible tip can be used for scraping.[20] The tip is ster-ilized in an alcohol flame between each scraping/inoculation. Other alternatives to the use of a spatula are a calcium alginate swab moistened with trypticase soy broth,[20] disposable #15 surgical blades, or disposable 18-gauge needles. Material should be obtained from both the rim and the center of the ulcer. If specimens cannot be obtained due to a deep infection, or there have been multiple negative cultures, a corneal biopsy can be performed.

Specimens are placed on a glass slide for staining. Common stains in cases of suspected bacterial keratitis include Gram stain and Giemsa stains. Other stains, discussed in Chapter 3, are used in cases where fungi and parasites are suspected.

Additional specimens are inoculated directly onto chocolate, blood, Sabouraud's, as well as thioglycollate broth. If acid-fast organisms are suspected, Lowenstein-Jensen agar should be inoculated. If *Acanthamoeba* is suspected, nonnutrient agar should be inoculated, which is then overlaid by *Escherichia coli, Pseudomonas*, or *Klebsiella* in the lab. Bacterial cultures are typically held for at least 1 week before being reported as "no growth," and cultures for atypical bacteria or fungi are held for 4 to 6 weeks.

After identifying the organism in the culture, antimicrobial susceptibility test-ing is performed. The results are reported both as "sensitive"/"resistant," and as a value of minimal inhibitory concentration (MIC). More effective antibiotics inhibit growth in a lower concentration, so their MIC is lower.

TREATMENT

Microbial keratitis can cause irreversible damage to the cornea, leading to vision loss. Severe cases can involve the entire eye. Deterioration can be quite rapid and is usually much faster than the time needed to obtain reliable pathogen identification and antimicrobial susceptibility results. Therefore, empiric antimi-crobial treatment is usually initiated and can be modified prior to the reporting of culture results as clinical and laboratory data accumulate.

There are many antibiotics available for the treatment of microbial keratitis. Antimicrobial agents (Table 2-2) can be classified based on chemical structure and proposed mechanism of action. In mild presumed bacterial keratitis, obtain-ing specimens for staining and cultures is optional and based on clinical signs and symptoms. Antimicrobial therapy may be commenced using a single broad-spectrum agent, usually a fourth-generation fluoroquinolone (gatifloxacin, besi-floxacin, moxifloxacin) or a highly concentrated third-generation fluoroquino-lone (levo-floxacin 1.5%). In severe presumed bacterial keratitis, after obtaining specimens for staining and cultures, empiric treatment with 2 agents is started.

Table 2-2

CLASSIFICATION OF ANTIMICROBIAL AGENTS BY MECHANISM OF ACTION

Agents That Inhibit Bacterial Cell Wall Synthesis

B-Lactams:
- Penicillin
- Cephalosporins
- Carbapenems

Vancomycin

Bacitracin

Cycloserine

Agents Affecting Bacterial Cell Membrane Permeability

Polymyxin

Polyene antifungal agents
- Nystatin
- Amphotericin B
- Natamycin (pimaricin)

Daptomycin

Agents That Disrupt Function of 30S or 50S Ribosomal Subunits to Reversibly Inhibit Protein Synthesis

Aminoglycosides
- Gentamicin
- Tobramycin

Chloramphenicol

Tetracyclines

Macrolides

Erythromycin

Azithromycin

Clindamycin

Streptogramins

Linezolid

Agents That Affect Bacterial Nucleic Acid Metabolism

Rifamycins
- Rifampin
- Rifabutin

Quinolones

Antimetabolites That Block Essential Enzymes of Folate Metabolism

Trimethoprim

Sulfonamides

Options include 2 commercially available topical antibiotics or 2 fortified antibiotics made at a compounding pharmacy, typically fortified cefazolin 50 mg/mL and fortified gentamicin or tobramycin 14 mg/mL. A typical regimen starts with 1 drop of each drug every 30 minutes to 1 hour, 24 hours a day. Decisions to replace the antibiotics with different compounds or to alter the frequency of administration are based on the clinical judgment of the ophthalmologist, who relies on the biomicroscopic appearance of the eye, the level of discomfort of the patient, and laboratory results.

When the clinical examination reveals improvement in the size of the epithelial defect, reduction in hypopyon size, clearing of infiltrate, reduction in conjunctival hyperemia, and reduction in discomfort, one can begin to taper the medication frequency. A positive microbial culture with known antimicrobial susceptibility to one of the antibiotics used may help the ophthalmologist decide to discontinue the other antibiotic agent, possibly replacing it with another antibiotic agent to which there is susceptibility. That agent should be of a different chemical group and preferably with a different mechanism of action. Deterioration under treatment should sometimes be managed by replacing the initially chosen antimicrobial regimen with another empiric combination (for instance, from cefazolin and gentamicin to vancomycin), or according to the laboratory data obtained (stained plates, microbiological identification, and antimicrobial susceptibility). If nonresponsive to treatment, other infectious organisms (fungi, *Acanthamoeba*, atypical bacteria), noncompliance, or even anesthetic abuse should be considered.

If unusual infectious organisms are suspected, consider reculturing on special media and obtaining special stains to aid in the identification of these organisms. Empiric therapy for these organisms may be started while waiting for microbiologic results.

Other agents commonly used in the treatment of microbial keratitis include oral analgesics (ie, acetaminophen and or prescription narcotics) and topical cycloplegics (ie, atropine sulfate 1%). Collagenase inhibitors (ie, acetylcysteine 20%) may be useful in the presence of a stromal melt.

Topical steroids have a controversial role in microbial keratitis. Steroids given during the healing period may have a role in reducing the inflammatory response, thereby reducing corneal scarring and preserving visual acuity. Although steroids can help reduce tissue damage by reducing the inflammatory response, they may also reduce the body's ability to eradicate the infectious agent. Steroids promote bacterial proliferation and stromal melting with potentially serious consequences, and steroids given during the healing period may have a role in reducing the inflammatory response, thereby reducing corneal scarring and preserving visual acuity. In general, steroids should not be given until it is clear that the active infection has been eradicated.

CONCLUSION

Bacterial corneal infections represent one of the few situations in ophthalmology where prompt treatment is essential for optimal results. Every ophthalmologist should be sensitive to the signs and symptoms of microbial keratitis, especially because bacterial corneal infections can rapidly cause severe visual loss or even loss of the entire eye. Fortunately, with timely and proper management, the degree of vision loss in severe infections can often be reduced.

REFERENCES

1. Erie JC, Nevitt MP, Hodge DO, Ballard DJ. Incidence of ulcerative keratitis in a defined population from 1950 through 1988. *Arch Ophthalmol.* 1993;111:1665-1671.

2. Seal DV, Kirkness CM, Bennett HG, Peterson M, and the Keratitis Study Group. Population-based cohort study of microbial keratitis in Scotland: incidence and features. *Contact Lens Anterior Eye.* 1999;22(2):49-57.

3. Upadhyay MP, Karmacharya PC, Koirala S, et al. The Bhaktapur Eye Study: ocular trauma and antibiotic prophylaxis for the prevention of corneal ulceration in Nepal. *Br J Ophthalmol.* 2001;85:388-392.

4. Gonzales CA, Srinivasan M, Whitcher JP, Smolin G. Incidence of corneal ulceration in Madurai district, South India. *Ophthalmic Epidemiol.* 1996;3:159-166.

5. Whitcher JP, Srinivasan M. Corneal ulceration in the developing world—a silent epidemic. *Br J Ophthalmol.* 1997;81:622-623.

6. Whitcher JP, Srinivasan M, Upadhyay MP. Corneal blindness: a global perspective. *Bull World Health Organ.* 2001;79(3):214-221.

7. Leibowitz HM. Bacterial keratitis. In: Leibowitz HM, ed. *Corneal Disorders: Clinical Diagnosis and Management.* Philadelphia, PA: WB Saunders; 1984:353.

8. Arffa RC. Infectious ulcerative keratitis. In: Arffa RC, Grayson M, eds. *Grayson's Diseases of the Cornea.* St. Louis, MO: CV Mosby; 1991:163-164.

9. Wilson L. Bacterial corneal ulcers. In: Duane TD, ed. *Clinical Ophthalmology.* Vol 4. Hagerstown, MD: Harper & Row; 1976.

10. Abbott RL, Zegans M, Kremer PA. Bacterial corneal ulcers. In: Tasman W, Jaeger EA, eds. *Duane's Clinical Ophthalmology on CD.* Vol 4. Philadelphia, PA: Lippincott Williams & Wilkins; 2005.

11. Cruz OA, Sabir SM, Capo H, Alfonso EC. Microbial keratitis in childhood. *Ophthalmology.* 1993;100:192-196.

12. Mah-Sadorra JH, Yavuz SGA, Najjar DM, Laibson PR, Rapuano CJ, Cohen EJ. Trends in contact lens–related corneal ulcers. *Cornea.* 2005;24:51-58.

13. Luchs JI, Cohen EJ, Rapuano CJ, Laibson PR. Ulcerative keratitis in bullous keratopathy. *Ophthalmology.* 1997;104:816-822.

14. Najjar DM, Aktan SG, Rapuano CJ, Laibson PR, Cohen EJ. Contact lens-related corneal ulcers in compliant patients. *Am J Ophthalmol.* 2004;137(1):170-172.

15. O'Brien TP. Bacterial keratitis. In Krachmer JH, Mannis MJ, Holland EJ, eds. *Cornea.* Vol 2. St. Louis, MO: Mosby; 1997:1144-1148.

16. Jones DB. Pathogenesis of bacterial and fungal keratitis. *Trans Ophthalmol Soc UK.* 1978; 98:367-371.

17. Jones DB. Polymicrobial keratitis. *Trans Am Ophthalmol Soc.* 1981;79:153-167.

18. Marangon FB, Miller D, Alfonso EC. Impact of prior therapy on the recovery and frequency of corneal pathogens. *Cornea.* 2004;23:158-164.

19. Charnock C. Are multidose over-the-counter artificial tears adequately preserved? *Cornea.* 2006;25:432-437.

20. Benson WH, Lanier JD. Comparison of techniques for culturing corneal ulcers. *Ophthalmology.* 1992;99:800-804.

21. Chambers HF. General principles of antimicrobial therapy. In: Brunton LL, Parker KL, Buxton ILO, Blumenthal DK, eds. *Goodman & Gilman's The Pharmacological Basis of Therapeutics.* 11th ed. Online ed. McGraw-Hill.

22. Henderer JD, Rapuano CJ. Ocular pharmacology. In: Brunton LL, Parker KL, Buxton ILO, Blumenthal DK, eds. *Goodman & Gilman's The Pharmacological Basis of Therapeutics.* 11th ed. Online ed. McGraw-Hill.

23. Benson WH, Lanier JD. Current diagnosis and treatment of corneal ulcers. *Curr Opin Ophthalmol.* 1998;9(4):45-49.

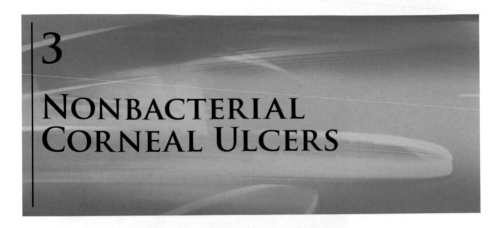

3

NONBACTERIAL CORNEAL ULCERS

David M. Sachs, MD; Henry D. Perry, MD; and Eric D. Donnenfeld, MD

Historically, ulceration of the cornea has been divided into several distinct categories including but not limited to bacterial, viral, fungal, parasitic, and non-infectious or sterile. Corneal ulcers are a multifactorial problem where a careful history and clinical evaluation go a long way toward finding the correct diagnosis. When coupled with a thorough laboratory evaluation consisting of, but not limited to, corneal smears and cultures plated directly on the appropriate media, the correct diagnosis is made in the majority of cases. Occasionally, corneal biopsy or cytological evaluation of the fluid in a contact lens case or the contact lens itself is needed to secure the diagnosis.

FUNGAL ULCERS

Residents and practitioners alike bristle at the mention of mycotic keratitis. Surprisingly, mycotic keratitis is probably the easiest subject in suppurative keratitis to master. Knowing that the filamentous molds such as *Fusarium* and *Aspergillus* and yeasts such as *Candida* represent more than 80% of the cases of mycotic keratitis often helps the clinician narrow his focus of possible etiologic agents. Furthermore, corneal scrapings are diagnostic in more than 85% of cases (Figure 3-1).[1] Smears stained with periodic acid Schiff (PAS) or Gomori methenamine silver (GMS) give the best chance of a positive result, but even a Gram-stained slide will typically yield positive results in fungal cases. Such smears will demonstrate the 45 degree branching septate hyphae of *Aspergillus* and the pseudohyphae and budding yeasts of *Candida*. Clinically, molds are more aggressive, tend to be recalcitrant to medical treatment, and often require surgical intervention, whereas yeasts are more indolent and usually respond to medical therapy.

The incidence of fungal ulcers in the United States varies significantly depending on local climatic and geographic features. In the humid climate of the Southern United States, fungal keratitis accounts for as much as 35% of microbial keratitis, compared to only 1% in the temperate climate of New York.[2] Trauma is another important risk factor for fungal keratitis. Fungal keratitis is significantly more common among agricultural workers, and corneal injury secondary to

Trattler WB, Majmudar PA, Luchs JI, Swartz TS, eds.
Cornea Handbook (pp. 23-36)
© 2010 SLACK Incorporated

Figure 3-1. Giant cell with clusters of varying sized yeasts, most with prominent capsules consistent with *Cryptococcus neoformans* (600X Papanicolaou) (Green micro).

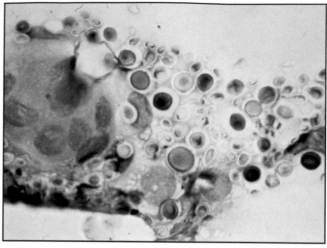

organic material such as thorns or tree branches is responsible for up to 44% of cases of fungal keratitis.[2] Ocular surface disease, recurrent epithelial erosions, dry eye, and neurotrophic keratitis also increase the risk for fungal keratitis. Topical steroid use leading to local immunosuppression and systemic immuno-suppression secondary to diabetes and human immunodeficiency virus (HIV) are also important risk factors for fungal keratitis.[2]

Contact lens use has become an increasingly important cause of fungal kera-titis, especially in the United States. A study in Philadelphia found that approxi-mately 30% of patients with fungal keratitis were contact lens wearers.[3] Recently there has been an outbreak in *Fusarium* keratitis thought to be associated with ReNu MoistureLoc (Bausch & Lomb, Rochester, NY) soft contact lens solution.[4,5] This epidemic began in 2005 in Asia and by May of 2006, 165 confirmed cases had occurred in the United States and 75 more were suspected.[2,6] This was a greater than 7-fold increase in the documented annual cases of *Fusarium* keratitis compared to previous years.[3,7] Unfortunately, many of these cases required kera-toplasty. A better understanding of the approach to mycotic keratitis may have allowed for earlier and more effective treatment. The exact cause for this *Fusarium* outbreak is still unclear because inspectors were unable to identify *Fusarium* from the ReNu Moisture Loc production facility. Since the outbreak, Bausch & Lomb has removed ReNu Moisture Loc from the market.[2]

The clinical picture of a relatively quiet eye with an adherent hypopyon points to mycotic keratitis (Figure 3-2). Obtaining a good history from the patient and maintaining a high index of suspicion will also help in the early diagnosis of fungal keratitis. Treatment with topical and systemic antifungals is often effective early in the disease. However, despite initial enthusiasm with each new antifun-gal treatment, specific therapy is lacking. Medical therapy for mycotic keratitis is problematic because fungal elements, especially molds, penetrate into the deepest layers of the cornea in order to avoid the polymorphonuclear leukocyte infiltration (Figure 3-3). Histopathology reveals the presence of hyphae in, and anchored to, Descemet's membrane. This is often the reason for an adherent hypopyon at a relatively early stage of the infection. This also explains why, in established infections, surgery is the rule rather than the exception, even in patients treated with intracameral antifungals. The management of these cases

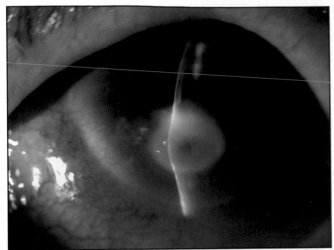

Figure 3-2. *Candida albicans* corneal ulcer showing prominent descemetocele with less than expected inflammation given severity of the infection.

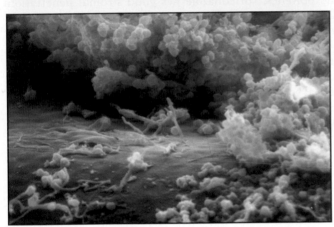

Figure 3-3. Fungus (*Aspergillus fumigatus*) penetrating corneal endothelium and anchoring a characteristic adherent hypopyon. (Scanning electron 800X.)

postkeratoplasty is difficult and may include topical nonsteroidal anti-inflammatory therapy (NSAIDs) and topical Cyclosporin A in an effort to limit the use of corticosteroids as much as possible.[8] The latter is thought to potentiate fungal recurrence in the host or graft.[9]

Currently, natamycin (a polyene) is the only antifungal agent approved by the US Food and Drug Administration (FDA) for topical ophthalmic use. Unfortunately, because of its large molecular size, it has poor penetration into the corneal stroma, and intermittent epithelial debridement is recommended to increase stromal concentration. Amphotericin B, another polyene, has been shown to be successful in treating *Aspergillus*, and clinical studies have shown it to be superior in treating *Candida* compared to natamycin. In severe keratitis, amphotericin B is also available for subconjunctival, intracameral, and intravitreal use. Unfortunately, like natamycin, amphotericin B has poor stromal penetration and also requires frequent epithelial debridement.[2,10,11]

Azoles including intraconazole, clotrimazole, ketoconazole, and fluconazole are commonly used as adjuvant therapy because they are generally less effective than the polyenes. Voriconazole is a new azole with broad spectrum activity against both filamentous fungi and yeast including *Fusarium*, *Aspergillus*, and

Figure 3-4. Herpes simplex dendrite using fluorescein stain. (Courtesy of Eric D. Donnenfeld, MD.)

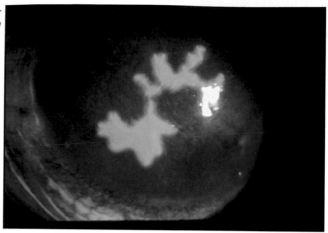

Candida.[2,10,11] Unlike the polyenes, voriconazole has good stromal penetration and great oral bioavailability, achieving therapeutic aqueous and vitreous levels after oral administration.[11] Recent literature has shown oral and topical voriconazole to have lower MIC against both *Aspergillus* and *Fusarium* compared to amphotericin B and natamycin.[10] Another study showed that 5 of 7 patients who failed conventional therapy with amphotericin B and natamycin were successfully treated with topical and oral voriconazole.[11]

VIRAL CORNEAL ULCERS

Herpes simplex virus keratitis is by far the most common viral infection in the United States and the most important cause of corneal blindness. HSV is a DNA virus in the herpes virus family, which also includes varicella zoster virus (VZV) and Epstein-Barr virus. The vast majority of the population has been exposed to HSV, although the primary infection is usually subclinical. The virus remains dormant in the trigeminal ganglion but may reactivate along the fifth cranial nerve, usually in the form of cold sores or fever blisters. Occasionally the reactivation occurs in the portion of the fifth cranial nerve that subserves the anterior segment of the eye, in the form of herpes ocular disease. One-half million Americans have herpes keratitis in the United States. The most common presentation is a dendritic epithelial keratitis (Figures 3-4, and 3-5), which responds well to topical and/or systemic antivirals but recurrences will occur in 25% of patients and then successive episodes occur at a rate of 50%.[12,13] Of great concern is the development of disciform keratitis. In this type of keratitis there is usually central corneal edema lined by keratic precipitates. Disciform keratitis may be chronic and lead to permanent scarring and loss of vision. Disciform keratitis may rarely become necrotizing, which characteristically results in a descemetocele and perforation. Rapid treatment with antivirals and steroids may halt its progression, but cyanoacrylic adhesives and surgery such as therapeutic keratoplasty may often be required. Several studies such as the Herpetic Eye Disease Study (HEDS) have shown that our preconceived notions of the benefits of steroids in stromal disease are not warranted in terms of final visual acuity in patients with disciform keratitis.[14] Use of steroids does continue to be the standard of care. The prophylactic use of acyclovir orally has been shown to decrease the recurrence rate by almost half for both

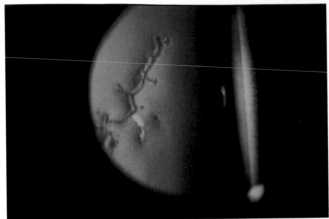

Figure 3-5. Herpes simplex dendrite seen in retroillumination. (Courtesy of Eric D. Donnenfeld, MD.)

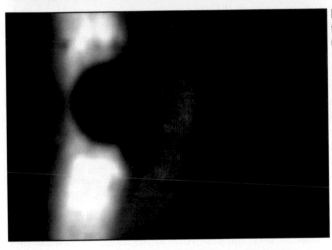

Figure 3-6. Stromal herpetic keratitis. (Courtesy of Tracy S. Swartz, OD, MS.)

epithelial keratitis and stromal disease.[15] Topical antivirals such as trifluridine are the mainstay of treatment of HSV epithelial keratitis. The dosage is typically every 2 hours initially, followed by a tapering dose over the subsequent 10 to 14 days. Trifluridine carries considerable epithelial toxicity and its use should be limited to a maximum of 21 days of intensive therapy. In cases of stromal disease, topical trifluridine may be used for longer periods of time (2 to 4 times a day), but the practitioner should be observant for medicamentosa. Topical steroids should not be used in cases of epithelial keratitis because they may potentiate viral replication. Their use should be reserved for stromal HSV keratitis (Figure 3-6), and even then only in conjunction with topical or oral antivirals.

Herpes zoster keratitis may also present as either a dendritic epithelial keratitis or a disciform keratitis, but because it is usually found in association with the classic skin lesions, the diagnosis is easily made. One difference between the epithelial keratitis of VZV and HSV is that the dendrites associated with VZV infection are lacking the classic terminal bulbs found with HSV keratitis. A common outcome of keratitis from both VZV and HSV is a decrease in corneal sensation. This can be tested for using a Cochet-Bonnet aesthesiometer or grossly by using a cotton wisp from a cotton swab applicator. Zoster corneal ulcers may also occur in up to 3% of cases associated with herpes simplex. Treatment of viral corneal ulcers is often directed at the use of local and systemic medications that are specific for viral infections. The 2 newer systemic antivirals, famciclovir and valacyclovir, have been shown to have at least equal efficacy and greater potency than acyclovir in treating superficial and deep forms of viral keratitis due to herpes simplex and may be of value in treating acute herpes zoster keratitis.[16]

Topical trifluridine has no activity against varicella zoster virus and therefore its use is not required. The mainstay of therapy is topical steroids and oral antiviral medications.

Parasitic Ulcers

Worldwide, there are numerous parasites that can cause keratitis. In the United States, parasitic keratitis is almost always caused by *Acanthamoeba* in a non-immune-compromised patient. *Acanthamoeba* is a ubiquitous protozoan parasite that has become an increasing public health concern since its first description in the early 1970s. *Acanthamoeba* exist in 2 forms in the environment: the motile trophozoite, and the dormant cyst (Figure 3-7). Both forms are found in infected human corneas, but only the trophozoite is infectious. The dormant cysts are very resistant to environmental stressors such as heat and cold, making medical treatment difficult. The classic double-walled cysts can be easily identified using calcofluor white or acridine orange stains (Figure 3-8).

The initial epidemic began in contact lens wearers who used homemade saline solution using salt tablets that were commercially available.[17] Recent epidemics have been linked to swimming while wearing contact lenses, either in fresh water, salt water, or swimming pool water. Until recently, *Acanthamoeba* keratitis (AK) had been a relatively rare occurrence. The annualized incidence of AK in the United States had been estimated to be approximately 2 cases per one million contact lens wearers. This number dramatically increased from 2003 to 2006, when 63 cases were identified in the Chicago area alone. More than 60% of these cases reported use of AMO Complete MoisturePlus (Abbott Medical Optics, Santa Ana, CA) contact lens solution.[18] Like the case with ReNu Moisture Loc contact lens solution and *Fusarium* keratitis, the mechanism for how AMO Complete MoisturePlus put its users at increase risk for infection is unknown. It is extremely disturbing, however, that in the last 2 years there have been 2 epidemic-like increases in incidences of previously uncommon infections.[18,19]

A retrospective study of the 63 cases of AK in Chicago also found 3 hygiene-related variables that significantly increased the risk of AK independent of the use of Complete MoisturePlus contact lens solution. These included reuse of contact lens solution, lack of rubbing the lenses while cleaning, and showering while wearing the contact lenses.[18,19]

Under normal circumstances, *Acanthamoeba* is not infective to the human cornea unless there is an insult to the corneal epithelium. *Acanthamoeba* infections are 10 times more common in contact lens wearers and may present bilaterally. Contact lens use may compromise the ocular surface, which allows for infection by the parasite. In addition, both the trophozoites and the cysts adhere to the surface of contact lenses, which further increases the risk of infection.[18] Another common association is with a recent history of hot tub use. Unless specifically treated for *Acanthamoeba*, organisms actually increase in hot tubs.

Current laboratory diagnostic techniques, which rely on corneal staining and cultures, have had limited yield, often leading to a delay in diagnosis. Tandem

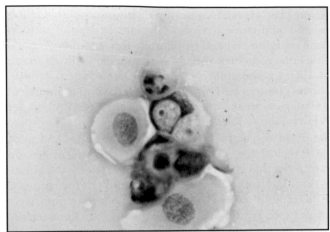

Figure 3-7. Papanicolaou stained smear showing a partially encysted trophozoite and also classic cysts. (600X oil.)

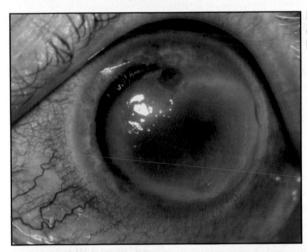

Figure 3-8. Ring ulcer in a patient with acanthamoebic keratitis eventually required keratoplasty. (Courtesy of Ramon Font.)

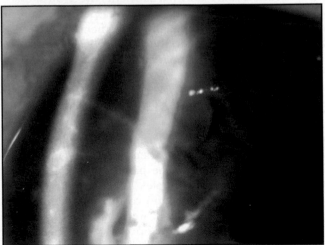

Figure 3-9. Acanthamoeba perineuritis. (Courtesy of Eric D. Donnenfeld, MD.)

scanning confocal microscopy (TSCM) is a noninvasive diagnostic tool that allows for both rapid quantitative and qualitative analysis of the entire cornea. Confocal microscopy can demonstrate both the cyst and trophozoite forms of *Acanthamoeba* as well as the characteristic enlarged corneal nerves in suspected AK. However, the greatest advantage of TSCM is the ability to make an immediate diagnosis. When compared to traditional cultures on *Escherichia coli* overlays on nonnutrient agar, which can take many days to weeks for positive growth, TSCM allows for earlier treatment and better visual outcomes.[20]

Clinically, the constellation of severe pain, corneal ring infiltrate, and poor response to medication are typical for AK (see Figure 3-8). Unrelenting and severe pain is a common symptom that is frequently found and reflects the organisms' random movements through tissues. Because passage through the cornea is easiest to navigate along the established pathways, *Acanthamoeba* randomly elect to migrate along nerve routes (see Figure 3-9). This explains the characteristic perineuritis, enlarged corneal nerves, and the ever-present pain as the organisms start digesting neural tissue.

In most cases the diagnosis is delayed by an average of 3 to 4 weeks, when a ring ulcer typically appears. Initially, the disease may often be confused with herpes simplex keratitis. Both may present as an epithelial keratitis and initially with *Acanthamoeba*, there may be a positive response to antiviral therapy, with relapse a possibility a few days to a week later. Corneal sensation may also be reduced in *Acanthamoeba*, further mimicking herpes simplex. Also in the second week the disease may affect deeper layers of the stroma, simulating a disciform keratitis. At 3 to 4 weeks, as perineuritis and ring ulcer become apparent, the correct diagnosis is usually made. However, therapy is much more effective if directed early in the course of the infection.[21] Keratoplasty is rarely needed if the condition is diagnosed in the first 14 days, underscoring the need for maintaining a strong clinical suspicion. Therapy through a quadruple approach is often successful. This includes Brolene (Sanofi-aventis, Bridgewater, NJ), Neosporin (Johnson & Johnson, New Brunswick, NJ), polyhexamethylene biguanide (or alternatively chlorhexidine 0.02%), and systemic itraconazole. These treatments have shown effectiveness against the trophozoite but are only partially effective against cysts. Newer biguanides (alexidine) and antifungal agents such as caspofungin appear to have a greater efficacy against the cysts.[17] If caught early, therapy is effective within a few weeks; if diagnosed at 4 weeks or later, therapy is typically prolonged (up to 6 months or longer) and keratoplasty may be required for visual rehabilitation[17,22] (Figure 3-10).

MANAGEMENT OF CORNEAL ULCERS

Our interest in management of noninfectious corneal ulceration became heightened and more focused in relationship to a patient with a severe corneal ulcer who was referred to us for definitive care. The patient was a 75-year-old male with a 50-year history of recurrent herpes simplex infections. His last episode failed to respond to topical antiviral therapy and corticosteroid treatment was initiated. Neosporin was added topically after 2 weeks when he failed to improve. Despite these medications, the patient developed a central ulcer with hypopyon. On initial exam, corneal scrapings showed a heavy concentration of encapsulated gram-positive diplococci consistent with *pneumococcus* (Figure 3-11).

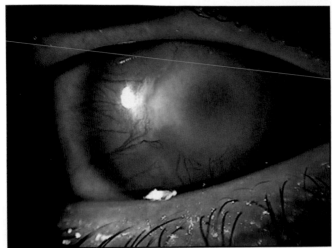

Figure 3-10. Acanthamoeba keratitis recurrence following a lamellar dissection for tissue sample, which positively identified the organism after two negative cultures. (Courtesy of Tracy S. Swartz, OD, MS.)

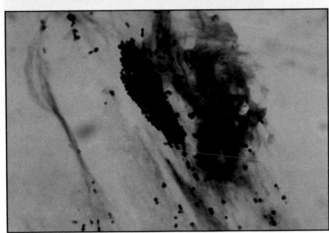

Figure 3-11. Photomicroscope picture under oil of gram-positive capsulated diplococcic consistent with *pneumococcus* (600X gram).

Corticosteroids were discontinued and topical and systemic penicillin therapy was started. The next day the patient had a total hypopyon with light perception vision and it appeared that the eye would not be salvaged. However, within a week the hypopyon cleared and there was a marked improvement. Then suddenly, increasing ulceration was noted, without increasing signs of inflammation. Smears and cultures were repeated and were negative. Was this recurrent herpes? Systemic tetracycline was prescribed because of rosacea-like facies and a hope that this treatment would help. The response was dramatic and within 48 hours the ulceration stopped and the corneal epithelium healed as the patient regained 20/80 visual acuity.

This case highlights several important aspects in the management of infectious keratitis. First, the value of corneal smears is evident because they provide an almost instantaneous diagnosis and allow the clinician to focus treatment in one direction. Obtaining corneal smears requires very little specialized equipment: a Kimura spatula (anvil-shaped is best), scored clean glass slides (cytology type), and a Koplin jar with methanol. The smear is taken using the spatula directly from the leading edge of the ulceration and then the material is directly inoculated on the appropriate media. Commonly used media are blood agar (bacteria and fungi), chocolate agar (bacteria), Sabouraud's dextrose without cycloheximide (fungi), and thioglycolate broth (anaerobes and microaerophilic organisms). In special cases, *E. coli* overlays can be performed on nonnutrient agar (*Acanthamoeba*), Lowenstein-Jensen for atypical mycobacteria, and brain heart infusion for fungi. Smears are placed immediately on clean, glass scored slides or cytology slides. The latter have a white central area upon which the corneal scraping is placed. By rapidly placing the smear on the glass slide and fixing in the methanol in the Koplin jar, you assure that the material noted on the final stained slides is from the cornea and that dust or other contaminants are not present. The most common stains in ophthalmic practice are the Gram's and Giemsa. We prefer the Papanicolaou over the

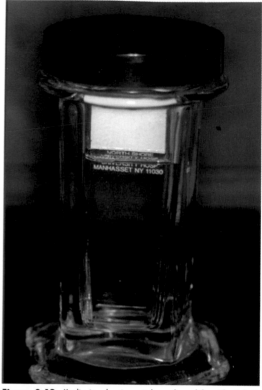

Figure 3-12. Koplin jar showing cytology glass slide with circle in methanol solution.

Giemsa because most labs do the Papanicolaou stain daily and the cytological parameters are more clearly noted, especially herpes inclusions. We always save a slide for special stains such as the Gomori methenamine silver (fungi) or calcofluor white (*Acanthamoeba*). Occasionally an acid-fast slide (Ziehl-Neelsen) is necessary for atypical mycobacteria and *Nocardia*, although the latter is seen well on Gram stain.

Laboratory evaluation is the key to success with the management of infectious corneal ulceration.[23,24] Personal communication with the microbiologist or pathologist who is evaluating the smears and cultures will help to insure accurate and rapid reports. This is especially important with respect to *Acanthamoeba* because most pathologists and microbiologists have little contact with this organism. If you are not suspicious, the diagnosis will be overlooked and not considered. Similarly, Gram stains alone may miss cases of fungal keratitis, whereas a periodic acid Schiff or Gomori methenamine silver stain may highlight these organisms. Fluorescent stains such as calcofluor white are especially helpful for *Acanthamoeba*, which can be found in up to 92% of smears when evaluated by this modality.[25]

Recent literature has also shown the importance of sectioning and culturing the contact lens in a contact lens-related ulcer. A recent study found that 66% of negative corneal scrapings were positive on contact lens cultures.[26] Identifying the causative agent more often will allow you to choose your antimicrobial agent more effectively. Contact lens use has become one of the leading risk factors for microbial keratitis. Although patients using soft contact lenses are at greatest risk, rigid gas-permeable lenses also increase the risk for infectious corneal ulcers. There also tends to be an increase prevalence of gram-negative rods as the causative agent in contact lens users compared to non-contact lens–related infectious keratitis. The most important factor in contact lens-related infectious ulcers appears to be the overnight wearing of soft contact lenses, with the risk increasing exponentially with the number of nights of continued wear.[26]

Another important feature of suppurative keratitis that can be gleaned from the above case is the initial worsening of the clinical situation when steroids are stopped. Topical corticosteroids are notorious for deluding clinicians into an initial benefit from their use. Unfortunately, their effect often masks and confuses clinical management. When the steroids are stopped in a case of suppurative keratitis, there is often a dramatic worsening of the patient's clinical appearance. Cessation of steroids is necessary to not only gauge the true extent of the corneal ulceration but also to allow the patient's immune system to aid in the fight to clear the infection. Some clinicians advocate starting steroids topically within 48 hours after initiating antibiotic therapy. However, there is no evidence to support the use of corticosteroids early in the course of the disease. Indeed, the body of evidence points out the overall deleterious effects of topical corticosteroids in infectious keratitis,[27-29] and it may be prudent to wait at least 1 week after initiation of antibiotics before corticosteroids are added.

Perhaps the most interesting aspect about the above case was the response to systemic tetracycline. According to Lorne Golub, DDS, PhD, a professor at the University of New York at Stonybrook School of Dental Medicine, systemic tetracyclines may have significant anticollagenolytic action in gingival disease.[30,31] After a series of collaborations, our group began to systematically investigate the effects of the tetracycline family of antibiotics on corneal ulceration.[32,33] One study showed that in the rabbit alkali burn model, systemic tetracycline prevented ulceration in 85% of the rabbits as opposed to the control group, where all of the rabbits ulcerated.[34] We then investigated doxycycline and found an increased effectiveness and through further study documented its beneficial effect in treating noninfectious corneal ulceration.[35] This conclusion was confirmed by several investigators and led to systemic doxycycline being used as the gold standard to treat noninfectious corneal ulceration and as adjunctive therapy in patients with other forms of suppurative keratitis.[36,37] More recently, interest has rekindled in a more potent collagenase inhibitor, Ilomast, which was developed to be used for noninfectious corneal ulceration and adjunctive therapy for corneal ulcers. Unfortunately, the original company abandoned the drug and it was never bought to market. Recently, the rights were purchased by Quick-Med.

Knowledge of the various etiologies of suppurative keratitis, as well as careful study of the many different diagnostic and therapeutic modalities, will help the clinician form a systematic approach to this common ocular condition. This will undoubtedly allow for quicker diagnosis and ultimately better patient outcomes.

REFERENCES

1. Chander J, Chakrabarti A, Sharma A, Saini JS, Panigarhi D. Evaluation of Calcofluor staining in the diagnosis of fungal corneal ulcer. *Mycoses.* 1993;36:243-245.
2. Ou JI, Acharya NR. Epidemiology and treatment of fungal corneal ulcers. *Int Ophthalmol Clin.* 2007;47(3):7-16.

3. Gorscak JJ, Ayres BD, Bhagat N, et al. An outbreak of *Fusarium* keratitis associated with contact lens use in the northeastern United States. *Cornea.* 2007;26:1187-1194.

4. Chang DC, Grant GB, O'Donnell K, et al. Multistate outbreak of Fusarium keratitis associated with use of a contact lens solution. *JAMA.* 2006;296:953-963.

5. Foroozan R, Eagle RC, Cohen EJ. Fungal keratitis in a soft contact lens wearer. *CLAO J.* 2000;26:166-168.

6. Iver SA, Tuli SS, Wagoner RC. Fungal keratitis: emerging trends and treatment outcomes. *Eye Contact Lens.* 2006;32:267-271.

7. Choi DM, Goldstein MH, Salierno A, Driebe WT. Fungal keratitis in a daily disposable soft contact lens wearer. *CLAO J.* 2001;27:111-112.

8. Perry HD, Doshi SJ, Donnenfeld ED, Bai GS. Topical cyclosporin A in the management of therapeutic keratoplasty for mycotic keratitis. *Cornea.* 2002;21:161-163.

9. Wright TM, Afshari NA. Microbial keratitis following corneal transplantation. *Am J Ophthalmol.* 2006;142:1061-1062.

10. Lalitha P, Shapiro BL, Srinivasan M, et al. Antimicrobial susceptibility of *Fusarium, Aspergillus,* and other filamentous fungi isolated from keratitis. *Arch Ophthalmol.* 2007;125:789-793.

11. Bunya VY, Hammersmith KM, Rapuano CJ, Ayres BD, Cohen EJ. Topical and oral Voriconazole in the treatment of fungal keratitis. *Am J Ophthalmol.* 2007;143:151-153.

12. Shuster JJ, Kaufman HE, Nesburn AB. Statistical analysis of the rate of recurrence of herpes virus ocular epithelial disease. *Am J Ophthalmol.* 1981;91:328-331.

13. Liesegang TJ. A community study of ocular herpes simplex. *Curr Eye Res.* 1991;10 (suppl):111-115.

14. Barron BA, Gee L, Hauck WW, et al. Herpetic Eye Disease Study. A controlled trial of oral acyclovir for herpes simplex stromal keratitis. *Ophthalmology.* 1994;101:1871-1882.

15. Herpetic Eye Disease Study Group. Oral acyclovir for herpes simplex virus eye disease: effect on prevention of epithelial keratitis and stromal keratitis. *Arch Ophthalmol.* 2000;118:1030-1036.

16. Nikkels AF, Pierard GE. Oral antivirals revisited in the treatment of herpes zoster: what do they accomplish? *Am J Clin Dermatol.* 2002;3:591-598.

17. Foulks GN. *Acanthamoeba* keratitis and contact lens wear: static or increasing problem. *Eye Contact Lens.* 2007;33:412-414.

18. Joslin CE, Tu EY, Shoff ME, et al. The association of contact lens solution use and *Acanthamoeba* keratitis. *Am J Ophthalmol.* 2007;144:169-180.

19. Acharya NR, Lietman TM, Margolis TP. Parasites on the rise: a new epidemic of *Acanthamoeba* keratitis. *Am J Ophthalmol.* 2007;144:292-293.

20. Parmar DN, Awwad ST, Petroll M, Bowman W, McCulley JP, Cavanagh D. Tandem scanning confocal corneal microscopy in the diagnosis of suspected *Acanthamoeba* keratitis. *Ophthalmology.* 2006;113:538-547.

21. Perry HD, Donnenfeld ED, Foulks GN, Moadel K, Kanellopoulos AJ. Decreased corneal sensation as an initial feature of *Acanthamoeba* keratitis. *Ophthalmology.* 1995;102:1565-1568.

22. Thebpatiphat N, Hammersmith KM, Rocha FN, et al. *Acanthamoeba* keratitis: a parasite on the rise. *Cornea.* 2007;26:701-706.

23. Pharmakakaris NM, Andrikopoulos GK, Papadopoulos GE, et al. Does identification of the causal organism of corneal ulcers influence the outcome? *Eur J Ophthalmol.* 2003;13:11-17.

24. Khanal B, Deb M, Panda A, Sethi HS. Laboratory diagnosis in ulcerative keratitis. *Ophthalmic Res.* 2005;37:123-127.

25. Wilhelmus KR, Osata MS, Font RL, Robinson NM, Janes DB. Rapid diagnosis of *Acanthamoeba* keratitis using calcofluor white. *Arch Ophthalmol.* 1986;104:1309-1312.

26. Das S, Sheorey H, Taylor HR, Vajpayee RB. Association between cultures of contact lens and corneal scraping in contact lens-related microbial keratitis. *Arch Ophthalmol.* 2007;125:1182-1185.

27. Wilhelmus KR. Indecision about corticosteroids for bacterial keratitis: an evidence-based update. *Ophthalmology.* 2002;109:835-842.

28. Wong T, Ormonde S, Gamble G, McGhee CN. Severe infective keratitis leading to hospital admission in New Zealand. *Br J Ophthalmol.* 2003;87:1103-1108.

29. Hollander DA, Clay EL, Sidikaro Y. Infectious crystalline keratopathy associated with intravitreal and posterior sub-Tenon triamcinolone acetonide injections. *Br J Ophthalmol.* 2006;90:656-657.

30. Golub LM, Ramamurthy NS, McNamara TF, et al. Further evidence that tetracyclines inhibit collagenase, crevicular fluid in human periodontal pockets and from other mammalian sources. *J Periodont Res.* 1985;20:12-23.

31. Golub LM, Ramamurthy N, McNamara TF, et al. Tetracyclines inhibit tissue collagenase activity. A new mechanism in the treatment of periodontal disease. *J Periodontal Res.* 1984;19:651-655.

32. Perry HD, Golub LM. Systemic tetracyclines in the treatment of noninfected corneal ulcers: a case report and proposed new mechanism of action. *Ann Ophthamol.* 1985;17:742-744.

33. Perry HD, Kenyon KR, Lamberts DW, et al. Systemic tetracycline hydrochloride as adjunctive therapy in the treatment of persistent epithelial defects. *Ophthalmology.* 1986;93:1320-1322.

34. Seedor JA, Perry HD, McNamara TF, et al. Systemic tetracycline treatment of alkali inhibits corneal ulceration in rabbits. *Arch Ophthalmol.* 1987;105:268-271.

35. Perry HD, Hodes LW, Seedor JA, et al. Effect of Doxycycline hyclate on corneal epithelial wound healing in the rabbit alkali model. *Cornea.* 1993;12:379-382.

36. Levy JH, Katz HR. Effect of systemic tetracycline on progression of *Pseudomonas aeruginosa* keratitis in the rabbit. *Ann Ophthalmol.* 1990;22:179-182.

37. McElvanney AM. Doxycycline in the management of pseudomonas corneal melting: two case reports and a review of the literature. *Eye Contact Lens.* 2003;29:258-261.

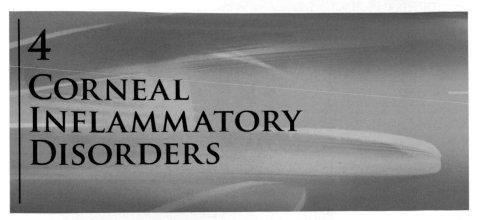

4

CORNEAL INFLAMMATORY DISORDERS

João Malta, MD; Fatima K. Ahmad, MD; Shahzad I. Mian, MD; and Alan Sugar, MD

The ocular immune response consists of a complex set of pathways that involve local and systemic reactions. The corneal epithelium, stroma, and endothelium can be involved in different types of inflammatory reactions, with resultant corneal disease. Corneal inflammation can result from trauma, neoplasia, systemic inflammation, an infectious agent, lid margin disease, or secondary to an immune-mediated hypersensitivity reaction. This chapter will focus on corneal inflammatory disorders involving the epithelium and stroma.

THYGESON'S KERATITIS

Thygeson's superficial punctate keratitis (TSPK) is an epithelial keratitis without associated systemic disease and is of unknown etiology. In 1950, Phillips Thygeson described a series of patients with multiple transient, punctate epithelial opacities, which he believed to represent a specific clinical entity.[1] The disease came to be known as Thygeson's superficial punctate keratitis, which is characterized by an insidious onset with spontaneous remissions and exacerbations for years and with good response to topical corticosteroid therapy.

Onset of TSPK can occur at all ages. In a series of 45 patients, Tabbara et al described patients ranging from 2.5 to 70 years with no gender predilection.[2] Patients can experience burning, photophobia, foreign-body sensation, tearing, and blurred vision. In the majority of cases (85% to 96%), there is bilateral involvement, although there is often asymmetry at presentation.[2,3] Though vision may be affected, visual acuity is often better than 20/30 during active disease.[3]

Slit-lamp examination typically reveals coarse, punctate, gray-white snowflake opacities in the corneal epithelium, measuring between 0.1 and 0.2 mm in diameter[4] (Figure 4-1). Although lesions can vary in number, between 3 and 20 lesions are reported in most cases,[1] which can occur anywhere in the cornea but typically affect the visual axis. There may also be associated subepithelial opacification, although this may represent stromal edema or a side effect of antiviral therapy.[2,5] During an acute attack, a raised center breaks through the epithelial surface

Trattler WB, Majmudar PA, Luchs JI, Swartz TS, eds.
Cornea Handbook (pp. 37-60)
© 2010 SLACK Incorporated

Figure 4-1. Thygeson's superficial keratitis: typical punctate gray-white snowflake opacities in the corneal epithelium.

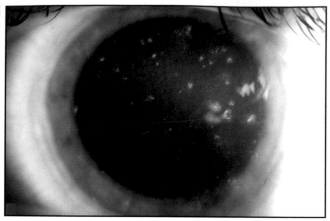

and stains irregularly with fluorescein. There is usually little to no conjunctival inflammation. Corneal sensation is mildly reduced or preserved.

The lesions are transient, can change position from week to week, and resolve on their own.[4,6] During remission, the inactive lesions are asymptomatic and appear flat with no epithelial staining. Recurrences are common, but the disease typically resolves within 3 years even when left untreated.[7] The duration is increased with use of corticosteroids and has been reported to last up to 41 years.[6,8] TSPK is considered benign, because the lesions do not lead to vascularization or scarring, and visual prognosis is very good.

The etiology of TSPK is unknown, although it is most likely immune-mediated. Thygeson suggested a viral etiology for TSPK due to the absence of bacteria, lack of response to antibiotics, and similarity of the lesions to those caused by viruses.[7] Braley et al isolated a virus from a patient with TSPK, and Lemp at al demonstrated varicella zoster virus from an 11-year-old patient with TSPK.[4,9] However, other attempts to isolate virus or viral DNA, including adenovirus, varicella zoster virus, HSV, and human papillomavirus (HPV) have been unsuccessful, suggesting that the previous findings may represent laboratory error.[5,6,10-13] It has also been suggested that TSPK could be caused by a latent viral infection in the anterior stroma.

Electron microscopic examinations of corneal epithelial cells of patients with TSPK have failed to reveal viral particles and mostly show cell necrosis.[6] In vivo confocal microscopy has shown that the lesions are characterized by clumps of enlarged, desquamating epithelial cells among normal epithelial cells.[14] There have also been abnormalities observed in the subepithelial nerve plexus, Bowman's layer, and anterior stroma, which could account for the subepithelial opacities observed clinically.[15] These findings correlate with histologic features, including intracellular and intercellular edema of the epithelium and exudates under the epithelium.[14] Conjunctival scrapings show occasional lymphocytes and monocytes.[16]

An immune mechanism for TSPK has been suggested given the presence of leukocytes without isolation of virus and response of the disease to topical corticosteroids. Darrell first reported that TSPK was associated with histocompatibility antigen HLA-DR3.[6] Patients with this haplotype were found to have a relative risk of 5.65 of developing TSPK in a study of 36 patients with the disease. HLA-DR3 is associated with other autoimmune diseases, including myasthenia gravis, Graves' disease and systemic lupus erythematosus. The presence of certain histocompatibility antigens, such as HLA-DR3, could influence the immunologic response to endogenous or exogenous antigens, including viral particles. However, this association has not been studied further in other patients with TSPK.

Topical corticosteroids have been shown to provide symptomatic relief and rapid resolution of lesions. Low-dose corticosteroids, including fluorometholone 0.1% and loteprednol 0.2%, have been shown to resolve TSPK lesions.[3] Steroids should be gradually tapered over several months, guided by clinical response. Recurrences are common when steroids are tapered, and their use may prolong the course of the disease.[2,17] Additionally, long-term use of corticosteroids is associated with increased IOP, cataract formation, and increased risk of infection. Bandage soft contact lenses can provide symptomatic relief for TSPK during acute attacks and reduce the need for topical steroid therapy.[10,17,18]

Trifluridine 1% has been shown to have a favorable effect in several cases of TSPK.[19] However, it has not been studied with controls. Idoxuridine may worsen the condition and is associated with the development of permanent subepithelial opacities.[5,7]

Topical cyclosporin A 2% (CsA) is an immunosuppressive agent that inhibits interleukin-2 and T-lymphocyte proliferation. Mononuclear cells, including T-lymphocytes, comprise the inflammatory response in TSPK and likely play an important role in pathogenesis of the disease. CsA has been studied prospectively in patients with TSPK, providing beneficial effects in the majority of adults (71.5%) receiving the medication.[20] However, chronic therapy is necessary in some patients and is not effective in children. The long-term side effects of CsA use are not known.

PRK may be considered a therapeutic option in myopic patients with TSPK.[21,22] In one case, PRK resulted in elimination of recurrent TSPK in the laser ablation zone but not the peripheral cornea.[22] The authors suggested that this was due to destruction of an inflammatory signal within the anterior stroma, which may be responsible for TSPK lesions. However, others have demonstrated recurrence of TSPK after PRK and laser-assisted subepithelial keratomileusis (LASEK), including lesions in the laser ablation zone.[21,23,24]

FILAMENTARY KERATITIS

Filamentary keratitis is characterized by filaments composed of mucus and degenerated epithelial cells adherent to the cornea.[25-28] Filamentary keratitis is often recurrent and can be difficult to treat.

Filamentary keratitis is associated with a variety of ocular and systemic conditions (Table 4-1). The most common presentation is secondary to aqueous tear deficiency, including keratoconjunctivitis sicca.[29-31] Sjögren's syndrome, an autoimmune disorder of exocrine glands, can lead to severe keratoconjunctivitis sicca.[32] Superior limbic keratoconjunctivitis (SLK) leads to a superior filamentary keratitis in up to one third of cases.[33,34] Corneal occlusion, including prolonged patching, ptosis, and contact lens overwear, is associated with filamentary keratitis.[35-38] Ocular trauma and surgery may contribute to development of filamentary keratitis. Filaments have been noted postoperatively after cataract surgery, particularly in patients with preexisting dry eye conditions.[39-42] Penetrating

Table 4-1

CAUSES OF FILAMENTARY KERATITIS

Keratoconjunctivitis sicca

- Sjögren's syndrome
- Rheumatoid arthritis
- Wegener's granulomatosis
- Systemic lupus erythematosus
- Graft-versus-host disease

Superior limbic keratoconjunctivitis

Corneal occlusion

- Prolonged patching
- Ptosis
- Essential blepharospasm

Trauma

- Abrasion
- Recurrent erosions
- Contact lens overwear or allergy

Ocular surgical procedures

- Cataract surgery
- Penetrating keratoplasty
- Photorefractive keratectomy
- Laser-assisted keratomileusis

Infectious

- Herpes simplex virus keratitis
- Adenoviral keratoconjunctivitis

Dermatologic conditions

- Atopic dermatitis
- Psoriasis
- Ectodermal dysplasia

Bullous keratopathy

Neurotrophic keratitis

Brain stem injury

Medications

- Anticholinergic drugs
- Topical medication toxicity (medicamentosa)

keratoplasty (PK) commonly results in filament formation, with 14% to 27% of postoperative cases developing filamentary keratitis.[40,43,44] Albietz et al noted filaments in patients with persistent epithelial defects following laser-assisted keratomileusis.[29] Loss of corneal sensation may play a role in development of postsurgical filamentary keratitis. Similarly, neurotrophic keratitis, herpetic keratitis, and brain stem injury[45] may contribute to filamentary keratitis. Other conditions associated with filamentary keratitis include ectodermal dysplasia and bullous keratopathy. Finally, medications including diphenhydramine hydrochloride have been implicated in development of corneal filaments, likely through anticholinergic effects.[46]

Filamentary keratitis is relatively uncommon except in high-risk patients with dry eye syndrome or postpenetrating keratoplasty. In a series of 67 patients with advanced keratoconjunctivitis sicca, Fraunfelder et al reported that 17 had corneal mucous plaques adherent to the cornea.[30] Given the correlation with Sjögren's syndrome, rheumatoid arthritis, and other connective tissue disorders, filamentary keratitis may present more commonly in middle-aged and older women. Depending on etiology, the condition can present unilaterally or bilaterally.

Filamentary keratitis presents with symptoms that range in severity from mild irritation to severe pain. Patients can experience foreign-body sensation, burning, photophobia, ocular pain, and increased blinking. Patient history can be helpful in identifying etiology, including previous medical and ocular history, prior surgery, or trauma.

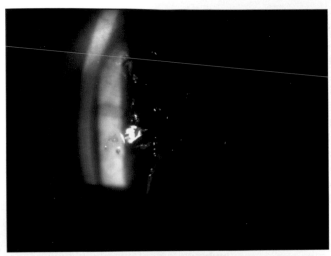

Figure 4-2. Filamentary keratitis: broad-based filaments adherent to the anterior cornea.

On slit-lamp examination, limbal hyperemia may be present. Presence of filaments adherent to the anterior cornea is diagnostic for filamentary keratitis. Filaments can range in size between 0.5 and 10 mm in length and may be fine strands or broad-based[26] (Figure 4-2). Rose bengal or lissamine green dye can be used to better visualize the filaments. Various clinical tests can be performed to make a diagnosis of dry eyes, including the Schirmer test or ocular surface staining. Corneal sensation may be decreased in many conditions that are associated with filamentary keratitis.

Although the exact mechanism is not known, filamentary keratitis is seen in a variety of pathological processes. Corneal filaments consist of a central core of epithelial cells surrounded by PAS-positive amorphous mucin-like material.[25,27,47] Impression cytology in filamentary keratitis secondary to blepharospasm has shown that corneal filaments are attached to superficial metaplastic epithelial cells.[47] Filaments are therefore likely to form in the setting of damaged epithelium and abnormal mucus tear film. Injury to surface epithelial cells can lead to exposure of intracellular keratins, which allows attachment of mucus.[48] Premature epithelial cell exfoliation and increased turnover causes incorporation of desquamated epithelial cells into the filament. Abnormal mucus production and increased viscosity of the tear film have been observed in conditions associated with filamentary keratitis.[49,50] Filaments may occur in dry eye syndrome due to altered components of the tear film and inflammation.

Early histopathologic analysis of filamentary keratitis demonstrates inflammatory cells and fibroblasts disrupting basal epithelial cells and the basement membrane, leading to focal areas of detachment.[26] This damage to the basal epithelial layer can contribute to degeneration of the epithelium seen in filamentary keratitis.

Surgical procedures such as cataract surgery and PK are thought to worsen dry eye, perhaps due to inflammation or decreased corneal innervation.[51] Ptosis and other occlusive processes may contribute to pathogenesis of filamentary keratitis due to prolonged contact between the eyelid and the cornea, which prevents mucin from being diffusely spread over the cornea with blinking.[37] Conversely, blepharospasm has also been observed to contribute to filamentary keratitis, perhaps through mechanical trauma.[47]

Filamentary keratitis is often recurrent and can be difficult to treat. Chronic disease can result in vascularization of the cornea.[52] Identification of the underlying cause can help in both treatment and prevention of the condition. Kazizaki et al described 2 cases of filamentary keratitis in the setting of blepharoptosis that improved after surgical correction.[37] Contact lens wear or any medication that can contribute to the disease should be discontinued.

In dry eye syndrome, lubricant therapy with artificial tear supplements is beneficial in treatment and prevention of filaments. Due to frequent dosing, nonpreserved tear supplements are suggested due to the toxicity of preservatives that can damage corneal epithelium and thereby exacerbate filamentary keratitis.[53,54] Artificial tears with electrolyte supplementation and moderate viscosity are suggested for promoting ocular health.[29] Punctal occlusion has been shown to improve filamentary keratitis in tear deficiency syndromes and can reduce frequency of artificial tear use.[55,56] Punctal occlusion with silicone plugs is generally well tolerated, but adverse effects include extrusion of plugs and foreign-body sensation.[57] Soft bandage contact lenses have also been used in treatment of filamentary keratitis and can help prevent trauma associated with blinking.[58,59] However, contact lens use can cause epithelial hypoxia and infectious keratitis and has been associated with filamentary keratitis.[29,60]

Mechanical removal of corneal filaments can provide symptomatic relief. This is performed with use of jeweler's or tying forceps at the slit lamp under topical anesthesia. Though this may be beneficial in the acute presentation, this does not prevent recurrence and may cause further trauma. Impression debridement with cellulose acetate filter paper may also be used to remove filaments with less damage to surrounding tissue.[61] N-acetylcysteine is a mucolytic agent that may help to dissolve filaments and loosen adherence of the filament. Topical application of 10% acetylcysteine has been reported to improve filamentary keratitis in keratoconjunctivitis sicca.[30] Acetylcysteine is not available commercially and should be refrigerated.

Hypertonic saline (sodium chloride, 5%) was beneficial in a series of patients with filamentary keratitis.[31] The hypertonic solution draws fluid from the cornea, improving adherence of the epithelium to the basement membrane. In a series of 19 patients, Hamilton and Wood saw resolution of filaments in 95% of cases where sodium chloride 5% was used 3 to 4 times daily. The treatment was less effective in patients with filaments secondary to keratoconjunctivitis sicca. Hypertonic saline is a safe, effective therapy but may not be the best agent in severe cases.

Because inflammation is thought to be a pathogenic factor in filament formation, anti-inflammatory agents have been used in the treatment of filamentary keratitis. Diclofenac sodium, a nonsteroidal anti-inflammatory drug, has been beneficial in improvement of filamentary keratitis and provides analgesia. In a randomized study of patients with filamentary keratitis secondary to Sjögren's syndrome, both diclofenac sodium 0.1% and sodium chloride 5% were efficacious.[62] Diclofenac sodium resulted in more rapid improvement in symptoms associated with filamentary keratitis, including ocular pain. Diclofenac sodium has also been beneficial in patients with filamentary keratitis after ophthalmic surgery.[40]

Topical corticosteroid therapy for treatment of filamentary keratitis has been evaluated in patients with Sjögren's syndrome–associated keratoconjunctivitis sicca. In a case series of 21 patients, 10 eyes were reported to have filamentary keratitis.[32] All 10 eyes showed resolution of filaments after treatment with topical nonpreserved methylpred-nisolone, with treatment duration ranging from 2 weeks to 7 months. Given the risks of therapy, however, including increased IOP and cataract formation, steroid therapy should be limited in duration and reserved for cases refractive to other therapies.

Topical cyclosporine is effective in treatment of dry eye disease.[63,64] It has also been described as possible therapy for SLC. In one case report of SLC, a patient was noted to have resolution of superior filamentary keratitis after a 6-week course of topical CsA 0.5% in combination with artificial tears.[33] Cyclosporine may provide benefit by modulating T-cell-mediated destruction of lacrimal glands.

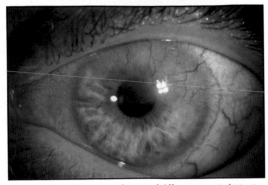

Figure 4-3. Ocular rosacea: chronic and diffuse conjunctival injection and marginal cornea vascular infiltration.

OCULAR ROSACEA

Rosacea is a common, idiopathic, chronic inflammatory disorder affecting both facial skin and the eye. The clinical presentation is most common in middle-aged women. The typical facial feature of advanced rosacea is rhinophyma or bulbous nose appearance caused by sebaceous gland hypertrophy.[65]

The pathogenesis of rosacea is unknown. The colonization of certain bacteria (*Staphylococcus epidermidis* and *Propionibacterium acnes*) on the eyelid margin produce lipases that appear to be indirectly responsible for meibomitis by altering the meibomian gland secretions near the gland orifices with a resultant change in the concentration of inflammatory free fatty acids in the tear film.[66] Vasomotor lability is easily induced and appears to be aggravated by coffee, tea, alcohol, spicy foods, hormonal changes, and anxiety.[67]

Ocular findings occur in about 50% of patients at some point in the course of their disease and the involvement is usually bilateral. Symptoms include burning, photophobia, redness, and foreign-body sensation. Blepharitis and meibomian dysfunction are the most common associated findings. The lid margins are hyperemic, thickened, telangiectatic, and, in some patients, staphylococcal lid infections can be demonstrated. The meibomian glands secrete excess sebum, and the orifices may be inspissated and inflamed with formation of chalazia and hordeola. Chronic and diffuse conjunctival injection may also occur.[68]

Corneal involvement is seen in approximately 5% to 30% of cutaneous rosacea patients and may be characterized by superficial punctate keratopathy, marginal vascular infiltration, subepithelial infiltrates, ulceration, and, in rare cases, corneal perforation (Figure 4-3). Chronic rosacea keratitis results in broad areas of pannus, usually inferior, with peripheral scars and stromal thinning. Keratitis sicca has also been described with ocular rosacea.[65]

Ocular findings include conjunctival and corneal infiltration with chronic inflammatory cells, including lymphocytes, epithelioid cells, plasma cells, and giant cells. An immunopathologic study of conjunctival inflammation suggested a type IV hypersensitivity reaction.[69]

Treatment of rosacea is palliative because no cure is currently available. Oral tetracycline or doxycycline may be required for daily maintenance, because antibiotic therapy is suppressive rather than curative.[70] The mechanism of action may be an effect on the secretion of sebum or influence on the interaction of the sebaceous glands with bacteria. Additional ocular therapy includes preservative free artificial tears, eyelid hygiene, and erythromycin ointment to help control blepharitis. Topical corticosteroids may be considered for conjunctivitis and keratitis; however, steroids must be used judiciously to avoid corneal melting and perforation.[71]

MARGINAL KERATITIS

Marginal keratitis, also termed *catarrhal infiltrate* or *ulcer*, represents a sterile hypersensitivity reaction to *Staphylococcus aureus* and most commonly occurs in the setting of longstanding staphylococcal blepharoconjunctivitis.[72]

Marginal keratitis typically affects adults with longstanding blepharitis, with cultures growing coagulase-positive *S. aureus*.[73] Thygeson reported in 1946 that *S. aureus* was isolated from the lids of 133 of 156 patients with catarrhal ulcers in the setting of chronic catarrhal conjunctivitis.[74] However, cultures from catarrhal ulcers were negative.[75] Furthermore, patients with recurrent marginal keratitis usually have negative lid cultures, which is likely due to treatment of a previous infection.[76]

Rabbits immunized and boosted with *S. aureus* have been shown to develop peripheral corneal infiltrates resembling catarrhal infiltrates in humans.[77,78] From these early animal models, it was suggested that delayed type hypersensitivity may play a role in development of marginal corneal disease, as it does with phlyctenulosis. However, when patients with marginal staphylococcal keratitis are tested for cell-mediated immunity to *S. aureus*, the majority have a normal response.[79] Superantigen toxins, which are expressed by some strains of *S. aureus*, are also not involved in development of marginal keratitis.[76]

Cytology of the lesions shows acute inflammation with neutrophils and corneal cell necrosis.[73,75] It is believed that the lesion is a result of an antigen–antibody reaction, which leads to immune complex deposition, complement activation, and neutrophil infiltration.[72,73] Catarrhal infiltrate is associated with elevated levels of C3 complement.[80] The peripheral cornea has been shown to have significantly higher levels of C1 complement compared to the central cornea.[73] Therefore, activation of the complement pathway could explain the distribution of the disease.

A sterile, peripheral keratitis has been reported following laser-assisted in situ keratomileusis (LASIK) in patients with chronic blepharitis and may represent a reactivation of marginal keratitis.[81-83] A sterile marginal keratitis has also been described in hypersensitivity reactions to topical eye medications, including phenylephrine, gentamicin, atropine, and dorzolamide.[84]

Staphylococcal blepharitis is relatively common, and up to one third of clinically quiet eyes have positive *S. aureus* cultures from lid margins.[72] However, not all patients with blepharitis develop corneal lesions. In a series of 116 patients with chronic blepharitis, Ficker et al reported that 37 had recurrent marginal keratitis.[79] In a series of 44 children aged 1 to 14 with staphylococcal blepharitis, 28 developed marginal infiltrates, and 4 had marginal ulcers.[85] The incidence of methicillin-resistant *S. aureus* (MRSA) has increased recently, and ocular isolates of MRSA increased from 18.3% in 2000 to 29.1% in 2005.[86]

Patients with sterile marginal keratitis typically have mild symptoms. They may experience pain, burning, foreign-body sensation, photophobia, redness, and irritation. In comparison to bacterial ulcers, the presentation is less severe, and this may delay presentation for treatment.[87] Signs of chronic blepharitis are usually present and include lid erythema, loss of lashes (madarosis), trichiasis, collarettes, plugging of meibomian gland openings, and conjunctival injection.

Catarrhal infiltrates occur in the peripheral corneal stroma and are separated from the limbus by an intervening 1-mm to 2-mm rim of normal corneal tissue. They most commonly originate at the 10-, 2-, 4-, and 8-o'clock positions (where lids cross corneal periphery) and are 1 to 2 mm in width. There can be one or multiple lesions, and these can form partial rings or crescents including circumferential involvement.

The infiltrate appears first, followed by epithelial breakdown and ulcer formation. As catarrhal ulcers heal, there may be neovascularization from the limbus. Recurrences are common, and often cultures from patients with recurrent marginal keratitis are negative, which reflects continued immunologic reaction without active infection.[76]

The first step is treatment of staphylococcal blepharitis with eyelid hygiene and antibiotic ointment. Topical aminoglycosides or fluoroquinolones can be used to treat the infection. Systemic antibiotics may be used in recurrent or severe cases. Macrolides, including erythromycin, and tetracycline have also been used successfully.[85,88] Tetracyclines should be avoided in children less than age 8 because they can cause dental abnormalities. Given the rise in community-acquired MRSA, which are usually resistant to erythromycin, cultures and sensitivities should be taken in cases refractory to therapy.[89]

In addition to blepharitis therapy, catarrhal infiltrates or ulcers are treated with topical corticosteroids. Prednisolone 1% or fluorometholone have been used effectively in treatment of catarrhal ulcers. The lesions of marginal keratitis respond rapidly to steroid treatment, which is helpful diagnostically. If there is concern for infection within the epithelial defect, corticosteroid therapy can be preceded by topical antibiotic therapy.

PHLYCTENULOSIS

Phlyctenulosis is an inflammatory, nodular reaction in the conjunctiva or cornea caused by a delayed-type hypersensitivity reaction to various pathogenic antigens. Epidemiology of the disease has changed over time, resulting in newer management strategies.

Phlyctenular keratoconjunctivitis (PKC) was described as early as 1722 by St. Yves. In the early 20th century, it was noted to commonly affect children who developed tuberculosis or those with a positive tuberculin skin test.[90-93] The Bacillus Calmette-Guérin (BCG) vaccine, a live attenuated vaccine derived from *Mycobacterium bovis*, also resulted in PKC in children 2 to 6 weeks after inoculation.[94] Multiple unsuccessful attempts were made to isolate the tubercle bacillus from phlyctenules, and injection of phlycten material into conjunctiva of apes did not produce disease.[91] It was concluded that phlyctenules were sterile nodules and likely represented a hypersensitivity reaction to tuberculin protein (Figure 4-4).

Figure 4-4. Corneal phlyctenule: peripheral white raised nodules surrounding neovascularization.

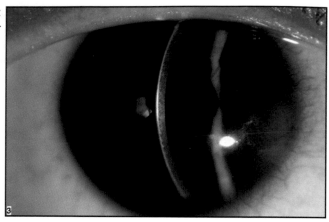

Other bacterial pathogens have also been described to be associated with PKC and represent a greater portion of phlyctenulosis cases today. *S. aureus*,[72,95] *Neisseria gonorrhea*, *P. acnes*,[96] and *Chlamydia*[97,98] have been implicated as etiologic agents in PKC. Mondino et al developed an animal model for phlyctenulosis by sensitizing and then challenging rabbits with *S. aureus*, with the antigen responsible for development of phlyctenulosis in this model being ribitol teichoic acid.[77]

Infection with parasites is an important cause of PKC in endemic regions. Specifically, infections with *Ascaris lumbricoides*, *Ancylostoma duodenale*, *Enterobius vermicularis*, and *Entamoeba histolytica* have been associated with PKC.[99] *Hymenolepis nana* (dwarf tapeworm) is common in patients with phlyctenulosis in Egypt.[100,101] *Pediculosis humanus capitis* (head louse) was noted in a population of Alaskan natives where PKC was common.[102] In addition, there have been reports of association of phlyctenulosis with viruses (herpes simplex virus),[103] fungi (*Candida albicans*),[92] and rosacea[104,105] (Table 4-2).

PKC represents a delayed type hypersensitivity reaction (DTH, type IV) to a variety of microbial antigens.[72,78] In animal experiments, implantation of tubercle bacilli into conjunctiva did not result in phlyctenulosis, but the disease could be replicated by sensitizing rabbits with tuberculin protein and reinjecting them.[91,106] Hypersensitivity reactions require prior exposure, or a sensitized state, in order for the immunologic response to be mounted.

Histology and immunohistochemistry of phlyctenules show an epithelial infiltrate of monocytes, macrophages, dendritic Langerhans cells, polymorphonuclear cells, and T-lymphocytes but few B-lymphocytes or plasma cells.[107] Immunocytology of scrapings from phlyctenules shows T-lymphocytes.[108] This is consistent with the inflammation associated with DTH, which is mediated by T cells and monocytes/macrophages. It is not understood why the disease manifests in a localized manner in the cornea and conjunctiva. Phlyctenulosis is associated with elevated levels of serum IgG and IgM, and IgA concentrations in human tears of patients with PKC are not different from matched controls.[109,110] This suggests that PKC is the result of systemic inflammation and not a local, mucosal response.

Phlyctenulosis is a disease predominantly affecting children and adolescents. Phlyctenular disease affects women more than men, with a ratio of approximately 2:1.[91] The prevalence of the disease has decreased dramatically with the

Table 4-2

CAUSES OF PHLYCTENULOSIS

Bacterial	*Mycobacterium tuberculosis*
	Staphylococcus aureus
	Neisseria gonorrhea
	Propionibacterium acnes
	Chlamydia
Fungal	*Candida albicans*
Parasitic	*Ascaris lumbricoides*
	Ancylostoma duodenale
	Enterobius vermicularis
	Entamoeba histolytica
	Leishmaniasis
	Hymenolepis nana
	Pediculosis capitis
Viruses	Herpes simplex virus
Other	Rosacea

eradication of endemic tuberculosis. It is believed that staphylococcal blepharitis is now a more common cause of PKC.[78] Though tuberculosis is less frequent in developed countries, it still remains a major cause of PKC throughout the world. In a prospective study of 112 patients in India in 2000, PKC was associated with tuberculosis in 76.7% of patients.[111] Pulmonary and lymph node tuberculosis are most commonly associated with PKC, although cutaneous, meningeal, and bone involvement have also been noted.[91,93,112]

Genetic factors may predispose patients to PKC. HLA-A26 and HLA-B35 have been associated with PKC and blepharitis in a population of Japanese patients.[96] McLean reported a high rate of phlyctenulosis among Eskimos of the Canadian eastern Arctic. This may be attributed to pediculosis capitis, which was also common in this population.[102]

Patients with PKC can present with tearing, foreign-body sensation, photophobia, redness, burning, or itching. If the cornea is involved, visual acuity may be affected and the patient can experience blepharospasm. In up to one half of cases, phlyctenulosis is bilateral at initial presentation.[93,96]

On examination, phlyctenules appear as white or pink raised nodules. They occur most commonly at the limbus but can also affect the cornea or bulbar conjunctiva (see Figure 4-4). A phlyctenule is typically between 1 and 3 mm in diameter.[96] Multiple phlyctenules can be present, as in miliary phlyctenulosis. There may be injection of the surrounding conjunctival vessels and neovascularization. Eyelids should be examined for blepharitis, meibomitis, or chalazia.

Corneal phlyctenules typically run a 2- to 3-week course, and some may resolve spontaneously.[93] In other cases, corneal phlyctenules ulcerate with erosion of the overlying corneal epithelium and stromal infiltration.[92,106] Phlyctenules can be mobile and tend to progress toward the center of the cornea.[113] Resolution of corneal ulcers can result in scarring with significant visual impairment and astigmatism.[114] Corneal perforation in staphylococcal PKC has been reported.[115]

Treatment of the underlying infection can improve symptoms of PKC.[100,116] Medical history, including exposure and travel history, will help guide which infectious testing should be performed. Though tuberculosis is less common, patients with even minimal risk should be referred for tuberculin skin test or chest X-ray. If parasitic disease is suspected, complete blood count may show eosinophilia, and appropriate testing should be performed. Corneal cultures may be helpful in diagnosis of other bacterial infections, including staphylococcal blepharitis or chlamydial infection.

In the case of mild PKC associated with blepharitis or meibomitis, eyelid hygiene with antibiotic–corticosteroid ointment should be initiated. Oral antibiotic therapy with macrolides (erythromycin) and tetracyclines has been reported to be an effective treatment for nontuberculous PKC, resulting in remission of the disease.[98,104,105] Systemic cephalosporin therapy was effective in treating PKC when associated with *P. acnes* meibomitis.[96]

When corneal phlyctenules are present, therapy with topical corticosteroids should be initiated to minimize inflammation and scarring. Corneal phlyctenules can be treated with prednisolone acetate 1% 6 times a day, or dexamethasone 0.1% 2 to 4 times a day.[85,114] Patients should be followed frequently, and the steroids can be tapered after a response is noted. Occasionally, patients become steroid dependent, and chronic steroid therapy is associated with adverse complications, including cataract formation, increased IOP, and infection.

CsA inhibits T-lymphocyte production of interleukin 2, which is essential in treating PKC. Topical application of CsA 2% has been shown to be an effective treatment in children with steroid-dependent PKC.[114] In a series of 11 patients with severe childhood PKC, cyclosporine could be withdrawn after 6 to 31 months of treatment with resolution of symptoms. This preparation has a higher concentration of CsA than Restasis (CsA 0.05%), and the long-term safety profile is not known. Other anti-inflammatory agents, such as methotrexate, have been shown to decrease inflammation and neovascularization in animal models of phlyctenular keratitis.[117] These agents do not yet have a role in the treatment of human disease.

If there is corneal ulceration or concern for infectious keratitis, the treatment regimen should be supplemented with topical antibiotic therapy. PK has been performed for treatment of corneal scarring secondary to inactive PKC with a favorable prognosis.[118,119]

INTERSTITIAL KERATITIS

Interstitial keratitis (IK) describes nonsuppurative inflammation of the corneal stroma, which may be associated with neovascularization, but does not specify etiology. Although syphilis is a common cause of IK, there are various other bacterial, viral, parasitic, and autoimmune causes (Table 4-3).

Bacterial Interstitial Keratitis: Syphilis

Syphilitic IK is classified as acquired or congenital. Acquired syphilis is divided into early (primary, secondary, and early latent < 2 years of infection) and late

Table 4-3

CAUSES OF INTERSTITIAL KERATITIS

Bacterial Infection	Parasitic Infection
Syphilis	Leishmaniasis
Tuberculosis	Onchocerciasis
Leprosy	Trypanosomiasis
Lyme disease	Cysticercosis
Brucellosis	Acanthamoeba
Chlamydia trachomatis	Microsporidiosis

Viral Infection	Systemic Disease
Herpes simplex virus	Cogan's syndrome
Herpes zoster virus	Sarcoidosis
Epstein-Barr virus	Lymphoma
Mumps	Kaposi's sarcoma
Rubeola	Mycosis fungoides
Measles	Incontinentia pigmenti
Influenza	Hidradenitis suppurativa
Small Pox	
Vaccinia	

(late latent > 2 years, and tertiary including gummatous, cardiovascular, and neurological involvement) syphilis.

In the United States, the estimated annual rates are 100 adults with acquired syphilis and 1 child with congenital syphilis per 1 million persons.[120] Fewer than 500 new cases of syphilitic IK occur each year.[121] The clinical presentation of IK in syphilis can be subcategorized as active keratitis and residual keratopathy.

Symptoms of active IK include pain, photophobia, epiphora, and blurred vision. Clinical findings may include peripheral or diffuse infiltrative stromal keratitis; deep, focal stromal keratitis with edema; multifocal or marginal stromal infiltrates; necrotizing stromal keratouveitis; and iritis. Although corneal endothelial function can be impaired, the epithelium usually remains intact.[122] Corneal neovascularization can be absent, minimal, or marked depending on the severity of inflammation and the use of anti-inflammatory drugs. Deep corneal blood vessels with superficial stromal inflammation can have the appearance of a "salmon patch." Once the cornea is vascularized, the inflammatory process begins to subside. Resolution usually starts peripherally, and the vessels slowly shrink, with many becoming all but invisible. Deeper vessels fade into tiny endothelial tubes that were formerly mistaken as phantom remnants and many continue to carry plasma. Stromal remodeling can alter surface topography where anterior stromal inflammation may result in flattening, whereas deep necrotizing keratitis may produce a steepened contour.[120]

Early congenital syphilis is a rare condition, with onset between birth and 2 years that may result in necrotizing stromal keratitis with bilateral opacification. Nonulcerative stromal keratitis is the most common and often the only inflammatory finding in late congenital syphilis.[123] Bilateral involvement is common, which may occur simultaneously but is often separated by several weeks or months.[124]

Figure 4-5. Syphilitic interstitial keratitis: residual stromal keratopathy with patchy stromal opacification, ridges in Descemet's membrane, and stromal ghost vessels.

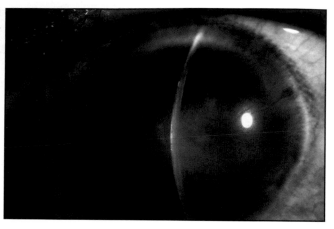

Approximately 5% to 15% of untreated cases of IK recur, generally with a milder reaction than the original episode. Approximately 10% of young children with syphilitic IK have chorioretinal scars (pigmentary chorioretinopathy), perivascular fibrotic sheathing, or paravascular pigmentation.[124]

IK is an uncommon manifestation of acquired syphilis typically presenting with a spontaneous, unilateral, nonulcerative stromal keratitis many years after a primary chancre. The clinical presentation has less neovascularization and resolves more quickly than congenital syphilis. Deep, focal stromal keratitis is typical; however, superficial punctate opacities, marginal ulcerative keratitis, and deep multifocal infiltrates can occur.[125] IK may be more likely if syphilis was acquired at a young age.[126]

Postsyphilitic stromal keratopathy presents with bilateral diffuse or patchy stromal opacification, ridges in Descemet's membrane, endothelial pleomorphism, stromal ghost vessels, iris atrophy, and iridoschisis (Figure 4-5). The postinflammatory endotheliopathy may predispose to corneal edema later in life, particularly after intraocular surgery. Peripheral anterior synechiae and posterior synechiae persist in one third of patients and contribute to pupillary distortion and anisocoria. Ocular hypertension and open and closed angle glaucoma may also occur 15 to 30 years after initial presentation.[127,128] Additional corneal findings include Salzmann's nodular degeneration and band keratopathy. Corneal sensation is typically intact.[129]

Regressed neovascularization appears as faint, translucent channels termed *ghost vessels*, in mid or deep stroma, which remain patent due to flow of plasma.[121] These channels can be visualized by indirect illumination, retroillumination, and specular reflection. They are also more commonly seen in congenital syphilis than in acquired syphilis.

Syphilitic keratitis is caused by an immune-mediated reaction, with an unknown antigenic stimulus. *Treponema pallidum* is unlikely to chronically infect the cornea. In fact, treponemes are not demonstrable in the cornea and aqueous humor as demonstrated by dark-field microscopy, special stains, rabbit infectivity, and molecular testing.[120] Histopathologic examination reveals a diffuse lymphocytic infiltrate with thickened corneal stroma.

Serologic testing for syphilis may be indicated for patients with bilateral stromal keratitis or keratouveitis; primary deep stromal keratitis with unknown etiology; sectoral stromal keratitis in childhood; stromal keratitis associated with pigmentary chorioretinopathy or other developmental stigmata of congenital syphilis; necrotizing stromal keratitis presenting with the skin rash of secondary acquired syphilis; and stromal keratitis associated with optic atrophy.

Two categories of serologic tests are assayed in the screening and evaluation of syphilis. Treponemal serologic tests detect immunoglobulins to *T. pallidum*. The most frequent tests used to detect antitreponemal antibodies are indirect immunofluorescence (FTA-ABS) and enzyme immunoassay (EIA and ELISA). The polymerase chain reaction (PCR) detects *T. pallidum* DNA or RNA. Nontreponemal tests (VDRL and RPR) detect immunoglobulins to mitochondrial membrane phospholipids. These anticardiolipin antibodies appear during early syphilis and gradually decrease in titer, ultimately disappearing in about a quarter of untreated individuals.[130] A treponemal test remains reactive for life in two thirds of patients with congenital syphilis and in 80% of adults treated for acquired syphilis. The titer of a nontreponemal test is used to assess disease activity and provides a measure for posttreatment comparison.[130]

Antibacterial treatment with intravenous penicillin G for systemic disease is recommended for children with congenital syphilis and adults with neurosyphilis. An alternative is procaine penicillin G 2.4 million units intramuscularly daily for 10 to 14 days, augmented with oral probenecid 500 mg orally 4 times daily. Systemic corticosteroid treatment is not needed for acute syphilitic keratitis.[131]

Corneal inflammation is treated with topical corticosteroids, which shorten the course of active syphilitic keratitis, reduce permanent opacification, and improve vision. Prednisolone 1% or dexamethasone 0.1% is usually given 4 to 8 times daily. A mydriatic-cycloplegic agent can be used for concomitant iridocyclitis. Topical antibiotics are not needed.[122]

PK is the preferred surgical procedure for treating residual corneal opacification. Deep lamellar keratoplasty is generally not recommended due to frequent involvement of Descemet's membrane and corneal endothelium. Surgical outcomes are good, with a 10-year corneal graft survival rate of 80%.[120]

Bacterial Interstitial Keratitis: Tuberculosis

Tuberculosis remains a significant infectious disease problem around the world and has recently reemerged as a public health concern in the United States. IK secondary to systemic *M. tuberculosis* infection is generally unilateral and occurs because of a localized immune response to tuberculin antigens. The inflammation may involve the anterior or posterior stroma, resulting in stromal vascularization, scarring, or thinning. Treatment involves systemic therapy for the underlying tuberculosis with isoniazid, rifampin, pyrazinamide, and streptomycin or ethambutol.[132] Ocular disease is treated with topical corticosteroids and cycloplegic medications.

Bacterial Interstitial Keratitis: Leprosy

In contrast to tuberculosis, corneal involvement in leprosy is generally bilateral. The presence of organisms throughout the stroma supports an infectious rather than an immunologic etiology. The ocular manifestations include punctate epithelial keratopathy, corneal hypesthesia, corneal pannus, corneal nerve involvement, and IK. Management of ocular disease includes topical corticosteroids and cycloplegic agents.[133]

Figure 4-6. Viral interstitial keratitis: immune stromal keratitis resulting in stromal scarring and corneal vascularization secondary to herpes simplex virus.

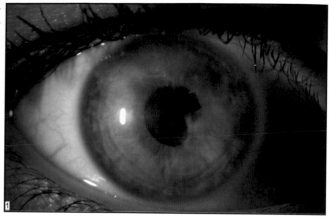

Bacterial Interstitial Keratitis: Lyme Disease

Lyme disease is caused by infection with the spirochete *Borrelia burgdorferi*. Keratitis is not a common feature of Lyme disease; however, the inflammation has an interstitial pattern. The clinical presentation is typically has bilateral, multiple poorly defined or nebular stromal opacities, rarely associated with stromal edema. Use of topical corticosteroids appears to prevent the progression of inflammation to vascularization and scarring.[134]

Viral Interstitial Keratitis

Immune stromal keratitis is a common chronic recurrent manifestation of HSV, occurring in 20% of patients with ocular HSV.[135] Viral IK may also occur secondary to herpes zoster, Epstein-Barr virus, mumps, and measles.

Stromal infiltration is the most common finding in recurrent immune stromal keratitis and can present as punctate stromal opacities, which represent antigen-antibody-complement (AAC) immune complexes. Others findings include central or paracentral localization, immune ring formation, and stromal neovascularization (Figure 4-6). The pattern of stromal inflammation may be focal, multifocal, or diffuse. Stromal infiltration is often accompanied by anterior chamber inflammation, ciliary flush, and significant discomfort.[136] Ghost vessels, lipid keratopathy, stromal scarring, and corneal thinning may occur. Corneal vascularization can decrease the success rate of penetration keratoplasty due to an increased risk of rejection.[137] The clinical course of immune stromal keratitis is chronic, with recurrent inflammation that can persist for years.

The mechanism of inflammation is thought to be due to retained viral antigen within the stroma. This antigen triggers the AAC cascade that results in intrastromal inflammation. Topical corticosteroids are required to treat acute and suppress chronic stromal inflammation. In addition, oral acyclovir 400 mg twice daily decreases risk of recurrent stromal keratitis.[138]

Parasitic Interstitial Keratitis

Leishmaniasis occurs due to a cutaneous or visceral infection with species of the protozoal genus *Leishmania*. The eyelids and the cornea can be affected in the facial form of leishmaniasis. IK can present with focal or diffuse stromal infiltration with characteristic deep vascularization. The ocular treatment involves systemic therapy with stibogluconate sodium and meglumine antimonite, which can also be used topically for keratitis.[139]

Onchocerciasis remains a significant health problem worldwide and a principal cause of infectious corneal blindness. The corneal manifestations include presence of live microfilariae, punctate epitheliopathy, subepithelial infiltration, stromal edema, scarring, and neovascularization. Systemic treatment with ivermectin is necessary.[140]

Cogan's Syndrome

Cogan's syndrome is defined as nonsyphilitic IK associated with vestibuloauditory disease manifested by a sudden onset of tinnitus, vertigo, nausea, and vomiting similar to Menière's disease.[141] Cogan's syndrome, in its classic description, represents the clinical manifestations of an immune response against an antigen present in both the corneal stroma and the inner ear.[142] Atypical Cogan's syndrome is defined by vestibuloauditory dysfunction and ocular inflammatory disease other than IK and iritis such as posterior uveitis, scleritis, episcleritis, disk edema, or orbital inflammation. This syndrome has been associated with a number of underlying systemic vasculitidies such as polyarteritis nodosa, Wegener's granulomatosis, and rheumatoid arthritis.

Cogan's syndrome commonly affects young adults, with onset on average at age 27.[143] IK associated with Cogan's syndrome presents with sudden onset, gradual resolution, and frequent recurrences over the course of the disease. The IK can be unilateral or bilateral with a patchy distribution. Symptoms include severe eye pain, tearing, redness, and photophobia. The anterior stroma may be involved in the earlier course of the disease, with corneal vascularization occurring later.[144] Other ocular findings include conjunctivitis, iritis, scleritis, and episcleritis.

Vestibuloauditory dysfunction is defined by nausea and vomiting associated with tinnitus, vertigo, and progressive loss of hearing. These symptoms usually occur no later than 1 to 6 months after the onset of ocular symptoms. The hearing loss can progress to total deafness within 3 months if left untreated.[145]

Cogan's syndrome is also associated with systemic vasculitis, predominantly involving large vessels (aortic insufficiency, aortitis, necrotizing large vessel, and polyarteritis nodosa),[146] in patients with antecedent upper respiratory illness.

The exact etiology of Cogan's syndrome remains unknown. Corneal histologic studies have demonstrated infiltration of the deep stromal layers with lymphocytes and plasma cells.[147] Other studies have also shown infiltration of the cochlea with plasma cells and lymphocytes in patients with atypical Cogan's syndrome.[148]

Patients may have leukocytosis and mild eosinophilia.[145] Most patients have elevated erythrocyte sedimentation rates, normal complement levels, and negative antinuclear antibodies.

Systemic corticosteroids are recommended to avoid severe and profound hearing loss. Patients are usually started on 2 mg/kg/day of prednisone for the first week and then slowly tapered, depending on the therapeutic response and development of adverse effects.[143] Ocular symptoms of IK and iritis tend to be relatively mild and treated with topical corticosteroids and cycloplegic agents, with most patients maintaining good visual acuity.

Prompt and prolonged immunosuppressive therapy is warranted for patients with Cogan's syndrome with an underlying active rheumatologic disease.

Corticosteroids alone and other immunosuppressive agents such as CsA, cyclophosphamide, tacrolimus, and tumor necrosis factor-alpha (TNF-α) inhibitors have been successfully used for the treatment of rheumatologic disease.[149,150]

CONCLUSION

Corneal inflammatory disorders have a variety of clinical presentations with involvement of different layers of the cornea. They also represent different immune-mediated hypersensitivity reactions that can result in chronic symptoms and a prolonged disease course if appropriate diagnosis and treatment are not initiated.

REFERENCES

1. Thygeson P. Superficial punctate keratitis. *J Am Med Assoc.* 1950;144:1544-1549.
2. Tabbara KF, Ostler HB, Dawson C, Oh J. Thygeson's superficial punctate keratitis. *Ophthalmology.* 1981;88:75-77.
3. Nagra PK, Rapuano CJ, Cohen EJ, Laibson PR. Thygeson's superficial punctate keratitis: ten years' experience. *Ophthalmology.* 2004;111:34-37.
4. Braley AE, Alexander RC. Superficial punctate keratitis: the isolation of a virus. *Trans Am Ophthalmol Soc.* 1951;49:283-296.
5. Jones BR. Thygeson's superficial punctate keratitis. *Trans Ophthalmol Soc UK.* 1963;83:245-253.
6. Darrell RW. Thygeson's superficial punctate keratitis: natural history and association with HLA DR3. *Trans Am Ophthalmol Soc.* 1981;79:486-516.
7. Thygeson P. Clinical and laboratory observations on superficial punctate keratitis. *Am J Ophthalmol.* 1966;61(pt 2):1344-1349.
8. Tanzer DJ, Smith RE. Superficial punctate keratitis of Thygeson: the longest course on record? *Cornea.* 1999;18:729-730.
9. Lemp MA, Chambers RW Jr, Lundy J. Viral isolate in superficial punctate keratitis. *Arch Ophthalmol.* 1974;91:8-10.
10. Sundmacher R, Press M, Neumann-Haefelin D, Riede U. Thygeson's superficial punctate keratitis. *Klin Monatsbl Augenheilkd.* 1977;170:908-916.
11. Reinhard T, Roggendorf M, Fengler I, Sundmacher R. PCR for varicella zoster virus genome negative in corneal epithelial cells of patients with Thygeson's superficial punctate keratitis. *Eye.* 2004;18:304-305.
12. Connell PP, O'Reilly J, Coughlan S, et al. The role of common viral ocular pathogens in Thygeson's superficial punctate keratitis. *Br J Ophthalmol.* 2007;91:1038-1041.
13. Schwab IR, Adrean SD. The superficial punctate keratitis of thygeson. In: Krachmer JH, Mannis MJ, Holland EJ, eds. *Cornea.* 2nd ed. Philadelphia, PA: Mosby; 2005.
14. Cheng LL, Young AL, Wong AKK, et al. In vivo confocal microscopy of Thygeson's superficial punctate keratitis. *Clin Exp Ophthalmol.* 2004;32:325-327.
15. Watson SL, Hollingsworth J, Tullo AB. Confocal microscopy of Thygeson's superficial punctate keratopathy. *Cornea.* 2003;22:294-299.
16. Thygeson P. Further observations on superficial punctate keratitis. *Arch Ophthalmol.* 1961;66:34-38.
17. Goldberg DB, Schanzlin DJ, Brown SI. Management of Thygeson's superficial punctate keratitis. *Am J Ophthalmol.* 1980;89:22-24.
18. Forstot SL, Binder PS. Treatment of Thygeson's superficial punctate keratopathy with soft contact lenses. *Am J Ophthalmol.* 1979;88:186-189.
19. Nesburn AB, Lowe GH III, Lepoff NJ, Maguen E. Effect of topical trifluridine on Thygeson's superficial punctate keratitis. *Ophthalmology.* 1984;91:1188-1192.

20. Reinhard T, Sundmacher R. Topical cyclosporin A in Thygeson's superficial punctate keratitis. *Graefes Arch Clin Exp Ophthalmol.* 1999;237:109-112.

21. Netto MV, Chalita MR, Krueger RR. Thygeson's superficial punctate keratitis recurrence after laser in situ keratomileusis. *Am J Ophthalmol.* 2004;138:507-508.

22. Fite SW, Chodosh J. Photorefractive keratectomy for myopia in the setting of Thygeson's superficial punctate keratitis. *Cornea.* 2001;20:425-426.

23. Jabbur NS, O'Brien TP. Recurrence of keratitis after excimer laser keratectomy. *J Cataract Refract Surg.* 2003;29:198-201.

24. Seo KY, Lee JB, Jun RM, Kim EK. Recurrence of Thygeson's superficial punctate keratitis after photorefractive keratectomy. *Cornea.* 2002;21:736-737.

25. Wright P. Filamentary keratitis. *Trans Ophthalmol Soc UK.* 1975;95:260-266.

26. Zaidman GW, Geeraets R, Paylor RR, Ferry AP. The histopathology of filamentary keratitis. *Arch Ophthalmol.* 1985;103:1178-1181.

27. Tabery HM. Filamentary keratopathy: a non-contact photomicrographic in vivo study in the human cornea. *Eur J Ophthalmol.* 2003;13:599-605.

28. Lohman LE, Rao GN, Aquavella JV. In vivo microscopic observations of human corneal epithelial abnormalities. *Am J Ophthalmol.* 1982;93:210-217.

29. Albietz J, Sanfilippo P, Troutbeck R, Lenton LM. Management of filamentary keratitis associated with aqueous-deficient dry eye. *Optom Vis Sci.* 2003;80:420-430.

30. Fraunfelder FT, Wright P, Tripathi RC. Corneal mucus plaques. *Am J Ophthalmol.* 1977;83:191-217.

31. Hamilton W, Wood TO. Filamentary keratitis. *Am J Ophthalmol.* 1982;93:466-469.

32. Marsh P, Pflugfelder SC. Topical nonpreserved methylprednisolone therapy for keratoconjunctivitis sicca in Sjogren syndrome. *Ophthalmology.* 1999;106:811-816.

33. Perry HD, Doshi-Carnevale S, Donnenfeld ED, Kornstein HS. Topical cyclosporine A 0.5% as a possible new treatment for superior limbic keratoconjunctivitis. *Ophthalmology.* 2003;110:1578-1581.

34. Theodore FH, Ferry AP. Superior limbic keratoconjunctivitis. Clinical and pathological correlations. *Arch Ophthalmol.* 1970;84:481-484.

35. Baum JL. The Castroviejo lecture. Prolonged eyelid closure is a risk to the cornea. *Cornea.* 1997;16:602-611.

36. Good WV, Whitcher JP. Filamentary keratitis caused by corneal occlusion in large-angle strabismus. *Ophthalmic Surg.* 1992;23:66.

37. Kakizaki H, Zako M, Mito H, Iwaki M. Filamentary keratitis improved by blepharoptosis surgery: two cases. *Acta Ophthalmol Scand.* 2003;81:669-671.

38. Unal M, Sarici A. Filamentary keratopathy caused by corneal occlusion by large-angle paralytic strabismus. *Cornea.* 2006;25:1105-1106.

39. Dodds HT, Laibson PR. Filamentary keratitis following cataract extraction. *Arch Ophthalmol.* 1972;88:609-612.

40. Grinbaum A, Yassur I, Avni I. The beneficial effect of diclofenac sodium in the treatment of filamentary keratitis. *Arch Ophthalmol.* 2001;119:926-927.

41. Jones RR, Maguire LJ. Corneal complications after cataract surgery in patients with rheumatoid arthritis. *Cornea.* 1992;11:148-150.

42. Ram J, Sharma A, Pandav SS, et al. Cataract surgery in patients with dry eyes. *J Cataract Refract Surg.* 1998;24:1119-1124.

43. Rotkis WM, Chandler JW, Forstot SL. Filamentary keratitis following penetrating keratoplasty. *Ophthalmology.* 1982;89:946-949.

44. Feiz V, Mannis MJ, Kandavel G, et al. Surface keratopathy after penetrating keratoplasty. *Trans Am Ophthalmol Soc.* 2001;99:159-168.

45. Davis WG, Drewry RD, Wood TO. Filamentary keratitis and stromal neovascularization associated with brain-stem injury. *Am J Ophthalmol.* 1980;90:489-491.

46. Seedor JA, Lamberts D, Bergmann RB, Perry HD. Filamentary keratitis associated with diphenhydramine hydrochloride (Benadryl). *Am J Ophthalmol.* 1986;101:376-377.

47. Kim JC, Chung H, Tseng SCG. Botulinum toxin treatment for filamentary keratitis associated with cornea. In: *Advances in Corneal Research: Selected Transactions of the World Congress on the Cornea IV.* New York, NY: Plenum Press; 1997.

48. Maudgal PC, Missotten L. Cytology of the superficial keratinised cells in experimental keratitis sicca. *Ophthalmologica.* 1978;176:113-119.

49. Tabery HM. Corneal surface changes in keratoconjunctivitis sicca. Part II: The mucus component. A non-contact photomicrographic in vivo study in the human cornea. *Eye.* 2003;17:488-491.

50. Whitcher JP. Clinical diagnosis of the dry eye. *Int Ophthalmol Clin.* 1987;27:7-724.

51. Li XM, Hu L, Hu J, Wang W. Investigation of dry eye disease and analysis of the pathogenic factors in patients after cataract surgery. *Cornea.* 2007;26(suppl 1):16-20.

52. Kowalik BM, Rakes JA. Filamentary keratitis—the clinical challenges. *J Am Optom Assoc.* 1991;62:200-204.

53. Adams J, Wilcox MJ, Trousdale MD, et al. Morphologic and physiologic effects of artificial tear formulations on corneal epithelial derived cells. *Cornea.* 1992;11:234-241.

54. Tripathi BJ, Tripathi RC, Kolli SP. Cytotoxicity of ophthalmic preservatives on human corneal epithelium. *Lens Eye Toxic Res.* 1992;9:361-375.

55. Tuberville AW, Frederick WR, Wood TO. Punctal occlusion in tear deficiency syndromes. *Ophthalmology.* 1982;89:1170-1172.

56. Diller R, Sant S. A case report and review of filamentary keratitis. *Optometry.* 2005;76:30-36.

57. Beisel JG. Treatment of dry eye with punctal plugs. *Optom Clin.* 1991;1:103-117.

58. Lemp MA. Bandage lenses and the use of topical solutions containing preservatives. *Ann Ophthalmol.* 1978;10:1319-1321.

59. Bloomfield SE, Gasset AR, Forstot SL, Brown SI. Treatment of filamentary keratitis with the soft contact lens. *Am J Ophthalmol.* 1973;76:978-980.

60. Dada VK. Contact lens induced filamentary keratitis. *Am J Optom Physiol Opt.* 1975;52:545-546.

61. Arora I, Singhvi S. Impression debridement of corneal lesions. *Ophthalmology.* 1994;101:1935-1940.

62. Avisar R, Robinson A, Appel I, et al. Diclofenac sodium, 0.1% (Voltaren Ophtha), versus sodium chloride, 5%, in the treatment of filamentary keratitis. *Cornea.* 2000;19:145-147.

63. Sall K, Stevenson OD, Mundorf TK, Reis BL. Two multicenter, randomized studies of the efficacy and safety of cyclosporine ophthalmic emulsion in moderate to severe dry eye disease. CsA Phase 3 Study Group. *Ophthalmology.* 2000;107:631-639.

64. Wilson SE, Perry HD. Long-term resolution of chronic dry eye symptoms and signs after topical cyclosporine treatment. *Ophthalmology.* 2007;114:76-79.

65. Yoo SH, Romano AC. Rosacea. In: Foster CS, Azar DT, Dohlman CH, eds. *Smolin and Thoft's The Cornea—Scientific Foundations and Clinical Practice.* Vol 1. Philadelphia, PA: Lippincott Williams & Wilkins; 2005.

66. Dougherty JM, McCulley JP, Silvany RE, Meyer DR. The role of tetracycline in chronic blepharitis. Inhibition of lipase production in staphylococci. *Invest Ophthalmol Vis Sci.* 1991;32:2970-2975.

67. Sadowsky AE. Dermatologic disorders. In: Krachmer JH, Mannis MJ, Holland EJ, eds. *Cornea—Fundamentals, Diagnosis and Management.* Vol 1. Philadelphia, PA: Mosby Elsevier; 2005.

68. Alvarenga LS, Mannis MJ. Ocular rosacea. *Ocul Surf.* 2005;3:41-58.

69. Hoang-Xuan T, Rodriguez A, Zaltas MM, et al. Ocular rosacea. A histologic and immuno-pathologic study. *Ophthalmology.* 1990;97:1468-1475.

70. Stone DU, Chodosh J. Oral tetracyclines for ocular rosacea: an evidence-based review of the literature. *Cornea.* 2004;23:106-109.

71. Stone DU, Chodosh J. Ocular rosacea: an update on pathogenesis and therapy. *Curr Opin Ophthalmol.* 2004;15:499-502.

72. Smolin G, Okumoto M. Staphylococcal blepharitis. *Arch Ophthalmol.* 1977;95:812-816.

73. Mondino BJ. Inflammatory diseases of the peripheral cornea. *Ophthalmology.* 1988;95:463-472.

74. Thygeson P. Marginal corneal infiltrates and ulcers. *Trans Am Acad Ophthalmol Otolaryngol.* 1946;51:198-209.

75. Hogan MJ, Diaz-Bonnet V, Okumoto M, Kimura SJ. Experimental staphylococcic keratitis. *Invest Ophthalmol.* 1962;1:267-272.

76. Jayamanne DG, Dayan M, Jenkins D, Porter R. The role of staphylococcal superantigens in the pathogenesis of marginal keratitis. *Eye.* 1997;11(Pt 5):618-621.

77. Mondino BJ, Adamu SA, Pitchekian-Halabi H. Antibody studies in a rabbit model of corneal phlyctenulosis and catarrhal infiltrates related to *Staphylococcus aureus. Invest Ophthalmol Vis Sci.* 1991;32:1854-1863.

78. Mondino BJ, Kowalski R, Ratajczak HV, et al. Rabbit model of phlyctenulosis and catarrhal infiltrates. *Arch Ophthalmol.* 1981;99:891-895.

79. Ficker L, Ramakrishnan M, Seal D, Wright P. Role of cell-mediated immunity to staphylococci in blepharitis. *Am J Ophthalmol.* 1991;111:473-479.

80. Imanishi J, Takahashi F, Inatomi A, et al. Complement levels in human tears. *Jpn J Ophthalmol.* 1982;26:229-233.

81. Ambrosio R Jr, Periman LM, Netto MV, Wilson SE. Bilateral marginal sterile infiltrates and diffuse lamellar keratitis after laser in situ keratomileusis. *J Refract Surg.* 2003;19:154-158.

82. Haw WW, Manche EE. Sterile peripheral keratitis following laser in situ keratomileusis. *J Refract Surg.* 1999;15:61-63.

83. Moshirfar M, Welling JD, Feiz V, et al. Infectious and noninfectious keratitis after laser in situ keratomileusis Occurrence, management, and visual outcomes. *J Cataract Refract Surg.* 2007;33:474-483.

84. Taguri AH, Khan MA, Sanders R. Marginal keratitis: an uncommon form of topical dorzolamide allergy. *Am J Ophthalmol.* 2000;130:120-122.

85. Viswalingam M, Rauz S, Morlet N, Dart JK. Blepharokeratoconjunctivitis in children: diagnosis and treatment. *Br J Ophthalmol.* 2005;89:400-403.

86. Freidlin J, Acharya N, Lietman TM, et al. Spectrum of eye disease caused by methicillin-resistant *Staphylococcus aureus. Am J Ophthalmol.* 2007;144:313-315.

87. Carmichael TR, Wolpert M, Koornhof HJ. Corneal ulceration at an urban African hospital. *Br J Ophthalmol.* 1985;69:920-926.

88. Meisler DM, Raizman MB, Traboulsi EI. Oral erythromycin treatment for childhood blepharokeratitis. *J AAPOS.* 2000;4:379-380.

89. Lee JE, Oum BS, Choi HY, Lee JS. Methicillin-resistant *Staphylococcus aureus* sclerokeratitis after pterygium excision. *Cornea.* 2007;26:744-746.

90. Hird RB. Phlyctenular disease and its relation to tuberculosis. *Br J Ophthalmol.* 1918;2:215-223.

91. Sorsby A. The aetiology of phlyctenular ophthalmia. *Br J Ophthalmol.* 1942;26:189-215.

92. Thygeson P. The etiology and treatment of phlyctenular keratoconjunctivitis. *Am J Ophthalmol.* 1951;34:1217-1236.

93. Carvill M. A contribution to the study of phlyctenular keratoconjunctivitis. *Trans Am Ophthalmol Soc.* 1929;27:314-334.

94. Damato FJ. B.C.G. vaccine and phlyctenular kerato-conjunctivitis. *Br J Ophthalmol.* 1951;35:416-418.

95. Thygeson P. Complications of staphylococcic blepharitis. *Am J Ophthalmol.* 1969;68:446-449.

96. Suzuki T, Mitsuishi Y, Sano Y, et al. Phlyctenular keratitis associated with meibomitis in young patients. *Am J Ophthalmol.* 2005;140:77-82.

97. Bialasiewicz AA, Holbach L. Phlyctenular keratoconjunctivitis in bacterial epibulbar infections [in German]. *Klin Monatsbl Augenheilkd.* 1987;191:260-263.

98.   Culbertson WW, Huang AJ, Mandelbaum SH, et al. Effective treatment of phlyctenular keratoconjunctivitis with oral tetracycline. *Ophthalmology.* 1993;100:1358-1366.

99.   Jaffery MP. Ocular diseases caused by nematodes. *Am J Ophthalmol.* 1955;40:41-53.

100. Al-Hussaini MK, Khalifa R, Al-Ansary AT, et al. Phlyctenular eye disease in association with Hymenolepis nana in Egypt. *Br J Ophthalmol.* 1979;63:627-631.

101. Hussein AA, Nasr ME. The role of parasitic infection in the aetiology of phlyctenular eye disease. *J Egypt Soc Parasitol.* 1991;21:865-868.

102. McLean CM. Phlyctenulosis in the Eskimos of the Canadian Eastern Arctic. *Can Med Assoc J.* 1963;89:1212-1213.

103. Holland EJ, Mahanti RL, Belongia EA, et al. Ocular involvement in an outbreak of herpes gladiatorum. *Am J Ophthalmol.* 1992;114:680-684.

104. Zaidman GW, Brown SI. Orally administered tetracycline for phlyctenular keratoconjunctivitis. *Am J Ophthalmol.* 1981;92:178-182.

105. Blaustein BH, Gurwood AS. Recurrent phlyctenular keratoconjunctivitis: a forme fruste manifestation of rosacea. *Optometry.* 2001;72:179-184.

106. Thygeson P, Diaz-Bonnet V, Okumoto M. Phlyctenulosis. Attempts to produce an experimental model with BCG. *Invest Ophthalmol.* 1962;1:262-266.

107. Abu el-Asrar AM, Van den Oord JJ, Geboes K, et al. Phenotypic characterization of inflammatory cells in phlyctenular eye disease. *Doc Ophthalmol.* 1988;70:353-362.

108. Abu el-Asrar AM, Geboes K, Maudgal PC, et al. Immunocytological study of phlyctenular eye disease. *Int Ophthalmol.* 1987;10:33-39.

109. Sen DK, Sarin GS. Immunoglobulin concentrations in human tears in ocular diseases. *Br J Ophthalmol.* 1979;63:297-300.

110. Tyagi RN, Thakur V, Gupta RM. Serum immunoglobulins in phlyctenulosis. *Indian J Ophthalmol.* 1977;25(2):3-4.

111. Rohatgi J, Dhaliwal U. Phlyctenular eye disease: a reappraisal. *Jpn J Ophthalmol.* 2000;44:146-150.

112. Singal A, Aggarwal P, Pandhi D, Rohatgi J. Cutaneous tuberculosis and phlyctenular keratoconjunctivitis: a forgotten association. *Indian J Dermatol Venereol Leprol.* 2006;72:290-292.

113. Taherian K, Shekarchian M, Taylor RH. Fascicular keratitis in children: can corneal phlycten be mobile? *Clin Exp Ophthalmol.* 2005;33:531-532.

114. Doan S, Gabison E, Gatinel D, et al. Topical cyclosporine A in severe steroid-dependent childhood phlyctenular keratoconjunctivitis. *Am J Ophthalmol.* 2006;141:62-66.

115. Ostler HB. Corneal perforation in nontuberculous (staphylococcal) phlyctenular keratoconjunctivitis. *Am J Ophthalmol.* 1975;79:446-448.

116. Al-Amry MA, Al-Amri A, Khan AO. Resolution of childhood recurrent corneal phlyctenulosis following eradication of an intestinal parasite. *J AAPOS.* 2008;12(1):89-90.

117. Rootman J, Bussanich N, Gudauskas G, Kumi C. Effects of subconjunctivally injected antineoplastic agents on three models of corneal inflammation. *Can J Ophthalmol.* 1985;20:142-146.

118. Smith RE, Dippe DW, Miller SD. Phlyctenular keratoconjunctivitis: results of penetrating keratoplasty in Alaskan natives. *Ophthalmic Surg.* 1975;6(3):62-6.

119. Smith RE, Dippe DW, Miller SD. Corneal transplantation in Alaska natives (excerpts). 1975. *Alaska Med.* 2006;48:61-63.

120. Wilhelmus KR. Syphilitic interstitial keratitis. In: Krachmer JH, Mannis MJ, Holland EJ, eds. *Cornea—Fundamentals, Diagnosis and Management.* Vol 1. 2nd ed. Philadelphia, PA: Mosby Elsevier; 2005.

121. Hariprasad SM, Moon SJ, Allen RC, Wilhelmus KR. Keratopathy from congenital syphilis. *Cornea.* 2002;21:608-609.

122. Kiss S, Damico FM, Young LH. Ocular manifestations and treatment of syphilis. *Semin Ophthalmol.* 2005;20:161-167.

123. Schwartz GS, Harrison AR, Holland EJ. Etiology of immune stromal (interstitial) keratitis. *Cornea.* 1998;17:278-281.

124. Klauder J, VanDoren E. Interstitial keratitis: analysis of five hundred and thirty-two cases with particular reference to standardization of treatment. *Arch Ophthalmol.* 1941;26:408-429.

125. Martinez JA, Sutphin JE. Syphilitic interstitial keratitis masquerading as staphylococcal marginal keratitis. *Am J Ophthalmol.* 1989;107:431-433.

126. Wilhelmus KR, Jones DB. Adult-onset syphilitic stromal keratitis. *Am J Ophthalmol.* 2006;141:319-321.

127. Matsuo T, Taira Y, Nagayama M, Baba T. Angle-closure glaucoma as a presumed presenting sign in patients with syphilis. *Jpn J Ophthalmol.* 2000;44:305-308.

128. Knox D. Glaucoma following syphilitic interstitial keratitis. *Arch Ophthalmol.* 1961;66:18-25.

129. Lee ME, Lindquist TD. Syphilitic interstitial keratitis. *JAMA.* 1989;262:2921.

130. Larsen SA, Steiner BM, Rudolph AH. Laboratory diagnosis and interpretation of tests for syphilis. *Clin Microbiol Rev.* 1995;8:1-21.

131. Goh BT. Syphilis in adults. *Sex Transm Infect.* 2005;81:448-452.

132. Helm CJ, Holland GN. Ocular tuberculosis. *Surv Ophthalmol.* 1993;38:229-256.

133. Lewallen S, Courtright P. A overview of ocular leprosy after 2 decades of multidrug therapy. *Int Ophthalmol Clin.* 2007;47:87-101.

134. Zaidman GW. The ocular manifestations of Lyme disease. *Int Ophthalmol Clin.* 1993;33:9-22.

135. Liesegang TJ. Herpes simplex virus epidemiology and ocular importance. *Cornea.* 2001;20:1-13.

136. Holland EJ, Brilakis HS, Schwartz GS. Herpes simplex keratitis. In: Krachmer JH, Mannis MJ, Holland EJ, eds. *Cornea—Fundamentals, Diagnosis and Management.* Vol 1. Philadelphia, PA: Mosby Elsevier; 2005.

137. Wilhelmus KR, Coster DJ, Donovan HC, et al. Prognosis indicators of herpetic keratitis. Analysis of a five-year observation period after corneal ulceration. *Arch Ophthalmol.* 1981;99:1578-1582.

138. Herpetic Eye Disease Study Group. Oral acyclovir for herpes simplex virus eye disease: effect on prevention of epithelial keratitis and stromal keratitis. *Arch Ophthalmol.* 2000;118:1030-1036.

139. Roizenblatt J. Interstitial keratitis caused by American (mucocutaneous) leishmaniasis. *Am J Ophthalmol.* 1979;87:175-179.

140. Hall LR, Pearlman E. Pathogenesis of onchocercal keratitis (River blindness). *Clin Microbiol Rev.* 1999;12:445-453.

141. Cogan DG. Syndrome of nonsyphilitic interstitial keratitis and vestibuloauditory symptoms. *Arch Ophthalmol.* 1945;33:144-149.

142. Helmchen C, Arbusow V, Jager L, et al. Cogan's syndrome: clinical significance of antibodies against the inner ear and cornea. *Acta Otolaryngol.* 1999;119:528-536.

143. Grasland A, Pouchot J, Hachulla E, et al. Typical and atypical Cogan's syndrome: 32 cases and review of the literature. *Rheumatology.* 2004;43:1007-1015.

144. Cobo LM, Haynes BF. Early corneal findings in Cogan's syndrome. *Ophthalmology.* 1984;91:903-907.

145. Haynes BF, Kaiser-Kupfer MI, Mason P, Fauci AS. Cogan syndrome: studies in thirteen patients, long-term follow-up, and a review of the literature. *Medicine (Baltimore).* 1980;59:426-441.

146. Cochrane AD, Tatoulis J. Cogan's syndrome with aortitis, aortic regurgitation, and aortic arch vessel stenoses. *Ann Thorac Surg.* 1991;52:1166-1167.

147. Whitcup SM, Smith JA. Nonsyphilic interstitial keratitis. In: Krachmer JH, Mannis MJ, Holland EJ, eds. *Cornea—Fundamentals, Diagnosis and Management.* Vol 1. Philadelphia, PA: Mosby Elsevier; 2005.

148. Fisher ER. Cogan's syndrome and systemic vascular disease. *Arch Pathol.* 1961;72:572.
149. Roat MI, Thoft RA, Thomson AW, et al. Treatment of Cogan's syndrome with FK 506: a case report. *Transplant. Proc.* 1991;23:3347.
150. Vaiopoulos G, Sfikakis PP, Skoumas B, et al. Lack of response to corticosteroids and pulse cyclophosphamide therapy in Cogan's syndrome. *Clin Rheumatol.* 1994;13:110-112.

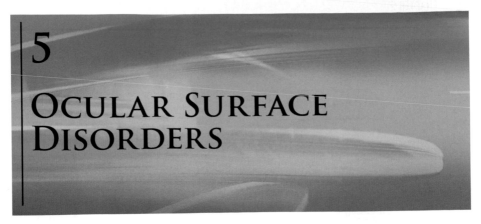

5

OCULAR SURFACE DISORDERS

Ahmad Kheirkhah, MD; V.-K. Raju, MD, FRCS, FACS;
and Scheffer C. G. Tseng, MD, PhD

The cornea, conjunctiva, and the limbus comprise tissues at the ocular surface. The primary function of the ocular surface is to provide clear vision, because the anterior surface of the cornea contributes more than two thirds of the total refractive power of the eye. To achieve this, maintain comfort, and prevent microbial invasion, the ocular surface must be covered by a stable tear film. The mechanism by which ocular surface health is ensured is built in the ocular surface defense that encompasses an intimate relationship between ocular surface epithelia and the pre-ocular tear film. In this chapter, we first discuss the ocular surface defense that governs how a stable tear film is formed when the eye is open and then describe some of the more important ocular surface diseases that develop due to a deficient ocular surface defense.

OCULAR SURFACE DEFENSE MECHANISMS

When the eye is open, the ocular surface health is dictated by a stable pre-ocular tear film. To maintain a stable tear film, the ocular surface employs a unique strategy of defense involving both compositional and hydrodynamic factors. Together they require the close participation of the ocular surface epithelia and all external adnexae including the lacrimal gland, the meibomian gland, and eyelids.[1] Compositionally, the normal tear film consists of mucins secreted by ocular surface goblet cells and nongoblet epithelial cells, aqueous tear fluids produced primarily from the lacrimal glands, and meibum lipids released by meibomian glands. Even if these normal tear components are present, a stable tear film cannot be formed without the kinetic movement of eyelid blinking that helps spread the tear components into a thin layer over the entire ocular surface. Eyelid blinking also facilitates the expression of meibum lipids to the lid margin, as well as the refreshment of tear fluid by clearing "old tears" into the nasolacrimal drainage system. The open-eye state needs to be intermittently turned off by eyelid closure in order to avoid unnecessary evaporation of the tear fluid and exposure of the ocular surface, which leads to dryness. The frequency of eyelid blinking and completeness of eyelid closure ensure the establishment of a stable tear film between blinks.

Trattler WB, Majmudar PA, Luchs JI, Swartz TS, eds.
Cornea Handbook (pp. 61-74)
© 2010 SLACK Incorporated

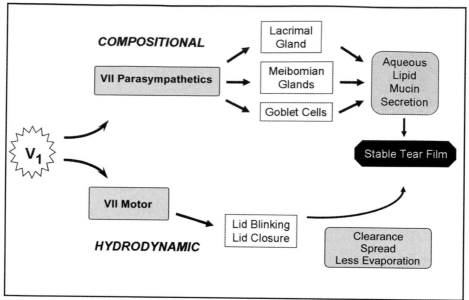

Figure 5-1. Neuroanatomic integration governing the stability of pre-ocular tear film. Both compositional and hydrodynamic factors for tear production, spreading, and maintenance are controlled by a neuroanatomic integration via 2 neural reflexes, both of which are triggered by corneal sensitivity mediated by the ophthalmic division of the trigeminal nerve (V_1).

Both compositional and hydrodynamic factors are controlled by neuroanatomic integration via 2 neural reflexes, both of which are triggered by corneal sensitivity mediated by the ophthalmic division of the trigeminal nerve (V_1) (Figure 5-1). The efferent limb of the reflex that controls the compositional factor is through the parasympathetic branch of the facial nerve (VII), and the reflex that controls the hydrodynamic factor is mediated by the motor branch of the facial nerve (VII). Through such neuroanatomic integration, activation of the compositional reflex induces secretion of all tear components, and activation of the hydrodynamic reflex induces eyelid blinking and closure. These 2 reflexes operate subconsciously and autonomously without eliciting conscious acknowledgment during most daily activities. As a result, the entire ocular surface and all external adnexae function as a single unit for a common purpose, to maintain a stable tear film, prevent tear evaporation, and facilitate tear clearance during the open-eye state.[1,2]

This concept refutes an older belief that all tearing is subdivided into basic and reflex tearing. Basic tearing was thought to be produced by accessory lacrimal glands, whereas reflex tearing was thought to be produced by the main lacrimal gland. Based on the concept described earlier, we believe that both basic and reflex forms of tearing are mediated by the same neuronal reflex and that the difference between the two is that the former is driven by minimal stimulation, whereas the latter is driven by maximal stimulation. The production of tears is controlled by sensory stimuli, which are derived from all of the ocular surface tissues (mostly cornea and lid margin/lashes) that are innervated by V_1. The amount of tearing varies according to the intensity of the summated sensory drive from both eyes.

Increased Eyelid Blinking Compensates for Unstable Tear Film

Under the normal open-eye situation, the tear film needs to be stable only during the time period between blinks. For an individual with normal compositional factor, the demand for a stable tear film increases when the blink rate slows or the exposure zone enlarges or a combination of both. Alternatively, when tear film stability is threatened by compositional deficiency, it can be compensated for by the increase of eyelid blinking rate or by the narrowing of the exposure zone (eg, via squinting or closing eyelids) or by a combination of both. In other words, compositional deficiency can be compensated by hydrodynamic factors.

The control of lid blinking, exerted by the motor branch of the facial nerve, is a complex task mediated by local neuronal reflexes driven by corneal and supraorbital touch (pain) and light stimuli and modified by supranuclear pathways. Deficiency in this neuronal control will diminish the compensatory mechanism of blinking. For example, the blink rate slows when one is engaged in concentrated visual tasks; eg, reading, knitting, watching TV/movies, or driving. As a result, symptoms of dry eye manifest, particularly on these occasions, and may even develop in normal individuals working on video display terminals when upgaze dominates.[3] One can conclude that the compositional factor works in concert with the hydrodynamic factor and that deficiency of one increases the demand for the other. Failure to meet such a demand by the other can lead to an unstable tear film. For this reason, the clinical workup should always be directed to exploring the status of all elements in these 2 factors to gain a full grasp of each patient's ocular surface defense. Failure to do so will provide incomplete information for understanding the pathogenesis of the patient's ocular surface problems.

Neurotrophic Keratopathy—Worst Form of Dry Eye

Based on scheme shown in Figure 5-1, the ocular sensitivity mediated by V_1 is the single most important driving force controlling the integrity of both compositional and hydrodynamic factors of the entire ocular surface defense. As corneal sensitivity decreases with age, there is a high prevalence of dry eye among elderly. Deficiency in ocular sensitivity is also the hallmark of the neurotrophic state. Because aqueous tear deficiency can take place as a result of the compositional factor and increased exposure can develop as a result of inadequate blinking, the worst form of dry eye (broadly defined herein as an unstable tear film) is found in patients with neurotrophic keratopathy. Indeed, the decreased corneal sensitivity noted in a number of disorders[4] is frequently associated with dryness-induced keratopathy. In a prolonged state of dry eye, epithelial defects with ulceration can develop and progress, resulting in severe complications. Such a pathologic effect, mediated via disturbance of ocular surface defense, is in fact a secondary neurotrophic effect on the ocular surface and is clinically indistinguishable from that of keratitis sicca due to aqueous tear deficiency. Denervation of the cornea can cause a primary neurotrophic effect to the corneal epithelium by depriving essential neurotrophic factors, or neurotrophins.

Exposure Keratopathy—A Commonly Neglected Entity

Exposure keratopathy results from desiccation of the ocular surface due to failure of hydrodynamic factors. This may result from incomplete or infrequent blinking, incomplete eyelid closure, and/or reduced Bell's phenomenon. Although incomplete eyelid closure is widely recognized as a cause for exposure keratopathy, other causes of this condition are commonly overlooked. Incomplete closure may cause keratopathy even in the presence of normal compositional factor, and the corneal involvement may be aggravated if protective Bell's phenomenon is diminished, leading to nocturnal exposure. However, in the presence of compromised compositional factor, exposure keratopathy may ensue more easily in eyes where reduced blink rate or incomplete blinking might not be as apparent.

Tear Clearance Represents Final Integration of Both Reflex Arcs

The final neuroanatomic integration of these 2 reflex arcs is also manifested in tear clearance, or rate of tear turnover. The "hydrodynamic" reflex arc that gives rise to lid blinking also generates a pump function to remove the tear fluid from the tear meniscus into the nasolacrimal drainage system.[5] The "compositional" reflex arc controls the production of aqueous tear fluid, and the volume dictates tear clearance. The latter also explains why decreased tear secretion in keratoconjunctivitis sicca is frequently associated with decreased clearance rates as measured by fluorophotometry.[6,7] By using fluorescein as a tracer, the tear clearance rate can also be measured by a modified method using serial Schirmer paper strips.[8,9] Such measurements are consistent with those measured by fluorophotometry[10] and are useful to diagnose the dry eye state more accurately.[8] Such measurement also distinguishes aqueous tear deficiency dry eye associated with Sjögren's syndrome from non-Sjögren's syndrome aqueous tear deficiency, based on the presence or absence of reflex tearing triggered by nasal stimulation.

Adequate tear clearance is important to allow constant refreshment of the tear components and effective elimination of debris and irritants that can potentially harm and irritate the ocular surface. Dysfunction in tear clearance, particularly when it is delayed, is common, often overlooked, and may be pathogenic in several ocular surface disorders.[9] Besides decreased tear secretion, delayed tear clearance can be induced by ineffective or decreased blinking (functional block) and mucosal inflammation and edema in nasolacrimal drainage system (partial anatomic block). The former is contributed to by such risk factors as old age, female gender, decreased corneal sensitivity, and lid laxity, including floppy lids. In the context of ocular surface defense, an unstable tear film leading to dry eye and delayed tear clearance leading to accumulation of inflammatory debris are the 2 major pathogenic process identified.

CLINICAL MANIFESTATION

The sensory supply of the both aforementioned reflexes is an input summation from areas innervated in both eyes by V_1 division, which include the cornea, lid margin/lashes, conjunctiva, and anterior nasal mucosa. Therefore, conditions reducing the sensation of these structures may create an unstable tear film. For example, reduced corneal sensation due to chronic contact lens wear, HSV keratitis, or LASIK; reduced lid and lash sensation due to chronic blepharitis with lash loss; reduced conjunctival sensation due to atopy, allergy, floppy lid, or conjunctivochalasis; and reduced nasal mucosa sensation due to nasal allergy can only increase the severity of reduced ocular sensitivity, leading to a neurotrophic state.

Table 5-1

ETIOLOGIC CAUSES OF NEUROTROPHIC KERATOPATHY

Infectious	Herpes simplex virus* Herpes zoster virus* Mycobacterium leprae
Toxic	Acid* Alkali* Carbon disulfide Hydrogen sulfide
Neurogenic	Inflammatory: cavernous sinus syndrome, orbital apex syndrome, Gradenigo syndrome Neoplasia: acoustic neuroma Vascular: aneurysm Surgical ablation of trigeminal nucleus or ganglion Congenital: familial dysautonomia (Riley-Day syndrome), Goldenhar-Gorlin syndrome, Mobius syndrome, familial corneal hypoplasia Trauma: facial or intracranial trauma to trigeminal nerve
Topical Medications	Beta-blockers,* anesthetics, diclofenac sodium
Corneal Dystrophies	Lattice, macular
Metabolic Disease	Diabetes mellitus,* vitamin A deficiency
Iatrogenic	Corneal surgery*: penetrating keratoplasty, lamellar keratoplasty, radial keratotomy, laser-assisted in situ keratomileusis, photorefractive keratectomy. Contact lens use* Ciliary nerve damage*: retinal photoablation, retinal surgery, choroidal inflammation
Miscellaneous	Aging* Adie's syndrome

*Common causes.

Dry eye after LASIK is due to cutting of the corneal nerves and is accentuated if any of these conditions is present. Therefore, it is important to consider all these conditions as risk factors of developing dry eye for patients undergoing LASIK.

In addition to the above factors, neurotrophic keratopathy may be caused by involvement of sensory nerves anywhere from terminal nerve endings in the cornea along its course to the trigeminal nerve ganglion. The common causes for reduced corneal sensation are listed in Table 5-1 and include increasing age, herpes simplex and herpes zoster virus infections, multiple ocular surgeries, chemical burns, systemic disease such as diabetes mellitus, and topical medications.

Clinically, neurotrophic keratopathy should be suspected in any patient presenting ocular surface symptomatic complaints disproportionately less than the clinical signs, or in those patients presenting with a decreased eyelid blink rate. In patients with neurotrophic keratopathy, 2 types of ocular changes may be seen. First, there are some primary effects in the cornea that may be followed by second-

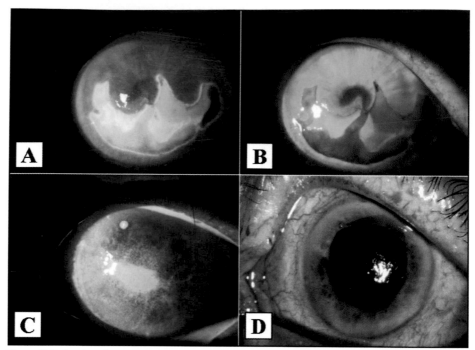

Figure 5-2. Rose bengal staining pattern in primary and secondary neurotrophic effects. In eyes with primary neurotrophic effect, rose bengal staining is confined to the epithelial defect (A and B); but in eyes with secondary neurotrophic effect, it extends beyond the defect to include the interpalpebral exposure zone of the conjunctiva (C and D).

ary effects in the ocular surface. Primary effect is intrinsic epithelial degeneration due to deprivation of neurotrophic factors (neurotrophins). Secondary effect is an unstable tear film or dry eye due to interruption of the 2 neural reflexes mediated by V_1. It is important to distinguish these 2 neurotrophic effects. To do so, the use of differential dye staining with fluorescein and rose bengal is advised. Although fluorescein detects the epithelial defect caused by both, rose bengal staining pattern is also helpful to differentiate the secondary effect from the primary effect. In eyes with primary neurotrophic effect, rose bengal staining is confined to the epithelial defect; but in eyes with secondary neurotrophic effect, it extends beyond that into the exposure zone of the conjunctiva, similar to that of Sjögren's syndrome (Figure 5-2). Following the dye staining, one can then use fluorescein clearance test (FCT) to verify the presence of the secondary effect by showing reduced tear secretion. Once detected, eyes with a secondary neurotrophic effect need punctal occlusion as the first step in the management of neurotrophic keratopathy. This point has been illustrated in the case example shown in Figure 5-3.

Exposure Keratopathy

Incomplete eyelid closure can be caused by neurogenic diseases such as seventh nerve palsy, cicatricial or restrictive eyelid diseases such as ectropion, previous blepharoplasty, and skin disorders such as Stevens-Johnson syndrome or xeroderma pigmentosum. Proptosis caused by thyroid orbitopathy or other inflam-

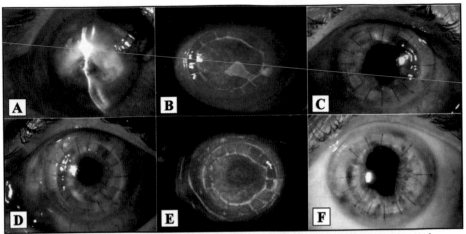

Figure 5-3. Case example of management of secondary neurotrophic effects. A 56-year-old man with a long history of recurrent herpetic keratitis developed corneal perforation that failed to be glued (A) and therefore underwent an emergency penetrating keratoplasty. Although there was no corneal epithelial defect at the first postoperative day, an epithelial defect was noted at day 7 after surgery (B). The rose bengal dye showed diffuse staining extending beyond the epithelial defect, suggestive of the presence of secondary neurotrophic effects (C). Fluorescein clearance test confirmed the presence of aqueous tear deficiency and thus directed to performing punctual occlusion by cauterization. One week later, the epithelial defect was healed (D and E). During 5 years of follow-up (F), the eye retained a smooth and stable corneal surface without any recurrent episodes of herpetic keratitis.

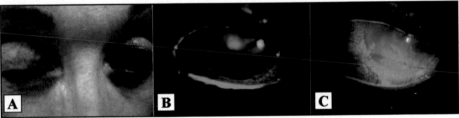

Figure 5-4. Exposure keratopathy due to incomplete blinking. This 60-year-old woman with a history of previous upper lid blepharoplasty had incomplete blinking in the left eye (A). Because of defective blinking, the inferior part of the cornea was not covered by the tear film most of the time (B). This resulted in desiccation of the corneal surface, leading to exposure keratopathy with punctuate epithelial erosion on the inferior corneal surface (C).

matory or infiltrative orbital diseases can also result in exposure keratopathy. Although reduced blink rate or incomplete blinking may be seen in old age or disease conditions such as Parkinson's disease, a common denominator is reduced corneal sensation.

Exposure keratopathy is characterized by a punctate epithelial keratopathy usually involving the most exposed inferior third of the cornea, although the entire corneal surface can be involved in more severe cases. Indeed, incomplete blinks leading to inferior corneal fluorescein staining patterns has been reported in 67% of all forms of exposure keratopathy (Figure 5-4).[11] Large, coalescent epithelial defects may ensue, leading to ulceration, melting, and perforation. Symptoms are similar to those associated with dry eye, including foreign-body sensation, photophobia, and tearing, unless there is an associated neurotrophic component resulting in corneal anesthesia. Most persistent corneal epithelial defects can be explained by the above-mentioned neurotrophic keratopathy that is complicated by factors that aggravate exposure or by factors that may damage the epithelium such as medication toxicity.

MANAGEMENT

Therapy of patients with ocular surface disorders requires an accurate initial evaluation directed to understanding the ocular surface defense governed by neuroanatomic integration of both hydrodynamic and compositional factors. After history taking, external examination may reveal the rate and completeness of blinking, presence of Bell's phenomenon, and completeness of eyelid closure. In cases of neurotrophic keratitis, medical and surgical history may point to the correct diagnosis by revealing the underlying cause (see Table 5-1). The clinical sign crucial to diagnosis is a decrease in corneal sensitivity. It is important to localize and quantify the loss of corneal sensitivity. A gross evaluation of corneal sensitivity may be performed with the tip of a cotton swab that has been drawn out, twisted, and then advanced slowly until it touches the central corneal zone. For a more accurate measure of corneal sensitivity, the simplest and most useful instrument is the Cochet-Bonnet esthesiometer, which records the patient's response at the touch of a nylon line (between 0 and 6 cm).

In all eyes with ocular surface disorders, tear function should be evaluated completely. FCT is of particular usefulness because it provides the following 3 important pieces of information regarding basic tearing, reflex tearing, and tear clearance.[9] For performing FCT, a drop of 0.5% proparacaine is first instilled into the eye and after a few seconds the conjunctival sac is dried. Then, 5 µL of 0.25% Fluoress solution (Akron, Inc, Buffalo Grove, IL) is applied to the eye and the patient is allowed to blink normally. At 10, 20, and 30 minutes after fluorescein application, Schirmer's paper is placed in the eye for only 1 minute. For the 30-minute point, cotton-tipped applicators are used to stimulate the anterior nasal mucosa in both sides. In normal individuals, the wetting length of the Schirmer's strips during FCT is more than 3 mm, increases after nasal stimulation, and has a normal clearance evidenced by disappearance of fluorescein in 15 minutes; ie, no fluorescein staining in the second strip (Figure 5-5A). In individuals with normal aqueous tear secretion but delayed tear clearance, the wetting length is more than 3 mm in all strips but the fluorescein is still present after 15 minutes (Figure 5-5B). In eyes having ATD dry eye with reflex tearing, the wetting length is less than 3 mm in the first and second strips but increases in the last strip due to reflex tearing, and the fluorescein clears by the second 20-min strip (Figure 5-5C). In eyes having severe ATD dry eye without reflex tearing, the wetting length is less than 3 mm in all strips and has delayed tear clearance as judged by fluorescein shown after 15 minutes using the second or third strip (Figure 5-5D). Therefore, delayed tear clearance is frequently found in eyes with severe dry eye because of the discontinuation of the tear meniscus to the punctum. Although this is a protective mechanism to conserve tears, delayed tear clearance also leads to stagnation of inflammatory cytokines/toxic medications in the tears.

The therapeutic strategy is formulated according to the dysfunctional elements identified in the ocular surface defense. Although frequent lubrication with artificial tears and lubricants is started in most cases with ocular surface diseases manifesting dry eye, the mainstay remains punctual occlusion, especially when ocular

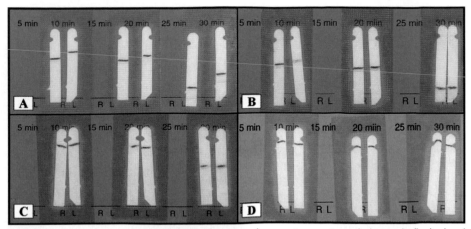

Figure 5-5. Fluorescein clearance test. Typical examples of normal aqueous tear secretion at the basic and reflex levels and normal tear clearance (A), normal aqueous tear secretion with delayed tear clearance (B), a patient with decreased aqueous tear secretion but with intact reflex tearing (C), a patient with decreased aqueous tear secretion but without reflex tearing (D). Note that severe aqueous tear deficiency is frequently associated with delayed tear clearance (D).

surface inflammation is controlled. Punctal occlusion by either plugs or cauterization for one or both puncta depends on the presence or absence of reflex tearing, which can be detected by FCT. If ATD dry eye still possesses reflex tearing, occlusion of only one punctum by plug can be started. In contrast, if severe ATD dry eye does not exhibit reflex tearing, occlusion of both puncta by cauterization can be considered. In addition, the choice between plug and cauterization is governed by the nature of the underlying lesion. When the underlying cause for ATD dry eye is temporary and reactive, plugs are sufficient, whereas cauterization is preferable if it is permanent and irreversible. The FCT can also be used to verify the effectiveness of punctual occlusion and whether there is suspicious recanalization following thermal cauterization.

Once punctual occlusion is performed, the eye becomes amenable for other measures such as insertion of a therapeutic bandage contact lens[12] or administration of autologous serum drops,[13] especially for eyes without reflex tearing. Once the compositional factor is augmented, one may begin to consider reducing exposure by taping the eyelid shut at bedtime (for nocturnal exposure), insertion of gold weights to the upper eyelid, or tarsorrhaphy by either Botox injection or sutures for daytime exposure. Finally, correction of eyelid/lash abnormalities, such as ectropion or trichiasis, is also important. For cases in which neurotrophic or exposure keratopathy failed to respond to the above measures and corneal ulceration persists, amniotic membrane transplantation can be used to improve the healing of the cornea. Conjunctival flaps may be reserved as a last resort in patients with limited visual potential and for those who refuse tarsorrhaphy for cosmetic reasons.

LIMBAL STEM CELL DEFICIENCY

As mentioned earlier, ocular surface health is dependent on the intimate relationship between tear film and the ocular surface epithelia, which are nonkeratinized and express mucins. Ultimately, such normal terminal differentiation of

Table 5-2

CORNEAL DISEASES MANIFESTING LIMBAL STEM CELL DEFICIENCY

Hereditary	Aniridia
	Keratitis associated with multiple endocrine deficiency
	Epidermal dysplasia (ectrodactyly—ectodermal dysplasia—clefting syndrome)
Acquired	Chemical or thermal burns, including mustard gas
	Stevens-Johnson syndrome, toxic epidermal necrolysis
	Multiple surgeries or cryotherapies to limbus
	Contact lens-induced keratopathy
	Severe microbial infection extending to limbus
	Antimetabolite uses (5-FU or mitomycin C)
	Radiation
	Chronic limbitis (vernal, atopy, phlyctenular)
	Peripheral ulcerative keratitis (Mooren's ulcer)
	Chronic bullous keratopathy
	Idiopathic

the ocular surface epithelium, a process that is coupled with cell desquamation as a result of apoptosis, must be compensated by the proliferation of epithelial stem cells. For the corneal epithelium, stem cells are located at the limbal basal layer.[14,15]

A number of ocular surface diseases may manifest limbal stem cell deficiency (LSCD) as a result of either destructive loss of the limbal epithelial stem cells or dysfunction of the limbal stroma (Table 5-2). They carry the hallmark of conjunctivalization of the cornea, where the conjunctival epithelium migrates to cover the corneal surface accompanied by vascularization, destruction of the basement membrane, chronic inflammation, and scarring of the cornea (Figure 5-6).[16] These limbal-deficient corneas show poor epithelial integrity manifested as irregular surface, recurrent erosion, or persistent ulcer. Patients with LSCD often suffer from severe photophobia and decreased vision and are poor candidates for conventional corneal transplantation, which only brings in short-lived corneal epithelial cells. Furthermore, preexisting corneal vascularization and inflammation increase the risk of allograft rejection.

For total LSCD, the transplantation of limbal stem cells is the only solution to improve the patient's symptoms and vision. Depending on the unilateral or bilateral involvement, the extent of LSCD involvement, and the patient's acceptance and expectations of the proposed treatment, several procedures of transplanting autologous or allogeneic limbal stem cells may be considered (see classification by Holland and Schwartz[17]).

Conjunctival Limbal Autograft

In this procedure, autologous limbal tissue with adjacent conjunctiva is harvested from the healthy fellow eye and transplanted to the diseased eye. Conjunctival limbal autograft (CLAU) is used to treat patients with unilateral LSCD. The sur-

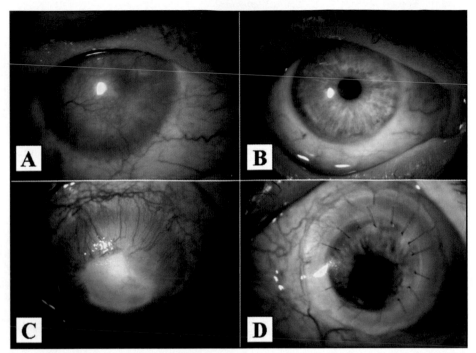

Figure 5-6. Surgical management of total limbal stem cell deficiency. For this eye with unilateral total limbal stem cell deficiency (LSCD) due to Stevens-Johnson syndrome (A), conjunctival limbal autograft (CLAU) taken from the fellow eye resulted in a smooth and stable corneal surface without systemic immunosuppression (B). For this patient with bilateral total LSCD due to chemical burn, presenting with persistent corneal epithelial defect in the left eye (C), keratolimbal allograft (KLAL) as a 360 degree ring, along with systemic immunosuppression and subsequent penetrating keratoplasty, resulted in a healed, smooth, and noninflamed ocular surface (D).

geon removes a lamellar graft encompassing a small portion of conjunctiva, the limbus, and the most peripheral portion of the cornea from one-third to one-half of the limbal circumference (see Figures 5-6A and 5-6B). Because CLAU uses an autologous tissue, there is no risk of immune rejection and hence no need for systemic immunosuppression. Besides limbal epithelial stem cells, CLAU also provides healthy, noninflamed conjunctiva. There have been some concerns when it is performed in an eye that may have subclinical LSCD.[18] This risk appears low if the donor eye is absolutely healthy.

Living-Related Conjunctival Limbal Allograft

In living-related conjunctival limbal allograft (lr-CLAL), allogeneic limbo-conjunctival tissue is harvested from a healthy eye of a patient's living relative and transplanted to the patient's diseased eye. Because lr-CLAL uses an allogeneic tissue, it is used to treat bilateral total LSCD.[19] Although lr-CLAL is obtained from living donors with some degree of histocompatibility, it does not completely obviate the necessity for systemic immunosuppression.

Cadaveric Keratolimbal Allograft

Cadaveric keratolimbal allograft (KLAL) is also used to treat bilateral total LSCD. Because KLAL does not include conjunctival tissue, however, it cannot help treat eyes that manifest additional active conjunctival inflammation and scarring such as symblepharon unless amniotic membrane transplantation is also used at the same time or before. KLAL is a better alternative in those patients who have LSCD but whose conjunctiva is normal, such as in aniridia, because there is no need to include donor conjunctiva. Because KLAL includes a 360 degree limbus, it can restore the entire limbal deficiency more so than lr-CLAL (Figures 5-6C and 5-6D).[20] Alternatively, this ring can be halved into 2 segments, and 3 segments from 2 donor eyes can be used for KLAL.[21] Like lr-CLAL, prolonged, if not indefinite, systemic immunosuppression is necessary. Therefore, the potential side effects derived from this long-term treatment must be considered.[22]

REFERENCES

1. Tseng SC, Tsubota K. Important concepts for treating ocular surface and tear disorders. *Am J Ophthalmol.* 1997;124:825-835.

2. Solomon A, Touhami A, Sandoval H, Tseng SCG. Neurotrophic keratopathy: basic concepts and therapeutic strategies. *Comp Ophthalmol Update.* 2000;3:165-174.

3. Tsubota K, Nakamori K. Effects of ocular surface area and blink rate on tear dynamics. *Arch Ophthalmol.* 1995;113:155-158.

4. Martin XD, Safran AB. Corneal hypoesthesia. *Surv Ophthalmol.* 1988;33:28-40.

5. Doane MG. Blinking and the mechanics of the lacrimal drainage system. *Ophthalmology.* 1981;88:844-851.

6. Mishima S, Gasset A, Klyce SD Jr, Baum JL. Determination of tear volume and tear flow. *Invest Ophthalmol.* 1966;5:264-276.

7. van Best JA, Benitez del Castillo JM, Coulangeon LM. Measurement of basal tear turnover using a standarized protocol. European concerted action on ocular fluorometry. *Graefes Arch Clin Exp Ophthalmol.* 1995;233:1-7.

8. Xu K-P, Yagi Y, Toda I, Tsubota K. Tear function index. A new measure of dry eye. *Arch Ophthalmol.* 1995;113:84-88.

9. Prabhasawat P, Tseng SCG. Frequent association of delayed tear clearance in ocular irritation. *Br J Ophthalmol.* 1998;82:666-675.

10. Xu K-P, Tsubota K. Correlation of tear clearance rate and fluorophotometric assessment of tear turnover. *Br J Ophthalmol.* 1995;79:1042-1045.

11. Abelson MB, Holly FJ. A tentative mechanism for inferior punctate keratopathy. *Am J Ophthalmol.* 1977;83:866-869.

12. Spraul CW, Lang GK. Contact lenses and corneal shields. *Curr Opin Ophthalmol.* 1997;8:67-75.

13. Tsubota K, Goto E, Shimmura S, Shimazaki J. Treatment of persistent corneal epithelial defect by autologous serum application. *Ophthalmology.* 1999;106:1984-1989.

14. Tseng SCG. Regulation and clinical implications of corneal epithelial stem cells. *Mol Biol Rep.* 1996;23:47-58.

15. Lavker RM, Sun T-T. Epidermal stem cells: properties, markers and location. *Proc Natl Acad Sci U S A.* 2000;97:13473-13475.

16. Puangsricharern V, Tseng SCG. Cytologic evidence of corneal diseases with limbal stem cell deficiency. *Ophthalmology.* 1995;102:1476-1485.

17. Holland EJ, Schwartz GS. The evolution of epithelial transplantation for severe ocular surface disease and a proposed classification system. *Cornea.* 1996;15:549-556.

18. Kenyon KR, Tseng SC. Limbal autograft transplantation for ocular surface disorders. *Ophthalmology.* 1989;96:709-722.

19. Rao SK, Rajagopal R, Sitalakshmi G, Padmanabhan P. Limbal allografting from related live donors for corneal surface reconstruction. *Ophthalmology*. 1999;106:822-828.

20. Tsubota K, Toda I, Saito H, Shinozaki N, Shimazaki J. Reconstruction of the corneal epithelium by limbal allograft transplantation for severe ocular surface disorders. *Ophthalmology*. 1995;102:1486-1496.

21. Holland EJ. Epithelial transplantation for the management of severe ocular surface disease. *Trans Am Ophthalmol Soc*. 1996;94:677-743.

22. Espana EM, Di Pascuale M, Grueterich M, Solomon A, Tseng SCG. Keratolimbal allograft for corneal surface reconstruction. *Eye*. 2004;18:406-417.

6

CORNEAL DYSTROPHIES

Sean Pieramici, MD; Natalie Afshari, MD; and Jodi I. Luchs, MD, FACS

Corneal dystrophies are a group of rare disorders characterized by the accumulation of abnormal deposits in the cornea. These dystrophies are inherited, usually bilateral, and are not associated with systemic diseases, prior eye conditions, or environmental factors. Most, but not all, of the dystrophies demonstrate an autosomal dominant inheritance pattern. Clinically, corneal dystrophies begin to develop after birth, slowly progressing throughout life. However, some dystrophies, such as Fuchs' endothelial corneal dystrophy, may not present until later in life.

The clinical manifestations of corneal dystrophies are directly related to the anatomical layer of the cornea involved. The anterior corneal dystrophies involve the corneal epithelium, epithelial basement membrane, and Bowman's layer of the cornea. These dystrophies most commonly cause recurrent corneal erosions (Figures 6-1 and 6-2) and irregular astigmatism. The stromal dystrophies, if more superficial, may cause recurrent corneal erosions, while dystrophies involving deeper layers of the stroma will cause more opacification, resulting in decreased vision. The posterior corneal dystrophies affecting Descemet's membrane and the endothelium result in corneal edema. As many of theses dystrophies progress, they can affect several layers of the cornea.

Histopathological findings using histochemical and electron microscopic techniques are known for many of the dystrophies. New developments in molecular genetics of the corneal dystrophies are now being discovered at an accelerating rate. These together have revolutionized our understanding of these conditions.

ANTERIOR CORNEAL DYSTROPHIES

Meesmann's Dystrophy

Meesmann's dystrophy is the only cornea dystrophy that exclusively affects the cornea epithelium. This is an extremely rare, bilateral, symmetric, autosomal dominant dystrophy with incomplete penetrance.[1] Clinically, this dystrophy presents in the first few years of life with tiny intraepithelial microcysts or vesicles seen best with retroillumination (Figures 6-3 and 6-4). The cysts are usually most

Trattler WB, Majmudar PA, Luchs JI, Swartz TS, eds.
Cornea Handbook (pp. 75-108)
© 2010 SLACK Incorporated

Figure 6-1. Recurrent corneal erosion, seen here accompanied by a small ulcer, is common among corneal dystrophies. (Courtesy of Tracy S. Swartz, OD, MS.)

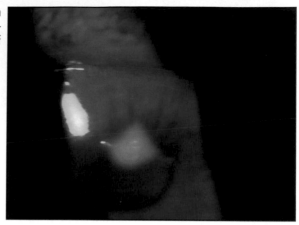

Figure 6-2. Recurrent corneal erosion. There is no frank epithelial defect, but the epithelial surface is irregular and picks up fluorescein dye over several minutes. Published with permission from Rapuano CJ, Luchs JI, Kim T, eds. *Anterior Segment: The Requisites in Ophthalmology.* New York, NY: Mosby Publishing; 2000. (Courtesy of Jodi I. Luchs, MD.)

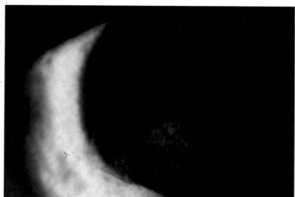

Figure 6-3. Meesman's dystrophy. Tiny intraepithelial gray-white dots are noted on direct illumination and illumination off the iris. Published with permission from Rapuano CJ, Luchs JI, Kim T, eds. *Anterior Segment: The Requisites in Ophthalmology.* New York, NY: Mosby Publishing; 2000. (Courtesy of Jodi I. Luchs, MD.)

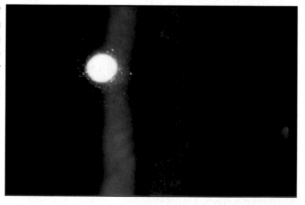

numerous in the interpalpebral area of the cornea. These clear cysts consist of cytoplasmic aggregates of keratin in the epithelial cells (originally described as "peculiar substance").[2]

Mutations in different keratin genes KRT3 on chromosome 12q13 and KRT12 on chromosome 17q12 have been shown to cause in Meesmann's dystrophy.[3] These mutations in the genes responsible for keratin filament assembly are believed to cause dysfunctional keratin formation.

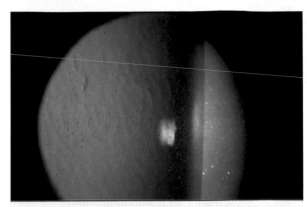

Figure 6-4. Meesman's dystrophy. Pinpoint dots are often best noted in retroillumination. Published with permission from Rapuano CJ, Luchs JI, Kim T, eds. *Anterior Segment: The Requisites in Ophthalmology.* New York, NY: Mosby Publishing; 2000. (Courtesy of Jodi I. Luchs, MD.)

The epithelial cysts can increase in number and density throughout life. Vision is usually unaffected in patients with Meesmann's dystrophy but can slightly diminish if the number of cysts increases, causing small irregularities on the corneal surface. Recurrent erosions are not a feature of this corneal dystrophy, unlike many of the other anterior corneal dystrophies. Most patients require no treatment, but lubrication of the corneal surface or soft contact lenses may be warranted for patients who experience intermittent symptoms related to minute erosions.[4]

Epithelial Basement Membrane Dystrophy

This dystrophy, also known as *map-dot-fingerprint dystrophy*[5] or *Cogan microcystic dystrophy*,[6] is the most common anterior corneal dystrophy. To date, there has been no genetic linkage established, and it is more often found sporadically in the population. However, epithelial basement membrane dystrophy (EBMD) has been classified as a dystrophy because the changes associated with this dystrophy occur more commonly in some families.[7] When found with a hereditary component, it is bilateral, autosomal dominant, often with incomplete penetrance. This dystrophy occurs more commonly in women than men.

Clinical appearance of this dystrophy varies based on the epithelial abnormalities encountered and are best seen by broad tangential beam and retroillumination (Figures 6-5, 6-6, and 6-7). Subtle EBMD changes can be seen using fluorescein stain, which will highlight negative staining over elevated areas of abnormal epithelium. The 3 most common clinical presentations are map lines, dots or microcysts, and/or fingerprint lines. Map-like changes, the most commonly encountered clinical presentation, are irregular grayish patches, sharply demarcated, with intervening clear zones. These epithelial changes take on the appearance of geographic borders seen on maps. Histopathology of these map-like changes show a thickened basement membrane extending into the epithelium. Microcystic changes are grayish white, irregular opacities of varying sizes resembling spheres with discrete edges. The dots are often seen adjacent to map line areas. Histopathologic findings of these microcysts show abnormal epithelial cells with microcysts, often containing intracellular and nuclear debris.[8,9] Fingerprint lines, the least commonly encountered clinical presentation, are thin parallel lines often arranged in a concentric pattern that resemble fingerprints. Histopathologic findings show thickened basement in parallel rows extending into the epithelium, similar to map-like changes.[8,9] Electron microscopy of this

Figure 6-5. Epithelial basement membrane dystrophy has a variable presentation, giving rise to its alternative name: map-dot-finger-print dystrophy. (Courtesy of Tracy S. Swartz, OD, MS.)

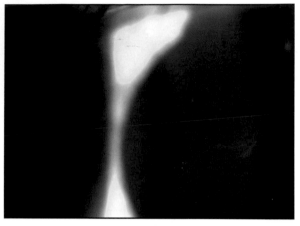

Figure 6-6. EBMD in retroillumination. Fingerprint lines, primarily seen superiorly and inferiorly, are highlighted in retroillumination. Published with permission from Rapuano CJ, Luchs JI, Kim T, eds. *Anterior Segment: The Requisites in Ophthalmology.* New York, NY: Mosby Publishing; 2000. (Courtesy of Jodi I. Luchs, MD.)

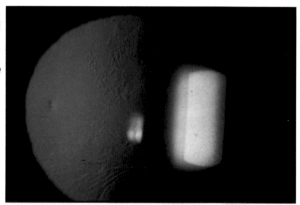

Figure 6-7. EBMD often presents with a negative fluorescein staining pattern illustrated here. Published with permission from Rapuano CJ, Luchs JI, Kim T, eds. *Anterior Segment: The Requisites in Ophthalmology.* New York, NY: Mosby Publishing; 2000. (Courtesy of Jodi I. Luchs, MD.)

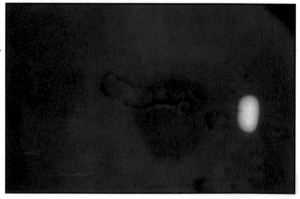

condition reveals poorly functioning adhesion complexes, hemidesmosomes, and anchoring fibrils.

Most patients with EBMD will remain asymptomatic. The primary symptoms related to this dystrophy are spontaneous recurrent corneal erosions and blurred vision, which usually do not occur until the third decade of life. Recurrent erosions are thought to be caused by poor epithelial cell attachment to the underlying abnormal basement membrane. Patients may experience extreme pain upon awakening as they open their eyelids, resulting in shearing effect of the weakened epithelium, causing a painful erosion. Any patient with recurrent corneal erosions and no prior history of trauma should have careful slit-lamp examination to look for any underlying EBMD. Blurred vision in EBMD is caused by irregular astigmatism resulting from an elevated corneal epithelial layer. This irregular astigmatism can often be documented by topography.

Treatment for EBMD is necessary only when patients are symptomatic. Recurrent corneal erosions are treated based on the severity of the attacks. For mild attacks, lubricating drops and ointments are employed, including 5% sodium chloride, which some physicians believe may promote tighter epithelial adhesions.[10] Patching the eye closed can also aid in epithelial healing. Lubricating ointments and patching at bedtime can also be used to prevent future corneal erosions. With more severe corneal erosions, a bandage contact lens can be placed to aid in healing and reduce the pain.[11] Antibiotic drops are usually applied concurrently with the bandage contact lens to reduce the infection risk.

In recalcitrant cases, superficial keratectomy (SK), anterior stromal puncture, and phototherapeutic keratectomy (PTK) may be employed.[12,13] SK works by mechanical debridement of loose epithelium and is thought to promote more normal epithelial adhesions as the new epithelium is laid down. Anterior stromal puncture using a 25-gauge or 27-gauge needle to place multiple small punctures into Bowman's layer is thought to promote tighter adhesions through microscopic scar formation. Anterior stromal puncture works better when areas of erosions are more focal and located outside the visual axis because scarring can occur. Some people feel that stromal puncture works better for recurrent erosions due to trauma because they tend to occur in the same location. PTK has become a more popular treatment choice for recurrent corneal erosions associated with EBMD. PTK works by both a mechanical debridement of the epithelial layer as well as excimer laser ablation of the basement membrane and superficial Bowman's, thereby potentially promoting stronger attachment of the new epithelial layer. Irregular astigmatism caused by EBMD can be treated by rigid gas permeable contact lenses, SK, or PTK.

Corneal Dystrophies of Bowman's Layer

Reis-Bücklers or corneal dystrophy of Bowman's type I (CDB-I) and Thiel-Behnke or corneal dystrophy of Bowman's type II[14] (CDB-II) share many similarities as well as some differences. Reis-Bücklers dystrophy (CDB-I) is an autosomal dominant dystrophy in which patients are born with normal appearing corneas. However, in the first and second decade of life, corneal opacification and scarring cause marked visual loss and recurrent corneal erosions lead to significant pain. CDB-I is synonymous with type III granular dystrophy.[14] Thiel-Behnke dystrophy (CDB-II) is also an autosomal dominant dystrophy with recurrent corneal erosions developing in the first and second decade of life. Decreasing visual acuity is seen later than with Reis-Bücklers dystrophy.

In both diseases, Bowman's layer is replaced with fibrocellular scar tissue. Clinically, a superficial grey-white reticular pattern is described in CDB-I and a honeycomb pattern of opacification is described in CDB-II (Figure 6-8). Despite these clinical differences, it is often impossible to distinguish one from the other by slit-lamp examination. Transmission electron microscopy better differentiates the two dystrophies. In Reis-Bucklers dystrophy, rod-like bodies are seen

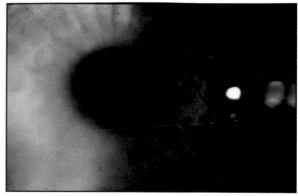

Figure 6-8. Corneal dystrophy of Bowman's membrane, type 1 (Reis-Bückler's dystrophy). The gray-white deposition is evident throughout the anterior cornea. Published with permission from Rapuano CJ, Luchs JI, Kim T, eds. *Anterior Segment: The Requisites in Ophthalmology.* New York, NY: Mosby Publishing; 2000. (Courtesy of Jodi I. Luchs, MD.)

deposited in Bowman's layer, whereas in Thiel-Behnke dystrophy, curly bodies are seen.[14] Molecular genetic studies have increased our knowledge of these two dystrophies. Both dystrophies are linked to mutations in BIGH3 on chromosome 5q31, the gene responsible for the formation of keratoepithelin.[15-17] Thiel-Behnke is also linked to a mutation on chromosome 10q23-24, though the gene product is currently unknown.[15-17]

Symptoms in these 2 dystrophies are related to recurrent corneal erosions and vision loss secondary to progressive corneal scarring. Initial management for both of these dystrophies is aimed at treating

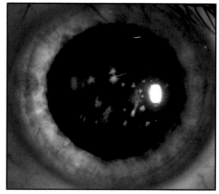

Figure 6-9. Granular dystrophy, as seen in the early stages. (Courtesy of J. Bradley Randleman, MD.)

recurrent corneal erosions similar for the treatment of recurrent erosions due to EBMD. If significant superficial corneal scarring or opacification occurs, then SK or more commonly PTK can be performed.[18,19] With deeper opacification and scarring, lamellar or penetrating keratoplasty is necessary. However, recurrence rates are high with these dystrophies after PK.

STROMAL CORNEAL DYSTROPHIES

Granular Dystrophy

Granular dystrophy is an autosomal dominant dystrophy characterized by the deposition of gray-white crumb like opacities in the anterior stroma (Figures 6-9 and 6-10). These lesions do not extend to the limbus, intervening stroma between the opacities remains clear, and vision is usually unaffected. This disease is usually slowly progressive, where the opacities may increase in number and size, coalesce, and further deepen in the stroma. With advancing disease, the intervening clear stroma becomes involved, resulting in reduction of vision.

Opacities in granular dystrophy are composed of eosinophilic hyaline deposits that stain with Masson trichrome[20] (Figure 6-11). Granular dystrophy has been

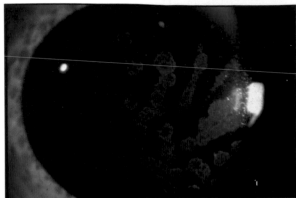

Figure 6-10. Granular dystrophy, gray-white opacities primarily involve the central cornea. The intervening spaces are clear. Published with permission from Rapuano CJ, Luchs JI, Kim T, eds. *Anterior Segment: The Requisites in Ophthalmology.* New York, NY: Mosby Publishing; 2000. (Courtesy of Jodi I. Luchs, MD.)

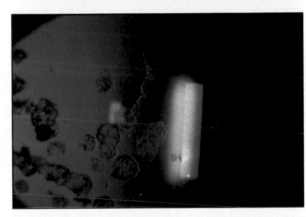

Figure 6-11a. Granular dystrophy, retroillumination. The clear spaces between the opacities are apparent. Published with permission from Rapuano CJ, Luchs JI, Kim T, eds. *Anterior Segment: The Requisites in Ophthalmology.* New York, NY: Mosby Publishing; 2000. (Courtesy of Jodi I. Luchs, MD.)

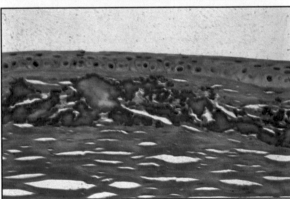

Figure 6-11b. Granular dystrophy, pathology. Masson trichrome stain revealing the hyaline deposits in the anterior stroma. Published with permission from Rapuano CJ, Luchs JI, Kim T, eds. *Anterior Segment: The Requisites in Ophthalmology.* New York, NY: Mosby Publishing; 2000. (Courtesy of Jodi I. Luchs, MD and Ralph C. Eagle, Jr., MD.)

linked to several mutations in BIGH3 on chromosome 5q31, along with lattice, Avellino, and CDB-I.[21] Mutations in the formation of keratoepithelin are responsible for this dystrophy.[15]

Granular dystrophy has been divided into 3 clinical types.[22] Type I is the most common form of granular dystrophy, described above, and occurs early in life with slow progression. Type II presents later, beginning around the second decade of life. Granular opacities type II are larger than type I and recurrent corneal erosions are rare. Type III causes more superficial disease and is synonymous with CDB-I.

Figure 6-12. Lattice dystrophy. (Courtesy of J. Bradley Randleman, MD.)

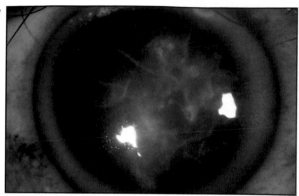

Figure 6-13. Lattice dystrophy. Numerous branching refractile lines are observed. Published with permission from Rapuano CJ, Luchs JI, Kim T, eds. *Anterior Segment: The Requisites in Ophthalmology.* New York, NY: Mosby Publishing; 2000. (Courtesy of Jodi I. Luchs, MD.)

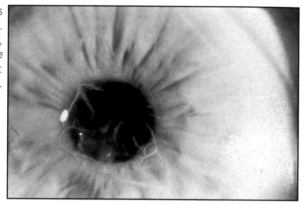

Most patients with granular dystrophy will not require treatment. Initial management, if warranted, is aimed at recurrent corneal erosions as described for EBMD. Treatment for visually significant superficial corneal disease includes SK, lamellar keratectomy, or more commonly PTK.[23] If the lesions are located more posterior and vision is severely reduced, penetrating keratoplasty may be performed. Recurrence after corneal transplant is common.[24]

Lattice Dystrophy

Lattice dystrophy, the most common of the stromal cornea dystrophies, is autosomal dominant with variable expression. The spectrum of corneal changes seen with this disease is large. Early on in this disease, discrete ovoid subepithelial deposits, white dots, and refractile lines are seen. The refractile lines or lattice lines as classically described are radially oriented with dichotomous branching near their central termination, which appears as glass-like branching lines in the stroma, seen best with retroillumination. As the disease progresses, patients can develop a fine anterior stromal haze (Figures 6-12 and 6-13). Later in the disease, opacities can coalesce and deepen in the stroma, taking on a ground glass appearance.

Lattice dystrophy is a primary localized corneal amyloidosis. These deposits stain orange-red with Congo red, and also demonstrate an apple green birefringence with a polarizing filter (Figures 6-14 and 6-15). Clinically and histologically, there are at least 4 types of lattice dystrophy. Type I is characterized by classic

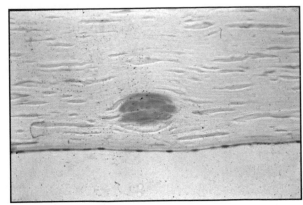

Figure 6-14. Lattice dystrophy. Congo red stain demonstrates deep corneal amyloid deposits. Published with permission from Rapuano CJ, Luchs JI, Kim T, eds. *Anterior Segment: The Requisites in Ophthalmology.* New York, NY: Mosby Publishing; 2000. (Courtesy of Jodi I. Luchs, MD and Ralph C. Eagle, Jr., MD.)

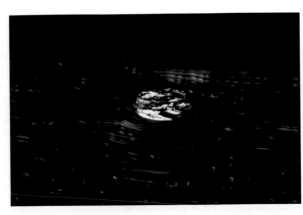

Figure 6-15. Lattice dystrophy, pathology. Apple green birefringence of the amyloid material is apparent using a polarizing filter. Published with permission from Rapuano CJ, Luchs JI, Kim T, eds. *Anterior Segment: The Requisites in Ophthalmology.* New York, NY: Mosby Publishing; 2000. (Courtesy of Jodi I. Luchs, MD.)

branching lattice lines with stromal haze.[25] There is no systemic amyloidosis. Type II lattice dystrophy or Meretoja syndrome is a systemic amyloidosis associated with corneal dystrophy.[26] Systemic findings include cranial and peripheral neuropathies, mask-like facies, and dermatologic changes. Type IIIa has a delayed onset but is inherited autosomal dominant. Type IIIb is autosomal recessive with symptoms delayed much later in life.[27] Lattice dystrophy types I and IIIa have been linked to mutations in BIGH3 on chromosome 5q31, along with granular, Avellino, and CDB-I.[21] Lattice dystrophy type II is associated with mutations in the gelsolin gene on chromosome 9q32-34.[28,29] Gelsolin is a precursor protein for amyloid.

Treatment for lattice dystrophy depends on the patient's symptoms. Recurrent corneal erosions, which often occur due to the predominance of anterior stromal involvement in lattice dystrophy, are managed in the usual fashion. If visual acuity is impaired due to superficial opacities and haze, then PTK can be used.[30] If opacities deepen into the stroma, lamellar and penetrating keratoplasty are needed. Recurrence of lattice dystrophy after corneal transplantation is more common than granular or macular dystrophy.[31]

Macular Dystrophy

Macular dystrophy, inherited in an autosomal recessive fashion, is the least common of the 3 classic stromal dystrophies (lattice, granular, and macular) but most severe clinically. Patients are born with clear corneas but begin to cloud between

Figure 6-16a. Macular dystrophy, pathology. The colloidal iron stain demonstrates the glycosaminoglycan (acid mucopolysaccharide) as blue deposits concentrated in the anterior cornea, but evident throughout the stroma. Published with permission from, Rapuano CJ, Luchs JI, Kim T, eds. *Anterior Segment: The Requisites in Ophthalmology.* New York, NY: Mosby Publishing; 2000. (Courtesy of Jodi I. Luchs, MD and Ralph C. Eagle, Jr., MD.)

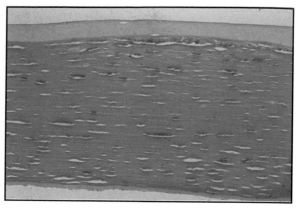

Figure 6-16b. Macular dystrophy. Published with permission from, Rapuano CJ, Luchs JI, Kim T, eds. *Anterior Segment: The Requisites in Ophthalmology.* New York, NY: Mosby Publishing; 2000. (Courtesy of Jodi I. Luchs, MD and Ralph C. Eagle, Jr., MD.)

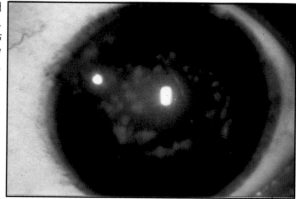

ages 3 and 9. The deposits start as central grey-white superficial stromal opacities, which over time will extend to the periphery and involve the entire thickness of the cornea stroma. Corneal guttata have also been observed in this dystrophy.[32] Patients experience progressive vision loss and irritation as the diseases worsens. Vision in this disease is severely affected by the third to fourth decade of life.

Macular dystrophy can be confused clinically with granular dystrophy early in its presentation. However, definite differences with macular dystrophy make the distinction possible, including recessive inheritance, full involvement of the cornea stroma, intervening haze between the opacities, and central corneal thinning.

The deposits seen in macular dystrophy are composed of GAGs, which stain with Alcian blue, colloidal iron, and PAS[33] (Figure 6-16). These GAGs accumulate within the stromal keratocytes and endothelial cells and subepithelium.

Macular dystrophy is divided into 2 types based on synthesis of keratan sulfate, an important component of corneal proteoglycans.[34] In the more common type I macular dystrophy, there is a lack of keratan sulfate synthesis and levels are not detectable in the cornea or in the patient's serum. In type II macular dystrophy there is production of keratan sulfate; however, it is synthesized 30% below the normal levels. Both types of macular dystrophy have been linked to chromosome 16q22.[35] Mutations on this chromosome location are found in the carbohydrate sulfotransferase-6 (CHST6) gene, which codes for the enzyme corneal N-acetylglucosamine-6-sulfotransferase.[36] This enzyme catalyzes the sulfation of keratan sulfate.

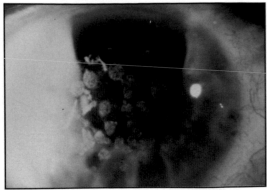

Figure 6-17. Avellino dystrophy. Lattice lines are seen among the more numerous granular dystrophy deposits. Published with permission from Rapuano CJ, Luchs JI, Kim T, eds. *Anterior Segment: The Requisites in Ophthalmology.* New York, NY: Mosby Publishing; 2000. (Courtesy of Jodi I. Luchs, MD.)

Treatment for macular dystrophy depends on the type of symptoms the patient experiences. Recurrent corneal erosions are managed in the typical fashion. Photophobia, a common complaint in macular dystrophy, may be relieved with tinted sunglasses. Vision loss resulting from superficial disease can be treated with PTK[30] and lamellar keratoplasty. However, due to the severe nature of this dystrophy, PK is often the treatment of choice, although recurrences in the grafts are often seen.

Avellino Dystrophy

Avellino dystrophy is a variant of granular dystrophy. Patients affected with Avellino dystrophy have clinical and histological granular dystrophy disease, as well as the presence of lattice lesions (Figure 6-17). Lattice lesions always develop after granular deposits are present and may not be seen early in the disease. The name of the dystrophy comes from Avellino, Italy, a city where 3 families affected with the disease originated. Avellino dystrophy is autosomal dominant and is linked to the R124H mutation in TGFβI gene.[22] Severity of the corneal deposits is dependent on the heterozygosity or homozygosity of this mutation.

Clinically, patients have a similar course to granular dystrophy and are treated in the same fashion. Recurrent corneal erosions are seen more commonly in patients with Avellino dystrophy than with classic granular dystrophy.

Schnyder's Crystalline Dystrophy

Schnyder's crystalline dystrophy is a rare autosomal dominant, slowly progressive stromal dystrophy that usually presents early in life but may not be apparent until much later. Early in the disease, minute yellow-white crystals are seen centrally in the anterior stroma (Figure 6-18). These crystal opacities accumulate just beneath Bowman's membrane and may take on several morphologies. Intervening stroma between the crystals is usually clear. Dense corneal arcus is frequently seen with the central deposits. A diffuse stromal haze may also be clinically evident in older patients with Schnyder's crystalline dystrophy (Figures 6-19 and 6-20).

It is important for clinicians to differentiate crystal deposits in Schnyder's crystalline dystrophy from other conditions causing crystal deposits, including multiple myeloma, cystinosis, gout, uremia, Waldenstrom's macroglobulinemia,

Figure 6-18. Schnyder's crystalline dystrophy. A dense central crystalline deposition is seen with a less dense surrounding halo. Published with permission from Rapuano CJ, Luchs JI, Kim T, eds. *Anterior Segment: The Requisites in Ophthalmology.* New York, NY: Mosby Publishing; 2000. (Courtesy of Jodi I. Luchs, MD.)

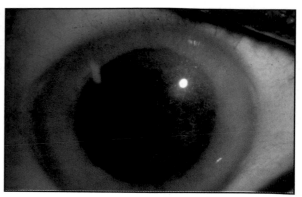

Figure 6-19. Schnyder's crystalline dystrophy. The dense central crystals are apparent. Published with permission from Rapuano CJ, Luchs JI, Kim T, eds. *Anterior Segment: The Requisites in Ophthalmology.* New York, NY: Mosby Publishing; 2000. (Courtesy of Jodi I. Luchs, MD.)

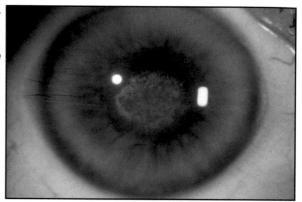

Figure 6-20. Schnyder's crystalline dystrophy. Central crystalline deposits with a prominent outer crystalline ring are seen. The dense arcus lipoides is also obvious. Published with permission from Rapuano CJ, Luchs JI, Kim T, eds. *Anterior Segment: The Requisites in Ophthalmology.* New York, NY: Mosby Publishing; 2000. (Courtesy of Jodi I. Luchs, MD.)

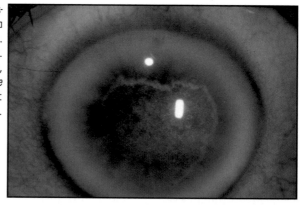

drugs, infectious crystalline keratopathy, and Bietti's peripheral crystalline dystrophy.

The exact pathogenesis of this disease is still unclear; however, a localized abnormality in cholesterol metabolism is suspected, which may be modified by systemic hyperlipidemia.[37] All patients with this dystrophy should have a fasting lipid profile done for the possibility of hyperlipoproteinemia or hyperlipidemia. Accumulations of cholesterol and neutral fats are seen throughout the corneal stroma as well as in the epithelium and Bowman's membrane.[38] Oil Red O stains the neutral fats.

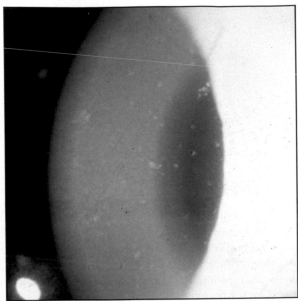

Figure 6-21. Fleck dystrophy. Multiple small, discrete, gray-white opacities are seen throughout the stroma. Published with permission from Rapuano CJ, Luchs JI, Kim T, eds. *Anterior Segment: The Requisites in Ophthalmology*. New York, NY: Mosby Publishing; 2000. (Courtesy of Jodi I. Luchs, MD.)

Most patients with Schnyder's crystalline dystrophy will maintain good vision without the need for intervention. However, as the disease progresses, visual acuity may be reduced significantly enough to warrant PTK, lamellar, or PK. Reoccurrences of this dystrophy have been seen after corneal transplantation.[39]

Gelatinous Drop-like Dystrophy

Gelatinous drop-like dystrophy is a rare autosomal recessive dystrophy that presents in the first decade of life and may initially resemble band keratopathy. As the disease progresses, corneal opacification increases as protuberant gelatinous masses accumulate in the subepithelium and anterior stroma. Symptoms include photophobia, lacrimation, foreign-body sensation, and decreased vision. These gelatinous masses are accumulations of amyloid deposits. Gelatinous drop-like dystrophy has been linked to mutations in the M1S1 gene located on chromosome 1p31.[40] M1S1 is a cell surface phosphoglycoprotein as well as a substrate for protein kinase C. Mutations in this gene lead to a truncated protein, which is thought to trigger amyloid formation in the cornea.[40] Patients with this disease are managed with lamellar and PK. Recurrences after corneal transplantation are high.

Fleck Dystrophy

Fleck dystrophy is a rare, autosomal dominant, nonprogressive stromal dystrophy often noted as an incidental finding on routine examination. Fleck dystrophy is characterized by widely scattered, discrete tiny white flecks seen throughout the entire corneal stromal and extending to the limbus (Figure 6-21). Intervening stroma between deposits is clear. This dystrophy is typically bilateral but often can be highly asymmetric or even unilateral. Ocular conditions such as central cloudy cornea, angiod streaks, keratoconus, limbal dermoid, pseudoxanthoma elasticum, and atopy have been associated with fleck dystrophy.[41]

Figure 6-22. Central cloudy dystrophy of François. Multiple central polygonal opacities are found in the posterior stroma. They appear identical to posterior crocodile shagreen but are considered a dystrophy when they are found in multiple members of a family. Published with permission from Rapuano CJ, Luchs JI, Kim T, eds. *Anterior Segment: The Requisites in Ophthalmology.* New York, NY: Mosby Publishing; 2000. (Courtesy of Jodi I. Luchs, MD.)

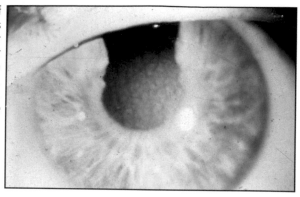

Histochemical analysis shows that certain keratocytes contain excessive GAGs and lipids.[42] The GAGs will stain with Alcian blue or colloidal iron, and the lipids will show staining with Sudan black and oil red O. The remainder of the stroma as well as Bowman's layer, Descemet's membrane, and endothelium are normal.

Patients with fleck dystrophy are asymptomatic with normal vision, requiring no treatment. On occasion, some patients may complain of mild photophobia.

Central Cloudy Dystrophy

Central cloudy dystrophy is an autosomal dominant, bilateral, symmetric dystrophy that is generally nonprogressive. Opacities appear as faint gray snowflake-like lesions located in the deep stromal layer (Figure 6-22). The margins of the lesions are ill-defined, and crack-like areas of clear stroma appear as a polygonal structure. Usually only the central two thirds of the cornea are affected, and the opacities are best seen with broad illumination or scleral scatter. Clinically, these opacities are identical to the opacities seen in crocodile shagreen.[43] However, crocodile shagreen does not follow a genetic pattern, is located more anteriorly in the stroma, and is present more in the periphery rather than centrally as in central cloudy cornea.

The pathogenesis of this dystrophy is unknown at this time, but abnormal collagen is thought to play the leading role.[44] No treatment is typically required.

Congenital Hereditary Stromal Dystrophy

Congenital hereditary stromal dystrophy (CHSD) is a rare, nonprogressive, autosomal dominant, congenital dystrophy that must be differentiated from other causes of corneal opacification. Clinically, opacities are seen as diffuse flaky or feathery clouding of the central anterior stroma. Stromal thickness is not increased in this dystrophy, unlike congenital hereditary endothelial dystrophy where corneal edema is present.

The pathogenesis of this dystrophy is still unknown, but abnormalities in collagen fibrils may play a role.[45] Endothelium may also play a role in the pathogenesis of this disease[45] because an abnormal anterior portion of Descemet's membrane is seen early in the disease. Significant opacification of the cornea as a result of this dystrophy warrants an early and aggressive intervention with penetrating keratoplasy to save useful vision and prevent dense amblyopia.

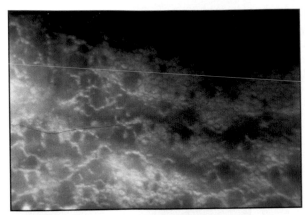

Figure 6-23. Specular micrograph of endothelial dystrophy. Specular microscopy reveals numerous irregular dark areas devoid of endothelial cells. Cells that can be seen are often larger and more varied in size (polymegethism) and shape (polymorphism). Published with permission from Rapuano CJ, Luchs JI, Kim T, eds. *Anterior Segment: The Requisites in Ophthalmology.* New York, NY: Mosby Publishing; 2000. (Courtesy of Jodi I. Luchs, MD and Ralph C. Eagle, Jr., MD.)

Pre-Descemet's Dystrophy

Pre-Descemet's dystrophy is a bilateral symmetric dystrophy with an unknown pattern of inheritance. Clinically, opacities are seen as discrete fine grey lesions taking on many morphologies, including dot-like, linear, semicircular, comma-shaped, and dendritic. These deposits are seen in the posterior stroma and may be diffuse, central, or form a ring. Opacities in this dystrophy are usually apparent around the fourth decade of life. This dystrophy can often be confused with cornea farinata, a degenerative disorder with similar opacities. However, corneal farinata tends to have finer opacities diffusely scattered throughout the stroma.

The pathogenesis of this dystrophy is unclear. However, pathological findings suggest the accumulation of lipofuscin-like material, which may be more consistent with a degenerative process related to aging.[46] No treatment is necessary.

Posterior Amorphous Stromal Dystrophy

Posterior amorphous stromal dystrophy is a rare, symmetric, bilateral, autosomal dominant corneal dystrophy characterized by posterior stromal opacification and diffuse corneal thinning. It may appear early, during the first decade of life, and be slowly progressive. Thinning may progress to a central corneal thickness of 300 µm with significant corneal flattening. Irregular astigmatism is not characteristic. Stromal opacification may present as patchy gray areas in the posterior stroma with indistinct borders located from limbus to limbus.

The pathology involves deposits of electron-dense fibrils and a thick collagenous layer posterior to Descemet's membrane. Focal disorganization and relative absence of keratocytes has also been described.[47]

POSTERIOR CORNEAL DYSTROPHIES

Fuchs' Endothelial Dystrophy

Fuchs' endothelial corneal dystrophy is a common progressive disorder more often affecting women than men. Endothelial dysfunction is the end result of this disease. The first signs of this dystrophy are asymptomatic corneal endothelial guttate excrescences (Figure 6-23). Guttate excrescences appear centrally at first and then spread peripherally on the posterior cornea, giving rise to the term "cor-

Figure 6-24. Corneal edema secondary to Fuchs' dystrophy. Published with permission from Rapuano CJ, Luchs JI, Kim T, eds. *Anterior Segment: The Requisites in Ophthalmology.* New York, NY: Mosby Publishing; 2000. (Courtesy of Jodi I. Luchs, MD and Ralph C. Eagle, Jr., MD.)

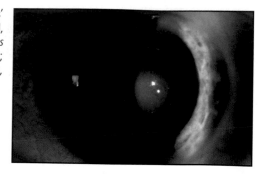

Figure 6-25. Fuchs' dystrophy. A large epithelial bulla is obvious on slit-beam examination. Published with permission from Rapuano CJ, Luchs JI, Kim T, eds. *Anterior Segment: The Requisites in Ophthalmology.* New York, NY: Mosby Publishing; 2000. (Courtesy of Jodi I. Luchs, MD and Ralph C. Eagle, Jr., MD.)

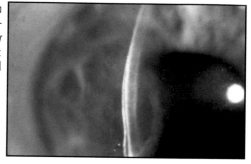

nea guttata." The findings may be best seen with retroillumination. Endothelial pigmentation may also occur as a fine dusting on the posterior surface. Guttate excrescences can coalesce to form a beaten metal appearance and Descemet's membrane may be thickened.

As the endothelial cells are further compromised, stromal edema results, heralding the onset of the symptomatic phase of the dystrophy (Figure 6-24). As edema worsens and the cornea thickens, vision becomes compromised. It is rare for patients with Fuchs' dystrophy to become symptomatic before age 50.[48] As the disease progresses, further corneal decompensation ensues, with marked stromal edema resulting in additional vision loss (Figure 6-25). Microcystic and bullous epithelial edema will result from continual progression of this dystrophy. Bullous keratopathy results in epithelial breakdown, causing irritation, pain, photophobia, scarring, and corneal neovascularization. Bullae can rupture, causing extreme pain from corneal erosions. Late stages of the disease show subepithelial fibrosis from chronic epithelial edema.

This dystrophy has been reported to have an autosomal dominant inheritance pattern but also may be sporadic. In some studies, this dystrophy has been linked to mutations in the COL8A2 gene on chromosome 1p34.3-p32.[49] The COL8A2 gene encodes a 703–amino acid alpha2 chain of type VIII collagen, a component of endothelial basement membrane. More recently, a late-onset Fuchs' corneal dystrophy has been linked to a new genetic locus 13pTel-13q12.13.[50] Further molecular genetic studies are needed to elucidate the genetic mutations behind this dystrophy.

The primary pathologic change seen in Fuchs' dystrophy is believed to be the endothelial cell that lays down abnormal Descemet's membrane (Figure 6-25). These abnormal cells are also thought to contain an abnormal pumping mechanism. Histochemical analysis of the cornea shows a thickened and sometimes redundant Descemet's membrane with a collagenous posterior layer.[51]

Both corneal pachymetry and specular microscopy are helpful in diagnosing Fuchs' dystrophy as well as following progression. Specular microscopy will show decreasing numbers of endothelial cells, as well as variation in shape (polymorphism) and size (polymegathism). These tests are helpful when deciding whether cataract surgery or other intraocular surgeries can proceed without resulting in corneal decompensation. Unfortunately, there are no absolute clinical findings that can predict which patients will develop cornea edema when asymptomatic.

Treatment of patients with Fuchs' endothelial dystrophy is aimed at reducing visually significant corneal edema. Medical management may include hypertonic saline solutions and ointments such as 5% sodium chloride, dehydration of the cornea with a blow dryer, and reduction in IOP. Lubricating drops and bandage contact lenses are used to treat bullous epithelial keratopathy in more advanced cases.

Penetrating keratoplasty has been the treatment of choice for patients with decreased vision in which medical therapy has failed. However, newer lamellar transplant techniques are replacing full-thickness cornea transplants. These innovative treatments, including deep lamellar endothelial keratoplasty (DLEK) and more recently DSEK, are becoming the new procedures of choice. Historically, PK for Fuchs' dystrophy meant an open sky procedure, transplantation of the entire cornea, extensive suturing, high amounts of astigmatism, and long visual recovery. Now with DSEK transplantation, most shortfalls of full-thickness corneal transplantation are avoided, including minimal suturing, minimal induced astigmatism, small incision, posterior layer transplantation only, and a much faster visual recovery.

Posterior Polymorphous Dystrophy

Posterior polymorphous dystrophy is a bilateral, autosomal dominant dystrophy that encompasses a wide spectrum of corneal and anterior segment abnormalities but is often overlooked due to the benign nature of this disease. The clinical expression of this disease varies widely even in the same families. This dystrophy can present early in life with isolated vesicle-like lesions, which are seen in the majority of patients with this dystrophy. Other lesions include broad band lesions with scalloped edges and more diffuse grey opacities (Figures 6-26 through 6-28). Variable amounts of iridocorneal adhesions, correctopia, corneal edema, and fine peripheral anterior synechiae have been reported.[52] Elevated IOP was also found in about 14% of the patients with this dystrophy, either open or closed angle glaucoma.[52]

Posterior polymorphous dystrophy has been mapped to chromosome 20p11.2-q11.2.[53] This region is also linked with congenital hereditary endothelial dystrophy.[54] Mutations have also been found in the homeobox gene located at the 20p11.2-g11.2 site.[55] Mutations in the VSX1 gene have also been associated with keratoconus.[56]

Pathogenesis of this disease revolves around abnormal endothelial cells that take on properties of epithelial cells. These abnormal cells manifest proliferative properties, showing rapid growth. Abnormalities in Descemet's membrane such as thickening are also present. Iridocorneal endothelial syndrome (ICE) shows similar changes to posterior polymorphous dystrophy both clinically and in its pathogenesis, although ICE is a unilateral condition.

Most patients with this dystrophy are asymptomatic and have stable disease throughout their lives. Corneal edema, if present, is managed in a similar fashion

Figure 6-26. Posterior polymorphous dystrophy. A scalloped edge band is seen in the periphery. Published with permission from Rapuano CJ, Luchs JI, Kim T, eds. *Anterior Segment: The Requisites in Ophthalmology.* New York, NY: Mosby Publishing; 2000. (Courtesy of Jodi I. Luchs, MD.)

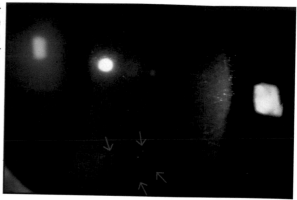

Figure 6-27. Posterior polymorphous dystrophy. The same eye as in Figure 6-26 is examined in retroillumination. The irregularities are easily visualized. Published with permission from Rapuano CJ, Luchs JI, Kim T, eds. *Anterior Segment: The Requisites in Ophthalmology.* New York, NY: Mosby Publishing; 2000. (Courtesy of Jodi I. Luchs, MD.)

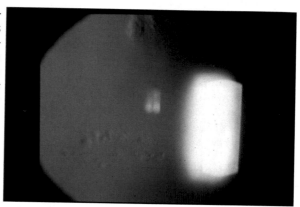

Figure 6-28. Posterior polymorphous dystrophy. Retroillumination using the red reflex easily demonstrates a central scalloped band. Published with permission from Rapuano CJ, Luchs JI, Kim T, eds. *Anterior Segment: The Requisites in Ophthalmology.* New York, NY: Mosby Publishing; 2000. (Courtesy of Jodi I. Luchs, MD.)

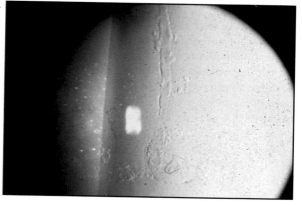

to Fuchs' dystrophy. Corneal transplant or glaucoma surgery may be necessary in more severe cases. Prognosis of a successful PK is diminished significantly with the presence of peripheral anterior synechiae or elevated IOP. This dystrophy may reoccur in grafts.[57]

Congenital Hereditary Endothelial Dystrophy

Congenital hereditary endothelial dystrophy (CHED) is a rare endothelial dystrophy that causes extensive corneal clouding at birth or shortly thereafter. There are no other anterior or posterior segment abnormalities found. Corneal edema is from limbus to limbus, and the entire stromal is involved. The corneal in this disease is markedly thickened. Epithelial edema is also present.

This dystrophy is divided into 2 types based on inheritance patterns. Patients with autosomal recessive inheritance present at birth with severe corneal clouding and develop sensory nystagmus due to severe vision loss. Patients with autosomal dominant disease present with normal corneas at birth. Corneal clouding begins in the first few years of life. Better vision is retained, so no associated nystagmus is experienced.

CHED is a diagnosis of exclusion. Other causes of corneal clouding must be excluded before this diagnosis is made, including congenital glaucoma, congenital infections, forceps injury, CHSD, and metabolic diseases. CHED maps to chromosome 20p along with posterior polymorphous dystrophy.[53,54] Endothelial dysfunction appears to be the primary problem in this disease. Histopathologically, endothelial cells are absent, reduced in number, or show evidence of significant degeneration.[58]

The prognosis and treatment for this dystrophy depends on the type of CHED. Patients with autosomal recessive disease tend to do poorly and require PK early in life. Patients with autosomal dominant disease tend to retain better vision because the corneal edema tends to slowly progress. PK is required later in life, and prognosis for vision is better in this group.

In summary, differentiation between corneal dystrophies is important for proper patient education and management. Anterior segment photography may aid in management to document progression, in addition to evaluation of best corrected vision. Many dystrophies recur in grafts, and newer technologies that avoid PK may be beneficial in these patients.

CORNEAL DEGENERATIONS

Corneal degenerations are age-related changes in the cornea, not related to heredity, that may occur due to aging, mineral deposition, or medications. Degenerations related to the aging process are typically painless, not visually significant, and require no treatment, but it is important to differentiate them from other corneal conditions that may pose a risk for vision loss when untreated.

Corneal Degenerations Related to Aging

Arcus Senilis

Arcus senilis, or corneal arcus, is an asymptomatic bilateral lipid deposition in the peripheral corneal stroma. The white to yellowish colored deposition typically begins inferiorly, increases superiorly, and finally progresses nasally and temporally. There is clear zone between the limbus and the ring of lipid deposition. An hourglass pattern of deposition in the stroma is typical, with denser lipid deposition in the anterior and posterior stroma. The borders are also characteristically sharper peripherally and less distinct centrally (Figure 6-29). If mild to moderate corneal thinning develops in the clear zone, it is called *furrow degeneration* and is not progressive or vision threatening.

Arcus senilis may be found in 60% of men between the ages of 40 and 60 years and nearly 100% of men over age 80.[59] It may occur later in females and earlier

Figure 6-29. Arcus senilis. Published with permission from Rapuano CJ, Luchs JI, Kim T, eds. *Anterior Segment: The Requisites in Ophthalmology.* New York, NY: Mosby Publishing; 2000. (Courtesy of Jodi I. Luchs, MD.)

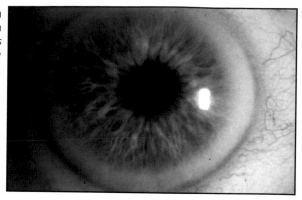

Figure 6-30. Limbal girdle of Vogt. Published with permission from Rapuano CJ, Luchs JI, Kim T, eds. *Anterior Segment: The Requisites in Ophthalmology.* New York, NY: Mosby Publishing; 2000. (Courtesy of Jodi I. Luchs, MD.)

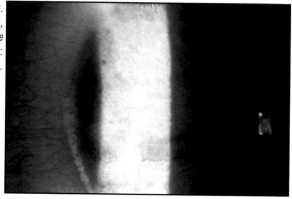

in African Americans. Though generally age-related and not clinically significant, arcus senilis may indicate a lipid abnormality (hyperlipoproteinemia and hypercholesterolemia) when found in patients under age 35 to 40 years.[60] Therefore, when noted in a young patient, a lipid/cholesterol workup is indicated. Unilateral arcus senilis is associated with carotid artery disease that is more severe on the side without the deposition, and carotid studies are indicated in these cases.

Limbal Girdle of Vogt

The limbal girdle of Vogt is a narrow, white opacity adjacent to the limbus nasally and temporally (Figure 6-30). The lack of a clear zone between the limbal girdle and the limbus differentiates this from arcus. At its central edge, it can have tiny irregular linear extensions. It is typically superficial, bilateral, and symmetric. This lesion is composed of elastotic degeneration, similar to that found in pinguecula and pterygia. The finding is not clinically significant.

Hassall-Henle Bodies

Hassall-Henle bodies are small, peripherally located, localized excrescences in Descemet's membrane. These are a normal aging change caused by an overproduction of basement membrane by peripheral endothelial cells and are sometimes referred to as *Descemet's warts.* Rarely noted in people under 25 years old, they increase with age and are common in patients over 65 years. Histopathologically, they are identical to central cornea guttata of endothelial dystrophy but do not cause progressive endothelial damage.[61]

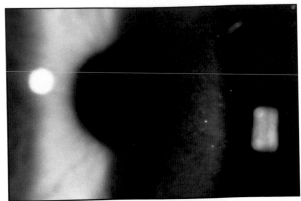

Figure 6-31. Cornea farinata. Thousands of dust-like dots are found in the posterior stroma. Published with permission from Rapuano CJ, Luchs JI, Kim T, eds. *Anterior Segment: The Requisites in Ophthalmology*. New York, NY: Mosby Publishing; 2000. (Courtesy of Jodi I. Luchs, MD.)

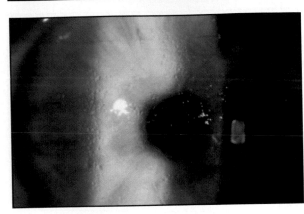

Figure 6-32. Polymorphic amyloid degeneration. Published with permission from Rapuano CJ, Luchs JI, Kim T, eds. *Anterior Segment: The Requisites in Ophthalmology*. New York, NY: Mosby Publishing; 2000. (Courtesy of Jodi I. Luchs, MD.)

Crocodile Shagreen

Crocodile shagreen is characterized by a mosaic pattern of polygonal gray-white opacities, separated by relatively clear spaces. It occurs centrally and incidence increases with age. The anterior form occurs at the level of Bowman's membrane and superficial stroma, whereas the posterior form is found in the deep stroma and Descemet's membrane and may be related to central cloudy dystrophy of Fran François as discussed previously.[62] Histologically, irregularities in the collagen lamellae are noted centrally. Pachymetry is normal. Acuity is not affected and no treatment is necessary.

Cornea Farinata

Cornea farinata is characterized by bilateral, fine, pinpoint opacities in the posterior stroma. The deposits resemble flour in color and size; hence the name *farinata*, which means "flour" in Latin. They are best seen as dust-like dots upon retroillumination (Figure 6-31). Histopathologically, they are composed of a lipofuscin-like substance. Acuity is not affected and no treatment is necessary.

Polymorphic Amyloid Degeneration

Polymorphic amyloid degeneration (PAD) is a primary localized degenerative form of amyloid deposition in the cornea, greater posteriorly and centrally, although they may present throughout the cornea. It is generally seen in patients older than 50 years and is typically bilateral but may be asymmetric.[63] Though the deposits appear gray-white on direct illumination (Figure 6-32), deposits are best

Figure 6-33. Terrien's marginal degeneration. Note the lipid deposition at the central edge of the opacity and the intact epithelium. Published with permission from Rapuano CJ, Luchs JI, Kim T, eds. *Anterior Segment: The Requisites in Ophthalmology.* New York, NY: Mosby Publishing; 2000. (Courtesy of Jodi I. Luchs, MD.)

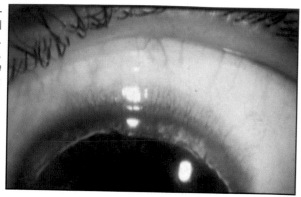

Figure 6-34. Terrien's marginal degeneration. Note the area of thinning. Published with permission from Rapuano CJ, Luchs JI, Kim T, eds. *Anterior Segment: The Requisites in Ophthalmology.* New York, NY: Mosby Publishing; 2000. (Courtesy of Jodi I. Luchs, MD.)

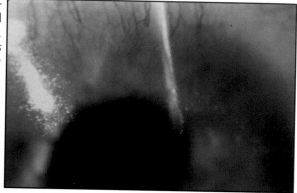

seen with retroillumination, where they appear refractile. Opacities may resemble dots, commas, or singular or branching lines reminiscent of lattice corneal dystrophy. Unlike lattice degeneration, they are not clinically significant, do not cause recurrent erosions or decreased vision, and no treatment is required.

Degenerations Unrelated to Aging

Terrien's Marginal Degeneration

Terrien's marginal degeneration is an inflammatory degenerative disorder that causes peripheral corneal thinning and is occasionally associated with inflammation. It typically presents between the ages of 20 and 40 years, affects more men than women, is bilateral but asymmetric, and is normally slowly progressive.

Early on, white opacities in the periphery can be seen, which coalesce into an arc of corneal thinning (Figures 6-33 and 6-34). The involved cornea is vascularized with radial vessels from the limbus. Epithelium remains intact. At the central extension of the thinning is a line of yellow-white lipid deposition. Corneal involvement progresses circumferentially but may involve the central cornea. In most patients the eyes are white and quiet, with little active inflammation. However, some patients have recurrent episodes of peripheral keratitis, which may be associated with episcleritis.[64] The active inflammatory process tends to respond to topical corticosteroids but these should be used judiciously. The involved area may progress to severe corneal thinning, which may protrude forward but rarely perforates.

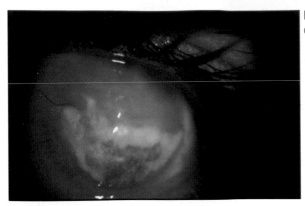

Figure 6-35. Band keratopathy. (Courtesy of Tracy S. Swartz, OD, MS.)

Significant corneal thinning peripherally may create irregular astigmatism. When the thinning is primarily superiorly or inferiorly, against-the-rule astigmatism results and causes blurred vision. When necessary, a gas-permeable or hybrid contact lens significantly improves acuity. In rare cases, the bulging associated with severe corneal thinning may cause foreign-body sensation. Corneal hydrops or perforation can rarely occur with minor trauma or even spontaneously. When surgical treatment is required, an inlay crescentic, lamellar, or full-thickness corneal graft may stabilize the condition.

Calcific Band Keratopathy

Calcific band keratopathy, or simply band keratopathy, involves calcium deposition at the level of Bowman's membrane. It is a slowly progressive condition typically occurring in the interpalpebral zone. It usually begins as a gray-white opacity nasally and temporally, progressing across the central cornea in a band-shaped pattern (Figure 6-35), although rarely it may initially present centrally. It has a distinct peripheral edge, with a clear zone between the deposition and the limbus. Small holes within the deposition occur where corneal nerves penetrate Bowman's membrane. It may appear in a thin, diffuse, relatively uniform strip across the cornea or in thick discrete plaques. If the calcium deposition progresses centrally towards the visual axis, visual acuity may be affected.

Calcific band keratopathy has numerous causes. Disorders with chronic inflammatory processes, such as uveitis, especially juvenile rheumatoid arthritis, interstitial keratitis, and phthisis are the most common etiology. Other causes include hypercalcemia due to renal failure, hyperphosphatemia without hypercalcemia, chronic mercury exposure such as from preservatives in ophthalmic preparations, silicone oil in aphakic patients, and primary hereditary band keratopathy. Patients with gout can develop a similar-looking band of deposition consisting of yellow-pigmented urate deposits in the epithelium.

In patients with poor visual potential, who are fortunate enough not to develop painful symptoms, the cosmetic appearance may be the chief complaint.

The first step in management of calcific band keratopathy is to determine the underlying cause and treat if indicated. Lubricating ointments may significantly improve the ocular discomfort symptoms when visual prognosis is poor. The best treatment for band keratopathy involves calcium chelation or chemical removal of the calcium.[65,66] This procedure can be performed at the slit-lamp in the office or under the operating microscope in the minor procedure room. Using topical

Figure 6-36. Spheroidal degeneration. Elevated yellow-white globular deposits have become confluent to cover the inferocentral cornea. Published with permission from Rapuano CJ, Luchs JI, Kim T, eds. *Anterior Segment: The Requisites in Ophthalmology.* New York, NY: Mosby Publishing; 2000. (Courtesy of Jodi I. Luchs, MD.)

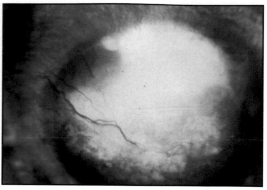

anesthesia, followed by insertion of an eyelid speculum, the epithelium overlying the entire area of calcium deposition is removed with a blunt spatula or sharp blade (such as a #15 Bard-Parker blade).

A cellulose sponge is prepared by soaking it with diluted disodium ethylene diamine tetraacetic acid (EDTA; Endrate 150 mg/mL). The EDTA is diluted 1:4 with normal saline. The cellulose sponge is then rubbed against the calcium deposits until they are completely dissolved. Note that one should not use calcium EDTA. The cellulose sponge is then applied to the cornea until the deposits are completely dissolved. The superficial calcium is readily removed, leaving Bowman's membrane intact. The time required to achieve complete calcium removal varies depending on the severity of the band keratopathy but can range from 5 to 45 minutes. Thick calcium plaques may require scraping prior to EDTA application. Superficial corneal scarring may be present beneath the calcium plaques, and scarring will not respond to chelating. Excimer laser PTK may be used to treat this residual corneal scarring but is less effective for primary treatment of calcium plaques than EDTA.[67]

Postoperatively, the eye is treated in the same manner as a large corneal abrasion. The band keratopathy may recur after treatment and patients should be educated that the procedure may be repeated when necessary.

Spheroidal Degeneration

Spheroidal degeneration refers to a disorder also termed *climatic droplet keratopathy, Labrador keratopathy, hyaline degeneration,* or *chronic actinic keratopathy.*[68-70] Climatic droplet keratopathy and chronic actinic keratopathy accurately describe the relationship of this disorder with sun exposure, but the condition also involves the conjunctiva, so the term *spheroidal degeneration* is preferred.

Clinically this condition presents initially with small, clear droplets grouped together under the epithelium of the cornea and/or conjunctiva. The droplets typically present peripherally and move centrally. As the disorder progresses, the droplets become discolored, becoming gray, white, yellow, and later gold or brown. Smaller droplets may coalesce and enlarge, becoming elevated. It is typically found interpalpebrally within exposed areas of cornea and conjunctiva (Figure 6-36). The droplets are usually smaller and fewer in number in the cornea compared to the conjunctivae. The condition is usually bilateral when the conjunctiva is involved. Unless the lesions are located centrally and dense, the patient is asymptomatic.

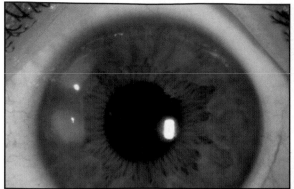

Figure 6-37. Salzmann's nodular degeneration. Published with permission from Rapuano CJ, Luchs JI, Kim T, eds. *Anterior Segment: The Requisites in Ophthalmology.* New York, NY: Mosby Publishing; 2000. (Courtesy of Jodi I. Luchs, MD.)

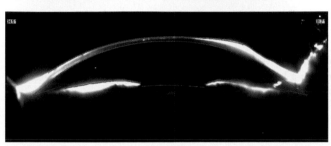

Figure 6-38. Salzmann's nodular degeneration as seen using Scheimpflug imaging. The nodules appear at the upper right of the image. (Courtesy of Tracy S. Swartz, OD, MS.)

It appears to be related to sun or ultraviolet light exposure, ocular dryness, and chronic exposure and may also be related to chronic corneal inflammation. Though usually bilateral, it may appear unilaterally if one eye has less actinic exposure, such as in cases of congenital ptosis. The droplets are composed of hyaline material histologically.

Treatment is considered when the opacities affect the vision. Larger elevated lesions may cause foreign-body sensation or even problems with cosmetic dissatisfaction. Conjunctival lesions can be directly excised. Elevated and anterior corneal lesions are removed via SK with a blade or excimer laser PTK. Deeper lesions may require a lamellar or penetrating keratoplasty.

Salzmann's Nodular Degeneration

Salzmann's nodular degeneration most commonly occurs in eyes with a chronic inflammatory condition, such as interstitial keratitis, vernal keratoconjunctivitis, and keratoconjunctivitis sicca. It may appear in eyes with no known history of keratitis and is typically bilateral but asymmetric. Salzmann's nodules occur more commonly in women and occur more frequently as patients age.

Clinically, white or gray-white elevated lesions are found on the corneal surface (Figures 6-37 and 6-38). The size, location, and elevation of the nodules vary, as does the condition of the underlying cornea, which may be scarred, vascularized, edematous, or normal. Iron pigment deposition surrounding the base of the nodule may be noted if the lesions are long-standing.

Histopathologically, the nodules are the result of hyalinized collagen deposition between the epithelium and stroma. Bowman's membrane may be intact or absent beneath the lesions.[71]

Patients are typically asymptomatic unless the lesions involve the visual axis, decreasing acuity. Elevated lesions may complicate contact lens wear or cause

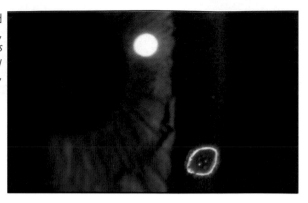

Figure 6-39. Coats' white ring. Published with permission from Rapuano CJ, Luchs JI, Kim T, eds. *Anterior Segment: The Requisites in Ophthalmology.* New York, NY: Mosby Publishing; 2000. (Courtesy of Jodi I. Luchs, MD.)

painful epithelial erosions. Symptomatic patients are treated with superficial keratectomy using a blade. Under topical or local anesthesia, the nodules are generally easily pealed off, leaving Bowman's membrane intact. If a smooth surface between Bowman's membrane and the lesion is lacking, an excimer laser PTK may be beneficial.[72] Rarely is a lamellar or penetrating keratoplasty indicated for deep stromal scarring beneath the nodules.

Coats' White Ring

Coats' white ring is typically an incidental finding in asymptomatic patients. A small, white, partial or complete oval or circle (generally 1 mm or less in diameter) can be seen in Bowman's membrane or the anterior stroma (Figure 6-39). Overlying epithelium is normal. The lesions are caused by previous metallic foreign bodies and are composed of iron deposition.[73]

Lipid Keratopathy

Lipid keratopathy presents in a more common secondary form and, rarely, a primary form. Secondary lipid keratopathy, or lipid degeneration, is related to corneal blood vessels or, less commonly, previous corneal necrosis. It is seen most commonly after corneal trauma or ulceration, or interstitial keratitis, including herpetic (simplex or zoster) keratitis. Severe corneal neovascularization secondary to corneal hypoxia from abusive contact lens wear may also cause lipid keratopathy.

Dense yellow-white lipid deposits appear in the stroma near the vascularization (Figure 6-40). A feathery appearance at the edge away from the blood vessel is typical, but fan-like patterns can develop at the ends of blood vessels. Refractile crystalline deposits in the stroma alone or in addition to the more dense opacities may be noted. Usually slow growing, they may take months to years to develop.

Clinical management requires treating the underlying condition. Addressing the etiology may improve the lipid deposition or control progression. Laser treatment of the corneal neovascularization to permanently occlude neovascularization can be attempted, but usually fails to improve the condition. Topical angiogenesis inhibitors have been attempted with mixed results. Corneal transplantation is discouraged even in severe cases, because vascularized corneas have an increased risk of graft rejection. If the neovascularization remains, the lipid may recur in the graft.

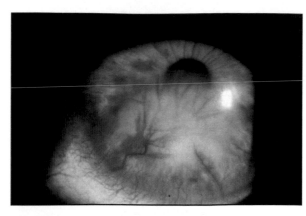

Figure 6-40. Lipid keratopathy. Published with permission from Rapuano CJ, Luchs JI, Kim T, eds. *Anterior Segment: The Requisites in Ophthalmology.* New York, NY: Mosby Publishing; 2000. (Courtesy of Jodi I. Luchs, MD.)

Iridocorneal Endothelial Syndrome

The term *iridocorneal endothelial* (ICE) syndrome comprises 3 related entities: (1) Chandler's syndrome, (2) essential iris atrophy, and (3) the iris nevus syndrome, all of which may present with degeneration of the cornea at various levels. The primary abnormality in these syndromes involves the endothelium, which may resemble posterior polymorphous dystrophy (PPMD) in appearance. However, whereas PPMD is hereditary, bilateral, and slowly progressive, ICE syndrome is sporadic, usually unilateral, and more rapidly progressive. Additionally, in the ICE syndrome, glaucoma and iris abnormalities, including peripheral anterior synechiae, iris atrophy, iris holes, and iris nodules, may be present. Histopathologic evaluation of ICE syndrome has found endothelial overgrowth in the anterior chamber.[74] The abnormal endothelial cells often have characteristics of epithelial cells, such as surface microvilli. These epithelial characteristics include loss of contact inhibition, allowing the endothelialization of the anterior segment to occur.[74] The 3 components of the ICE syndrome vary in their degree of corneal and iris pathology.

In Chandler's syndrome, corneal endothelial abnormalities are the most prominent. The posterior corneal surface has a hammered silver appearance, with a variable degree of corneal edema, from none to bullous keratopathy. Specular microscopic evaluation demonstrates patches of normal endothelial cells adjacent to patches of abnormal cells. Abnormal cells are larger than healthy cells, with dark bodies, white peripheries, and often a white central dot.[75]

The iris abnormalities are most notable in essential (or progressive) iris atrophy and iris nevus syndrome. In essential iris atrophy, broad-based peripheral anterior synechiae are present. The central iris is pulled toward the synechiae, leading to ectropion uveae, corectopia, iris atrophy and, eventually, hole formation on the opposite side. Gonioscopy reveals endothelialization of the anterior chamber angle, occasionally leading to angle closure glaucoma. The corneal endothelial cells migrate over the angle, cover the trabecular meshwork, and pull the iris, causing the peripheral anterior synechiae and iris holes in essential iris atrophy, leading to restriction of outflow and causing glaucoma.

Iris nevus syndrome, also called Cogan-Reese syndrome, is actually a misnomer. Endothelialization of the iris causes flattening of the normal iris crypt architecture and small knuckles of iris stroma protruding anteriorly through holes in the membrane, which appear to be nevi. It can also present as a diffusely flat pigmented area of heterochromia, resembling a large iris nevus.

Figure 6-41. An epithelial iron line in a post RK patient. Published with permission from Rapuano CJ, Luchs JI, Kim T, eds. *Anterior Segment: The Requisites in Ophthalmology.* New York, NY: Mosby Publishing; 2000. (Courtesy of Jodi I. Luchs, MD.)

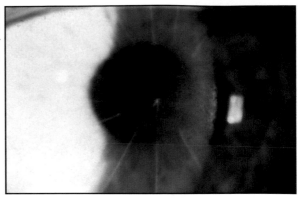

The clinical presentation of ICE syndrome varies. Chandler's syndrome typically presents with decreased vision and occasionally pain due to bullous keratopathy. Essential iris atrophy and iris nevus patients generally have good vision unless glaucoma develops. Initial diagnosis may occur on routine evaluation or when the patient reports an iris irregularity.

The management of ICE syndrome depends on the symptoms and clinical presentation. In Chandler's syndrome, corneal edema predominates. Topical hyperosmotics and intraocular pressure-lowering medications are used to control the edema. Severe corneal edema, reduced vision, or pain may require PK. In all 3 variants, glaucoma is a common problem that is difficult to treat and surgical treatment is often required. Trabeculectomies are frequently successful initially but blebs are subject to failure due to endothelialization. The control of the glaucoma in ICE syndrome is extremely important in maintaining a clear graft.

CORNEAL PIGMENTATIONS

Iron

Iron deposition in the cornea is a common finding. Most iron deposition occurs in the epithelial cells due to the accumulation of iron from the tear film. Numerous iron lines have been identified (Figure 6-41). A Hudson-Stahli line is a wavy horizontal line of iron deposition typically located where the lower eyelid meets the cornea and is associated with aging. Iron lines often occur at the base of corneal topographic abnormalities, such as Salzmann's nodules. A ring of iron deposition at the base of the cone in keratoconus is known as a *Fleischer ring.* The appearance of the ring varies with the severity of the keratoconus and may be small, large, complete, or incomplete. A Ferry line is an iron line at the anterior edge of a filtering bleb.[76] A Stocker line can be found at the head of a pterygium. Stellate iron patterns are also found after keratorefractive surgery, including radial keratotomy, PRK, and LASIK.

Siderosis is iron deposition within the eye, typically from an intraocular foreign body, but may also occur with systemic iron overload, such as in hemochromatosis. The iron can also deposit in the iris, causing heterochromia and mydriasis, and in the lens, causing a cataract. Metallic foreign bodies in the anterior chamber may cause yellow-brown iron pigment in the posterior stroma. Irreversible retinal degeneration can also occur with intraocular foreign bodies.

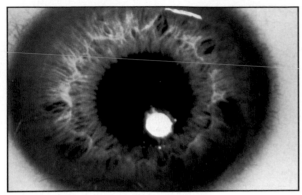

Figure 6-42. Kayser-Fleischer ring. Published with permission from Rapuano CJ, Luchs JI, Kim T, eds. *Anterior Segment: The Requisites in Ophthalmology.* New York, NY: Mosby Publishing; 2000. (Courtesy of Jodi I. Luchs, MD.)

Melanin

Epithelial pigment lines that run from the limbus centrally are termed *striate melanokeratosis.* It occurs most commonly in patients with dark skin or following ocular trauma or inflammation. Rarely, corneal melanin results from a conjunctival melanoma.

Copper

Copper deposition in the eye presents as a gray-green discoloration of Descemet's membrane and is also called *ocular chalcosis.* It is usually related to an intraocular copper foreign body. If the copper content of the foreign body is greater than 85%, a severe suppurative endophthalmitism may result.

A Kayser-Fleischer ring is a yellow-brown or gray-green discoloration at the level of Descemet's membrane, is found in the corneal periphery (Figure 6-42), and may be identified in angle structures in early stages using gonioscopy in the inferior cornea. It is found in Wilson's disease, an autosomal recessive disorder resulting in systemic copper accumulation. It can also be associated with chronic active hepatitis, progressive intrahepatic cholestasis, primary biliary cirrhosis, and multiple myeloma.[77] Systemic treatment with chelating agents such as d-penicillamine can be monitored by observing the disappearance of the Kayser-Fleischer ring.

Gold

Gold deposition in the cornea, termed *corneal chrysiasis,* has been associated with systemic gold treatment for rheumatoid arthritis. The deposits are yellow-brown, generally at the level of deep stroma and Descemet's membrane. Patients are asymptomatic and no treatment is required. The deposits may be reversible with discontinuation of treatment.

Silver

Silver deposition in the eye is called *argyrosis* and may be noted in asymptomatic patients. Silver-containing topical medications such as Argyrol are rarely used today. A diffuse gray discoloration of the conjunctiva and eyelid skin is characteristic. Descemet's membrane develops a gold-gray appearance in the periphery.

REFERENCES

1. Meesman A, Wilke F. Klinische und anatomische untersuchungen uber eine bisher unbekannte, dominant verebte epitheldystrophie der hornhaut. *Klin Monatsbl Augenheilkd.* 1939;103:361-369.

2. Kuwabara T, Cicarelli EC. Meesman's corneal dystrophy. A pathological study. *Arch Ophthalmol.* 1964;71:676-682.

3. Coleman CM, Hannush S, Covello SO, et al. A novel mutation in the helix termination motif of keratin K12 in a US family with Meesman corneal dystrophy. *Am J Ophthalmol.* 1999;128:687-691.

4. Bourne W. Soft contact lens wear decreases epithelial microcysts in Meesman's corneal dystrophy. *Trans Am Ophthalmol Soc.* 1986;84:170-181.

5. Trobe JD, Laibson PR. Dystrophic changes in the anterior cornea. *Arch Ophthalmol.* 1972; 87:378-382.

6. Cogan DG, Donaldson DD, Kuwabara T, Marshall D. Microcystic dystrophy of the corneal epithelium. *Trans Am Ophthalmol Soc.* 1964;63:213.

7. Laibson PR, Krachmer JH. Familial occurrence of dot (micro-cystic) map fingerprint dystrophy of the cornea. *Invest Ophthalmol.* 1975;14:397-400.

8. Rodrigues MM, Fine B, Laibson PR, Zimmerman L. Disorders of the corneal epithelium: a clinical pathological study of dot, geographic and fingerprint patterns. *Arch Ophthalmol.* 1974;92:475-482.

9. Cogan DG, Kuwabara T, Donaldson DD, Collins E. Microscopic dystrophy of the cornea. A partial explanation for its pathogenesis. *Arch Ophthalmol.* 1974;92:470-474.

10. Hykin PG, Foss AE, Pavesio C, Dart JKG. The natural history and management of recurrent corneal erosion; a prospective randomized trial. *Eye.* 1994;8:35-40.

11. Williams R, Buckley RJ. Pathogenesis and treatment of recurrent erosion. *Br J Ophthalmol.* 1985;69:435-437.

12. Wood TO, Griffith ME. Surgery for corneal epithelial basement membrane dystrophy. *Ophthalmic Surg.* 1988;19:20-24.

13. Mclean EN, MacRae SM, Rich LF. Recurrent erosion: treatment by anterior stromal puncture. *Ophthalmology.* 1986;93:784-788.

14. Küchle M, Green WR, Volcker HE, Barraquer J. Reevaluation of corneal dystrophies of Bowman's layer and the anterior stroma (Reis-Bücklers' and Thiel-Behnke types): a light and electron microscopic study of eight corneas and a review of the literature. *Cornea.* 1995; 14:333-354.

15. Munier FL, Korvatska, Djemai A, et al. Kerato-epithelin mutations in four 5q31-linked corneal dystrophies. *Nat Genet.* 1998;62:320-324.

16. Mashima Y, Nakamura Y, Noda K, et al. A novel mutation at codon 124 (R124L) in the *BIGH3* gene is associated with a superficial variant of granular dystrophy. *Arch Ophthalmol.* 1999;117:90-93.

17. Dighiero P, Drunat S, D'Hermies F, et al. A novel variant of granular corneal dystrophy caused by association of 2 mutations in the TGFBI gene-R124L and DeltaT125-DeltaE126. *Arch Ophthalmol.* 2000;118:814-818.

18. Rapuano CJ, Laibson PR. Excimer laser phototherapeutic keratectomy. *CLAO J.* 1993;19:235-240.

19. Dinh R, Rapuano CJ, Cohen EJ, Laibson PR. Recurrence of corneal dystrophy after excimer phototherapeutic keratectomy. *Ophthalmology.* 1999;106:1490-1497.

20. Jones ST, Zimmerman LE. Histopathologic differentiation of granular, macular, and lattice dystrophies of the cornea. *Am J Ophthalmol.* 1961;51:394.

21. Sommer JR, Wong F, Klintworth GK. Phenotypic variations of corneal dystrophies caused by different mutations in the BIGH3 gene (ARVO abstract 2347). *Invest Ophthalmol Vis Sci.* 1998;39(suppl):513.

22. Weidel EG. Granular corneal dystrophy: two variants. In: Ferraz de Oliveira FN, ed. *Ophthalmology Today. Proceedings of the Eight Congress of the European Society of Ophthalmology.* Amsterdam: Excepta Medica; 1989:617-619. International Congress Series; No.803.

23. Hahn TW, Sah WJ, Kim JH. Phototherapeutic keratectomy in nine eyes with superficial corneal diseases. *Refract Corneal Surg.* 1993;9:115.

24. Lyons CJ, McCartney AC, Kirkness CM, Ficker LA, Steele AD, Rice NS. Granular corneal dystrophy. Visual results and pattern of recurrence after lamellar or penetrating keratoplasty. *Ophthalmology.* 1994;101:1812-1817.

25. Durand L, Resal R, Burillion C. Focus on an anatomoclinical entity: Biber-Haab-Dimmer lattice dystrophy. *J Fr Ophthalmol.* 1985;8:729.

26. Donders PC, Blanksma LJ. Meretoja syndrome. Lattice dystrophy of the cornea with hereditary generalized amyloidosis. *Ophthalmologica.* 1979;178:173.

27. Hida T, Tsubota K, Kigasawa K, Murata H, Ogata T, Akiya S. Clinical features of a newly recognized type of lattice corneal dystrophy. *Am J Ophthalmol.* 1987;104:241-248.

28. de la Chapelle A, Kere J, Sack GH Jr, et al. Familial amyloidosis caused by asparagine or tyrosine substitution for aspartic acid at residue 187. *Nat Genet.* 1992;2:157-160.

29. de la Chapelle A, Kere J, Sack GH Jr, Tolvanen R, Maury CP. Familial amyloidosis, Finnish type:G654—a mutation of the gelsolin gene in Finnish families and an unrelated American family. *Genomics.* 1992;13:898-901.

30. Stein HA, Cheskes A, Stein RM, eds. Phototherapeutic keratectomy. In: *The Excimer: Fundamentals and Clinical Use.* Thorofare, NJ: SLACK Incorporated; 1994.

31. Meisler DM, Fine M. Recurrence of clinical signs of lattice corneal dystrophy (type 1) in corneal transplants. *Am J Ophthalmol.* 1984;97:210.

32. Pouliquen Y, Dhermy P, Renard G, Giraud JP, Savoldelli M. Combined macular dystrophy and cornea guttata: an electron microscopic study. *Graefe's Arch Clin Exp Ophthalmol.* 1980;212:149-158.

33. Jones ST, Zimmerman LE. Histopathologic differentiation of granular, macular, and lattice dystrophies of the cornea. *Am J Ophthalmol.* 1961;51:394.

34. Yang CJ, SundarRaj N, Thonar EJ, Klintworth GK. Immunohistochemical evidence of heterogeneity in macular corneal dystrophy. *Am J Ophthalmol.* 1988;106:65-71.

35. Vance JM, Jonasson F, Lennon F, et al. Linkage of a gene for macular corneal dystrophy to chromosome 16. *Am J Hum Genet.* 1996;58:757-762.

36. Akama TO, Nishida K, Nakayama J, et al. Macular corneal dystrophy type I and type II are caused by distinct mutations in a new sulfotransferase gene. *Nat Genet.* 2000;26:237-241.

37. Burns RP, Connor W, Gipson I. Cholesterol turnover in hereditary crystalline corneal dystrophy of Schnyder. *Tran Am Ophthalmol Soc.* 1978;76:184-196.

38. Rodrigues MM, Kruth HS, Krachmer JH, Willis R. Unesterified cholesterol in Schnyder's crystalline dystrophy of the cornea. *Am J Ophthalmol.* 1987;104:157-163.

39. Lisch W, Weidle EG, Lisch C, Rice T, Beck E, Utermann G. Schnyder's dystrophy. Progression and metabolism. *Ophthalmic Paediatr Genet.* 1986;7:45-56.

40. Tsujikawa M, Kurahashi H, Tanaka T, et al. Identification of the gene responsible for gelatinous drop-like corneal dystrophy. *Nat Genet.* 1999;21:420-423.

41. Purcell JJ Jr, Krachmer JH, Weingeist TA. Fleck corneal dystrophy. *Arch Ophthalmol.* 1977;95:440-444.

42. Nicholson DH, Green WR, Cross HE. A clinical and histopathological study of Francois-Neetans speckled corneal dystrophy. *Am J Ophthalmol.* 1977;83:554-560.

43. Goodside V. Posterior crocodile shagreen. *Am J Ophthalmol.* 1958;46:748-750.

44. Krachmer JH, Dubord PJ, Rodrigues MM, Mannis MJ. Corneal posterior crocodile shagreen and polymorphic amyloid degeneration. *Arch Ophthalmol.* 1983;101:54-59.

45. Witschel H, Fine BS, Grutzner P, McTigue JW. Congenital hereditary stromal dystrophy of the cornea. *Arch Ophthalmol.* 1978;96:1043-1051.

46. Curran RE, Kenyon KR, Green WR. Pre-Descemet's membrane corneal dystrophy. *Am J Ophthalmol.* 1974;77:711-716.

47. Johnson AT, Folberg R, Vrabec MP, Florakis GJ, Stone EM, Krachmer JH. The pathology of posterior amorphous corneal dystrophy. *Ophthalmology.* 1990;97:104-109.

48. Krachmer JH, Purcell JJ Jr, Young CW, Bucher KD. Corneal endothelial dystrophy. A study of 64 families. *Arch Ophthalmol.* 1978;96:2036-2039.

49. Biswas S, Munier FL, Yardley J, et al. Missense mutations in COL8A2, the gene encoding the alpha 2 chain of type VIII collagen, cause two forms of corneal endothelial dystrophy. *Hum Mol Genet.* 2001;10:2415-2423.

50. Sundin OH, Jun AS, Broman KW, et al. Linkage of late-onset Fuchs corneal dystrophy to a novel locus at 13pTel-13q12.13. *Invest Ophthalmol Vis Sci.* 2006;47:140-145.

51. Hogan MJ, Wood I, Fine M. Fuchs' endothelial dystrophy of the cornea. *Am J Ophthalmol.* 1974;78:363-383.

52. Cibis GW, Krachmer JA, Phelps CD, Weingeist TA. The clinical spectrum of posterior polymorphous dystrophy. *Arch Ophthalmol.* 1977;95:1529-1537.

53. Héon E, Mathers WD, Alward WL, et al. Linkage of posterior polymorphous dystrophy to 20q11. *Hum Mol Genet.* 1995;4:485-488.

54. Toma NM, Ebenezer ND, Inglehearn CF, Plant C, Ficker LA, Bhattacharya SS. Linkage of congenital hereditary endothelial dystrophy to chromosome 20. *Hum Mol Genet.* 1995;4:2395-2398.

55. Moroi S, Gokhale P, Schteingart M, et al. Clincopathologic correlation and genetic analysis in a case of posterior polymorphous corneal dystrophy. *Am J Ophthalmol.* 2003;135;461-470.

56. Harissi-Dagher M, Dana MR, Jurkunas UV. Keratoglobus in association with posterior polymorphous dystrophy. *Cornea.* 2007;26:1288-1291.

57. Boruchoff SA, Weiner MJ, Albert DM. Recurrence of posterior polymorphous dystrophy after penetrating keratoplasty. *Am J Ophthalmol.* 1990;109:323-328.

58. Pearse WG, Tripathi RC, Morgan G. Congenital endothelial corneal dystrophy: clinical, pathological, and genetic study. *Br J Ophthalmol.* 1969;53:577-591.

59. Cooke NT. Significance of arcus senilis in Caucasians. *J R Soc Med.* 1981;74:201-204.

60. Crispin S. Ocular lipid deposition and hyperlipoproteinaemia. *Prog Retin Eye Res.* 2002; 21:169-224.

61. Yanoff M, Fine BS. *Ocular Pathology: A Text and Atlas.* Philadelphia, PA: JB Lippincott; 1989.

62. Meyer JC, Quantock AJ, Kincaid MC, et al. Characterization of a central cloudiness sharing features of posterior crocodile shagreen and central cloudy dystrophy of François. *Cornea.* 1996;15:347-354.

63. Mannis MJ, Krachmer JH, Rodrigues MM, Pardos GJ. Polymorphic amyloid degeneration of the cornea: a histopathologic study. *Arch Ophthalmol.* 1981;99:1217-1223.

64. Austin P, Brown SI. Inflammatory Terrien's marginal corneal disease. *Am J Ophthalmol.* 1981;92:189-192.

65. Bokosky JE, Meyer RF, Sugar A. Surgical treatment of calcified band keratopathy. *Ophthalmic Res.* 1985;16:645-647.

66. Wood TO, Walker GG. Treatment of band keratopathy. *Am J Ophthalmol.* 1975;80:553.

67. O'Brart DP, Gartry DS, Lohmann CP, Patmore AL, Kerr Muir MG, Marshall J. Treatment of band keratopathy by excimer laser phototherapeutic keratectomy: surgical techniques and long term follow up. *Br J Ophthalmol.* 1993;77:702-708.

68. Rodgers FC. Clinical findings, course and progress of Bietti's corneal degeneration in the Dahlak islands. *Br J Ophthalmol.* 1973;57:657-664.

69. Young JD, Finlay RD. Primary spheroidal degeneration of the cornea in Labrador and northern Newfoundland. *Am J Ophthalmol.* 1975;79:129-134.

70. Dahan E, Judellson J, Welsh NH. Regression of Labrador keratopathy following cataract extraction. *Br J Ophthalmol.* 1986;70:737-741.

71. Wood TO. Salzmann's nodular degeneration. *Cornea.* 1990;9:17-22.

72. Kremer F, Aronsky M, Bowyer BL, et al. Treatment of corneal surface irregularities using biomask as an adjunct to excimer laser phototherapeutic keratectomy. *Cornea.* 2002;21:28-32.

73. Miller EM. Genesis of white rings in the cornea. *Am J Ophthalmol.* 1966;61:904-907.

74. Levy SG, et al. The histopathology of the iridocorneal-endothelial syndrome. *Cornea.* 1996;15:46-54.

75. Neubauer L, Lund O, Leibowitz HM. Specular microscopic appearance of the corneal endothelium in iridocorneal endothelial syndrome. *Arch Ophthalmol.* 1983;101:916-918.

76. Ferry AP. A "new" iron line of the superficial cornea. *Arch Ophthalmol.* 1968;79:142-145.

77. Frommer D, Morris J, Sherlock S, et al. Kayser-Fleisher rings in patients without Wilson's disease. *Gastroenterology.* 1977;72:1331-1335.

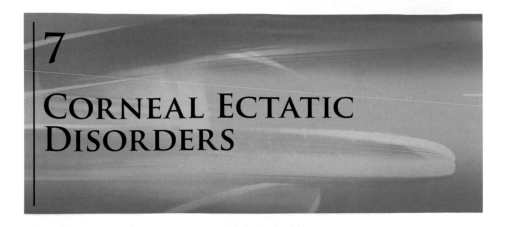

7

CORNEAL ECTATIC DISORDERS

J. Bradley Randleman, MD and Michelle B. Crosby, MD, PhD

There are a variety of clinical entities that present with progressive, noninflammatory corneal thinning. Of these, keratoconus and pellucid marginal corneal degeneration are by far the most frequently naturally occurring phenotypes. Keratoconus is a relatively common progressive noninflammatory corneal thinning disorder with a multifactorial etiology.[1] It has a variable presentation ranging from myopic astigmatism requiring spectacle correction only, to significant stromal thinning, corneal protrusion, and corneal scarring requiring corneal transplantation for visual rehabilitation. Pellucid marginal corneal degeneration (PCMD) is a less common but related ectatic corneal disease with similarities in clinical presentation and management strategies.[2] Progressive corneal thinning that occurs after keratorefractive surgery, commonly termed *postoperative corneal ectasia* or *keratoectasia*, shares similar physical and topographic features with naturally occurring ectatic disorders.[3]

In the past, the only effective methods for visual rehabilitation included rigid gas-permeable (RGP) contact lens wear or PK; however, recent insights into the mechanisms of ectatic corneal diseases and new less invasive treatment modalities have greatly expanded the available therapeutic alternatives.

INCIDENCE AND ETIOLOGY

The progression of keratoconus is based on the loss of the structural integrity and thinning of the corneal stroma, which can be genetic, biochemical, mechanical, or most likely multifactorial in origin. Keratoconus usually begins in puberty and progresses through adolescence, although there are reports of patients first presenting in their third through fifth decade of life.[1] The reported prevalence is 54.5 per 100000, with an incidence of 1 in 2000 in the general population. It can, however, be as high as 1 in 20 seeking refractive surgery, making accurate identification of this disease process vital to refractive surgeons and other physicians involved in the preoperative screening process.[4] There has been some research into keratoconus associated with connective tissue diseases, but the majority of patients, up to 96%, have isolated bilateral keratoconus.[1]

Trattler WB, Majmudar PA, Luchs JI, Swartz TS, eds.
Cornea Handbook (pp. 109-122)
© 2010 SLACK Incorporated

GENETIC FACTORS

A genetic component for keratoconus has been proposed but thus far has only been validated in rare cases, and no single "keratoconus gene" has been found. Therefore, isolated keratoconus without genetic association is by far the most prevalent clinical keratoconus manifestation.[5]

Previous studies have demonstrated rare dominantly inherited cases of keratoconus[6] and a higher incidence among monozygotic twins.[7] With the mapping of the human genome there has been slightly more progress into uncovering potential genetic targets[8-11]; however, many of the identified genes remain to be characterized for location, function, and clinical significance. Nielson and colleagues[9] found an upregulation of desmoglein 3 (DSG3) secretory leukocyte proteinase inhibitor (SLPI). Rabinowitz and colleagues[10] isolated a unique gene, designated KC6, and found an absence of aquaporin 5 (AQP5), which is normally expressed in human cornea; however, the significance of these remains undetermined.

BIOCHEMICAL FACTORS

The loss of collagen layers in keratoconus is thought to be due in part to a higher concentration of proteases that have migrated down from the subepithelial Bowman's layer.[12] This may lead to a signal transduction cascade involving interleukin-1 (IL-1), which induces keratocyte apoptosis in vitro and mediates upregulation of various matrix metalloproteinases (MMPs).[12,13] Mackiewicz and colleagues[13] found an upregulation in human trypsin-2 (TRY-2), which is responsible for cleaving type I collagen, and decreased expression of MMP-8, which has anti-inflammatory properties. Though intriguing, the ultimate significance of these findings is still unknown.

Another mechanism for the development of keratoconus involves repeated eye trauma such as chronic eye rubbing.[14-16] Keratoconus has been associated with atopy and may be secondary to eye rubbing related to keratoconjunctivitis sicca.[14-16] Certain patients may be self-causing repeated mild epithelial injury, allowing downward migration of subepithelial proteases, which contribute to stromal thinning. Jafri et al reported a series of cases with unilateral keratoconus secondary to unilateral eye rubbing or repeated minor trauma.[14] An increased incidence of keratoconus has also been seen in patients with Down syndrome and Leber's congenital amaurosis secondary to chronic eye rubbing.[14]

CLINICAL FINDINGS AND DIAGNOSIS

Early keratoconus may only be identifiable through topographic analysis or abnormal retinoscopy reflexes, whereas moderate to advanced keratoconus has several readily visible signs (Figure 7-1). Mild corneal warping induces a scissoring reflex and oil droplet sign on retinoscopy. As the corneal stroma thins, it takes on a conical shape and both the thinned stroma and "cone" may be apparent on slit-lamp biomicroscopy. Further signs include Vogt's striae, which are fine lines in the deep stroma caused by the stress on the cone that disappear with digital pressure. A Fleischer ring is representative of iron deposits in the epithelium at the base of the cone. Rizutti's sign is a conical reflection of light seen nasally when a light is directed across the cornea from the temporal side. Munson's sign, where

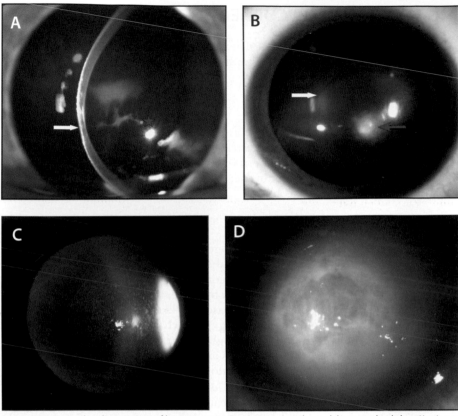

Figure 7-1. Various clinical presentations of keratoconus. (A) Demonstrates central corneal thinning and underlying Vogt's striae (white arrow), as well as deep scarring from previous Descemet's rupture (red star). (B) Demonstrates a prominent Fleischer ring (white arrow) and a paracentral subepithelial nodule from extended rigid gas permeable contact lens wear (red arrow). (C) Exhibits the shape and location of the cone with associated epithelial irregularities in retroillumination. (D) Demonstrates corneal hydrops.

the lower lid bulges on downgaze, is present in more advanced disease. Advanced disease can lead to scarring or corneal hydrops, which occurs due to sudden breaks in Descemet's membrane allowing an influx of aqueous humor into the thinned corneal stroma.

Pellucid marginal corneal degeneration is typically characterized by bilateral inferior thinning and against-the-rule corneal astigmatism, typically with the maximal area of corneal protrusion presenting superior to the area of maximal thinning.[2,17] The vast majority of patients with pellucid marginal corneal degeneration are myopic and have more than 5 diopters of astigmatism.[17,18]

Other less common ectatic phenotypes include keratoglobus and posterior keratoconus. Keratoglobus shares many features with keratoconus and pellucid marginal corneal degeneration, including bilateral manifestation; however, the classical appearance of keratoglobus is a more generalized "global" thinning and protrusion.[19] Further, keratoglobus typically presents at an earlier age. Posterior keratoconus is an extremely rare focal ectatic disorder localized to the posterior surface of the cornea. Posterior keratoconus represents a developmental abnormality and is almost always unilateral in occurrence and nonprogressive in nature.[20,21]

SCREENING FOR CORNEAL ECTATIC DISORDERS

Prior to clinical manifestations of disease, other diagnostic modalities, including confocal microscopy and topography, can facilitate identification of early keratoconus.

Confocal Microscopy

In vivo confocal microscopy of the cornea can potentially identify early keratoconic changes. Ucakhan et al[22] demonstrated enlarged subbasal nerves, increased reflectivity and irregular arrangement of stromal keratocytes, folds throughout the stroma and Descemet's membrane, and pleomorphic endothelial cells in patients with advanced keratoconus.

Topographic Features

Topographic patterns in keratoconus range from subtle to pronounced, depending on disease severity[23] (Figure 7-2), and subtle topographic abnormalities in early or subclinical (forme fruste) keratoconus can precede clinical findings or visual complaints by years. Though usually bilateral, topographic patterns can be highly asymmetric (Figure 7-3). In many cases it is likely that these patients, especially older patients with only subtle topographic changes, will never advance to clinically significant disease; thus, thorough topographic screening is especially important in refractive surgery practices to exclude patients with abnormal topographies from undergoing laser in situ keratomileusis (LASIK).

Initially described screening criteria to identify features of forme fruste keratoconus included an I-S value of 1.2 or greater, which is measured by comparing inferior K values at 5 points at 30 degree intervals 3 mm inferiorly to 5 corresponding points at 30 degree intervals 3 mm superiorly,[24] and a skewed radial axis.[25] There are now a variety of computer-generated screening criteria, including the KISA% index[26] and the Maeda/Klyce (KCI% and KPI) indices.[27] Other subtle changes, such as inferior steepening or asymmetric bowtie patterns that do meet the aforementioned criteria for forme fruste keratoconus, or significant between-eye asymmetry, may also be indicators in keratoconus suspects, and LASIK should also be avoided in these patients.[28,29]

Classic topographic features of pellucid marginal corneal degeneration include superior flattening with rapid increase in corneal power inferiorly, with the greatest steepening in the far periphery between 4 and 8 o'clock and a "crab-claw" appearance of central steepening that extends to the periphery[30] (Figure 7-4). However, atypical presentations with steepening in other corneal meridians have also been reported.[31]

Newer topographic systems utilize other corneal imaging techniques that may prove useful for patient evaluation. These include the Orbscan II (Bausch & Lomb, Rochester, NY), which utilizes slit-beam-based images, and the Pentacam (Oculus, Inc, Lynnwood, Wash), which utilizes Scheimpflug photography-generated images. A number of indices to identify keratoconus have been proposed for these instruments, including a "vertical D pattern" found in the keratometric map,[32] corneal thickness special profile and volume distribution,[33] posterior best-fit sphere radius and elevation,[34] absolute posterior float values,[35] and a combination of Orbscan II factors in a specific screening strategy.[36] Though promising,

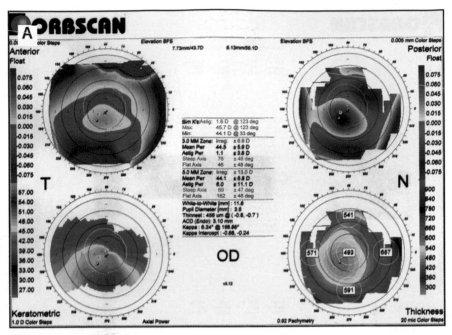

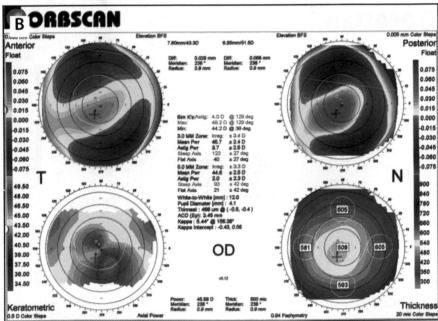

Figure 7-2. Topographic features in keratoconus. (A) Exhibits inferior steepening, an increased posterior float, and a thin central cornea consistent with early keratoconus. (B) Exhibits more advanced inferior steepening with a significantly skewed radial axis, thin central pachymetry, and elevation in the anterior and posterior float values.

these methods have yet to be validated on a large scale and, more importantly, have yet to prove more useful than placido-based imaging in identifying the earliest corneal abnormalities that are paramount for effective refractive surgical screening.

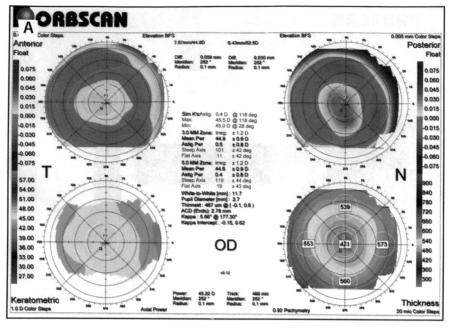

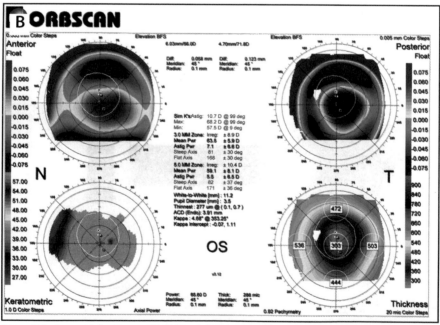

Figure 7-3. Asymmetric keratoconus. (A) (Right eye) displays a relatively normal keratometric pattern with only a thin central cornea and mild posterior float elevation. (B) (Left eye of same patient) demonstrates a grossly abnormally steep keratometric pattern, significant anterior and posterior float elevations, and a very thin central corneal thickness.

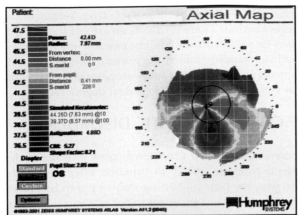

Figure 7-4. Topographic features of pellucid marginal corneal degeneration. The classical features demonstrated here include relative superior flattening, inferior steepening in the far periphery, and a "crab-claw" appearance of central steepening that extends to the periphery.

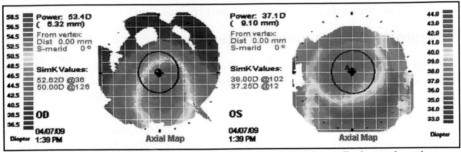

Figure 7-5. Ectasia following myopic laser-assisted in situ keratomileusis (LASIK). The right eye suffers from significant inferior steepening, and the left eye shows the typical central depression secondary to excimer ablation. (Courtesy of Tracy S. Swartz, OD, MS.)

POSTOPERATIVE CORNEAL ECTASIA

Corneal ectasia after LASIK is a progressive corneal steepening, usually inferiorly, with an increase in myopia and astigmatism, loss of uncorrected visual acuity, and often loss of best-corrected visual acuity that can present days to years after LASIK or PRK[37] (Figure 7-5). Ectasia has been reported in cases with preoperative forme fruste keratoconus[38,39] and pellucid marginal corneal degeneration.[40,41] Postoperative ectasia occurs most frequently in susceptible eyes with preoperative topographic abnormalities[29,38] but can rarely occur in patients without clear preoperative risk factors.[42,43]

Though there is great variability in the preoperative presentation of patients who develop ectasia, these patients tend to be younger, more myopic, have thinner corneas preoperatively, lower postoperative residual stromal bed thickness, and more frequently have abnormal preoperative topographies compared to the vast majority of patients who do not develop ectasia after keratorefractive surgery.

The earliest clinical manifestations of postoperative corneal ectasia can be subtle and require a high index of suspicion for diagnosis. Most patients experience increasing myopia and astigmatism that can be misinterpreted as simple regression. In these stages, topographic changes may also be quite subtle. It is imperative to avoid re-treatment in these individuals to prevent further corneal weakening.

Advanced postoperative ectasia is clinically indistinguishable from keratoconus or pellucid marginal corneal degeneration. There is usually an area of significant thinning and protrusion that can be seen with slit-lamp biomicroscopy with corresponding topographic alterations, including increasing corneal steepening and irregular astigmatism. Current management options for postoperative ectasia are similar to those for keratoconus and pellucid marginal corneal degeneration.

MANAGEMENT OF CORNEAL ECTATIC DISORDERS

Management of early keratoconus and PCMD generally begins with spectacle correction; however, most patients lose the ability to function effectively with spectacle correction only. In the past, the only remaining viable options included RGP contact lens fitting or PK; however, recent advances in contact lens materials and styles and other minimally invasive treatment modalities, such as intracorneal ring segments and collagen cross-linking, have proven effective for many patients in delaying or obviating the need for corneal transplantation.

Nonsurgical Management Strategies

Patients with early keratoconus or PCMD often present with increasing myopia and astigmatism. Keratoconus typically presents earlier in life, with a peak incidence in the early 20s,[44] whereas PCMD often presents later in life.[17]

Some patients with keratoconus are initially successfully fitted with spectacle correction, especially in their youth. However, once keratoconus manifests, it usually progresses past the point where spectacles will provide adequate visual acuity due to advanced corneal warpage with resultant irregular astigmatism and image distortion. Patients with PCMD are often spectacle intolerant early due to high astigmatism.

Soft contact lenses, especially toric lenses, may also temporarily provide functional visual acuity for patients with very mild keratoconus or PCMD; however, with more advanced irregular astigmatism and corneal warping these lenses fail to correct vision, and RGP contact lenses, either alone or in combination with other lenses, become necessary. They must be expertly fit to sit on the flatter superior portion of the cornea, clearing the apex of the cone, while maintaining good contact horizontally.[45] It is important not to fit the inferior steeper portion too tightly to prevent further warping.[45-48] In more advanced keratoconus, an aspheric lens-fitting approach may be necessary. In this case an RGP lens usually contains 3 or more spherical peripheral curves that allow for flattening as the periphery is approached.[45]

RGP lenses often provide excellent visual acuity for many years if the lenses can be tolerated. If centration or comfort is an issue, other lens options include a "piggyback" fit,[49] a "hybrid" lens,[50] a large-diameter semiscleral gas-permeable lens,[51] or a Rose K lens style.[52]

Combing soft and RGP lenses, or "piggybacking," utilizes high-DK soft silicone hydrogel lenses with high-DK RGP lenses, which allows adequate oxygen transmission even with 2 lenses in place and therefore is much safer than using older contact lens materials that function as barriers for adequate oxygen transmission.[49] Another lens style that can be effective for select patients are hybrid lenses, where the optical center is composed of RGP material, and the peripheral flange is made of a softer material to improve comfort and lens tolerability.[50] More recently there has been development of the Rose K RGP lens that is custom cut to fit each individual keratoconus patient based on topography.[52] They provide a more gradual posterior curve spherical change to allow for better optics and support of the cone. Often a variety of lenses must be tried to find a successful fit, and this is best accomplished by someone experienced at fitting keratoconic corneas.

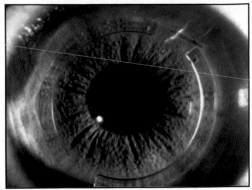

Figure 7-6. Intacs for keratoconus. The segments in this case were placed with the incision made at the steep preoperative meridian. A suture is still in place in the wound.

Surgical Management Strategies

In the past, once contact lenses became intolerable or ineffective in improving visual acuity, PK was the only viable option. PK is usually quite effective for visual rehabilitation and stable with a low incidence of graft rejection in keratoconus.[53] However, there are inherent risks associated with full-thickness corneal transplants, including graft dehiscence, graft failure, and the likely need for RGP lenses for optimal postoperative visual acuity. Recently, newer less-invasive alternatives, including intracorneal ring segments and collagen cross-linking, have become available that can postpone or potentially obviate the need for corneal transplantation.

Intracorneal Ring Segments

Originally designed and approved to treat low myopia, Intacs have recently been approved by the FDA and utilized for the treatment of keratoconus[54-56] and PCMD[57-60] (Figure 7-6). Intacs reduce myopia by an arc-shortening effect on the corneal stroma. The segments are implanted into the corneal stroma peripherally in an attempt to support the cone, flatten the central cornea, and improve vision.[54,61-63] There is some risk of infection,[64] but there is limited inflammatory potential. Intacs segments can be implanted through channels created mechanically or through the use of the femtosecond laser.[65] Some patients do not tolerate the segments for a variety of reasons, but if the segments erode through the cornea or become infected, they usually can be removed without incident, and if indicated a PK can still be performed. Intacs have also been successfully implanted for postoperative ectasia management.[66-68]

Because this is a relatively new technique, there is concern for stability of correction over time.[62] There is also discrepancy in the literature as to the most effective segment placement position, size, and symmetry, with some authors advocating symmetrical segments, asymmetrical segments,[54,55] or single segments inferiorly only[69] to support the cone.

Thus, though the optimal implantation technique, segment size, and orientation remain to be determined, Intacs implantation provides another option to keratoconus and PCMD patients that may improve vision or contact lens tolerance and may delay the need for PK. Another type of intracorneal ring segment, the Ferrara ring segment, may also be utilized for managing keratoconus; however, these devices are not currently available for use in the United States.[70]

Collagen Cross-Linking

One of the newest and most exciting therapies for keratoconus is the induction of stromal collagen cross-linking by using ultraviolet UVA light and riboflavin as described by Wollensak and colleagues.[71,72] This came about after Sady et al[73] and Seiler et al[74] noted a preponderance of advanced glycation end products in diabetics and their relative resistance to the development of advanced symptoms of keratoconus. They postulated that this was secondary to the innate ability to cross-link corneal collagen via these end products. Cross-linking corneal collagen hardens the cornea and stabilizes it from further degeneration. In the technique described by Wollensak and colleagues,[72] the epithelium is removed and riboflavin drops are applied to the cornea and exposed to UVA light for a period of 30 minutes. Collagen cross-linking occurs primarily in the anterior stromal bed. UVA light is also responsible for cataract development secondary to lens crystalline protein absorption; however, the calculated UVA exposure to the lens with this technique appears to be minimal. UVA light may also be potentially toxic to the corneal endothelium if corneal thickness is less than 400 µM; thus, corneal pachymetry measurements are essential prior to treatment. Collagen cross-linking may be utilized in isolation or in combination with intracorneal ring segments.[75] However, this therapy is currently not FDA-approved for use in the United States.

There is currently limited long-term data on the risks and stability of this procedure. However, the promise of corneal cross-linking is exciting as a means to improve the curvature and integrity of the keratoconic cornea.

Corneal Transplantation

It is estimated that 10% to 20% of keratoconic or PCMD eyes will eventually require corneal transplantation. PK is currently the "gold standard" surgical option. This procedure usually results in an acceptable outcome for most patients despite a potentially lengthy visual recovery time and probable need for RGP contact lenses for best corrected visual acuity postoperatively.[16,53,76-78] Following PK, patients are often left with a high degree of astigmatism, with or without suture adjustment or removal. There are several other potential long-term complications associated with PK, including graft rejection, wound dehiscence, infection, and the development of glaucoma and cataracts, many of which are influenced by the need for long-term topical steroids.[53]

Despite all of these potential problems, keratoconus patients undergoing PK usually enjoy successful postoperative course with good visual recovery and long-term stability.[53,78]

A newer variant on corneal transplantation is DALK via the big-bubble technique.[79,80] This technique transplants only the anterior stroma while preserving the patient's endothelium and Descemet's membrane. After incomplete trephination of the host cornea, an intrastromal injection of air by a blunt-tipped needle dissects the stroma away from Descemet's membrane. All host stroma is removed, and only the host's Descemet's membrane and endothelium remain intact. The donor cornea is trephinated to fit and is attached to the patient's cornea after the donor endothelium and Descemet's membrane has been removed. Potential advantages of this technique include preserving the healthy host endothelium and a reduced chance of graft rejection. The disadvantages include the technically challenging nature of the procedure, the potential need to convert to PK if microperforations in host Descemet's occur, and increased chance for scarring if incomplete separation occurs with the injection of the "big bubble," because layers of host stromal collagen remain. Poorer visual outcomes have been reported when manual removal of remnant lamellae was required.[79,80] It will be important to look at the long-term stability and complications associated with DALK and compare these to PK in order to effectively counsel keratoconus patients about their surgical options.

CONCLUSION

Keratoconus and PCMD are relatively common corneal disease processes, which are multifactorial in origin and variable in presentation and severity. The most advanced stages of disease result in extreme corneal warping and scarring, which require corneal transplantation. However, a variety of management alternatives are available for less severe disease manifestations, including a variety of contact lens-fitting strategies, intracorneal ring segments, and the promise of collagen cross-linking, which may halt or reverse the progression of the disease. As more is discovered regarding the molecular and biomechanical mechanisms underlying these ectatic corneal diseases, even more therapies may become available and provide better options for visual rehabilitation for affected patients.

REFERENCES

1. Rabinowitz YS. Keratoconus. *Surv Ophthalmol*. 1998;42:297-319.
2. Krachmer JH. Pellucid marginal corneal degeneration. *Arch Ophthalmol*. 1978;96:1217-1221.
3. Randleman JB, Woodward M, Lynn MJ, Stulting RD. Risk assessment for ectasia after corneal refractive surgery. *Ophthalmology*. 2008;115:37-50.
4. Wilson SE, Klyce SD. Screening for corneal topographic abnormalities before refractive surgery. *Ophthalmology*. 1994;101:147-152.
5. Rabinowitz YS. The genetics of keratoconus. *Ophthalmol Clin North Am*. 2003;16:607-620.
6. Falls HF, Allen AW. Dominantly inherited keratoconus. *J Genet Hum*. 1969;17:317-324.
7. Parker J, Ko WW, Pavlopoulos G, et al. Videokeratography of keratoconus in monozygotic twins. *J Refract Surg*. 1996;12:180-183.
8. Li X, Rabinowitz YS, Tang YG, et al. Two-stage genome-wide linkage scan in keratoconus sib pair families. *Invest Ophthalmol Vis Sci*. 2006;47:3791-3795.
9. Nielsen K, Heegaard S, Vorum H, et al. Altered expression of CLC, DSG3, EMP3, S100A2, and SLPI in corneal epithelium from keratoconus patients. *Cornea*. 2005;24:661-668.
10. Rabinowitz YS, Dong L, Wistow G. Gene expression profile studies of human keratoconus cornea for NEIBank: a novel cornea-expressed gene and the absence of transcripts for aquaporin 5. *Invest Ophthalmol Vis Sci*. 2005;46:1239-1246.
11. Tang YG, Rabinowitz YS, Taylor KD, et al. Genomewide linkage scan in a multigeneration Caucasian pedigree identifies a novel locus for keratoconus on chromosome 5q14.3-q21.1. *Genet Med*. 2005;7:397-405.

12. Wilson SE, He YG, Weng J, et al. Epithelial injury induces keratocyte apoptosis: hypothesized role for the interleukin-1 system in the modulation of corneal tissue organization and wound healing. *Exp Eye Res.* 1996;62:325-327.

13. Mackiewicz Z, Maatta M, Stenman M, et al. Collagenolytic proteinases in keratoconus. *Cornea.* 2006;25:603-610.

14. Jafri B, Lichter H, Stulting RD. Asymmetric keratoconus attributed to eye rubbing. *Cornea.* 2004;23:560-564.

15. Krachmer JH. Eye rubbing can cause keratoconus. *Cornea.* 2004;23:539-540.

16. Owens H, Gamble G. A profile of keratoconus in New Zealand. *Cornea.* 2003;22:122-125.

17. Sridhar MS, Mahesh S, Bansal AK, et al. Pellucid marginal corneal degeneration. *Ophthalmology.* 2004;111:1102-1107.

18. Tzelikis PF, Cohen EJ, Rapuano CJ, et al. Management of pellucid marginal corneal degeneration. *Cornea.* 2005;24:555-560.

19. Cameron JA. Keratoglobus. *Cornea.* 1993;12:124-130.

20. Krachmer JH, Rodrigues MM. Posterior keratoconus. *Arch Ophthalmol.* 1978;96:1867-1873.

21. Rao SK, Padmanabhan P. Posterior keratoconus. An expanded classification scheme based on corneal topography. *Ophthalmology.* 1998;105:1206-1212.

22. Ucakhan OO, Kanpolat A, Ylmaz N, Ozkan M. In vivo confocal microscopy findings in keratoconus. *Eye Contact Lens.* 2006;32:183-191.

23. Wilson SE, Lin DT, Klyce SD. Corneal topography of keratoconus. *Cornea.* 1991;10:2-8.

24. Rabinowitz YS, McDonnell PJ. Computer-assisted corneal topography in keratoconus. *Refract Corneal Surg.* 1989;5:400-408.

25. Rabinowitz YS. Videokeratographic indices to aid in screening for keratoconus. *J Refract Surg.* 1995;11:371-379.

26. Rabinowitz YS, Rasheed K. KISA% index: a quantitative videokeratography algorithm embodying minimal topographic criteria for diagnosing keratoconus. *J Cataract Refract Surg.* 1999;25:1327-1335.

27. Maeda N, Klyce SD, Smolek MK, Thompson HW. Automated keratoconus screening with corneal topography analysis. *Invest Ophthalmol Vis Sci.* 1994;35:2749-2757.

28. Binder PS, Lindstrom RL, Stulting RD, et al. Keratoconus and corneal ectasia after LASIK. *J Refract Surg.* 2005;21:749-752.

29. Randleman JB, Woodward M, Lynn MJ, Stulting RD. Risk assessment for ectasia after corneal refractive surgery. *Ophthalmology.*

30. Maguire LJ, Klyce SD, McDonald MB, Kaufman HE. Corneal topography of pellucid marginal degeneration. *Ophthalmology.* 1987;94:519-524.

31. Rao SK, Fogla R, Padmanabhan P, Sitalakshmi G. Corneal topography in atypical pellucid marginal degeneration. *Cornea.* 1999;18:265-272.

32. Abad JC, Rubinfeld RS, Valle MD, et al. Vertical D a novel topographic pattern in some keratoconus suspects. *Ophthalmology.* 2007.

33. Ambrosio R Jr, Alonso RS, Luz A, Coca Velarde LG. Corneal-thickness spatial profile and corneal-volume distribution: tomographic indices to detect keratoconus. *J Cataract Refract Surg.* 2006;32:1851-1859.

34. Quisling S, Sjoberg S, Zimmerman B, et al. Comparison of Pentacam and Orbscan IIz on posterior curvature topography measurements in keratoconus eyes. *Ophthalmology.* 2006;113:1629-1632.

35. Rao SN, Raviv T, Majmudar PA, Epstein RJ. Role of Orbscan II in screening keratoconus suspects before refractive corneal surgery. *Ophthalmology.* 2002;109:1642-1646.

36. Tabbara KF, Kotb AA. Risk factors for corneal ectasia after LASIK. *Ophthalmology.* 2006;113:1618-1622.

37. Randleman JB. Post-laser in-situ keratomileusis ectasia: current understanding and future directions. *Curr Opin Ophthalmol.* 2006;17:406-412.

38. Randleman JB, Russell B, Ward MA, et al. Risk factors and prognosis for corneal ectasia after LASIK. *Ophthalmology.* 2003;110:267-275.

39. Seiler T, Quurke AW. Iatrogenic keratectasia after LASIK in a case of forme fruste keratoconus. *J Cataract Refract Surg.* 1998;24:1007-1009.

40. Fogla R, Rao SK, Padmanabhan P. Keratectasia in 2 cases with pellucid marginal corneal degeneration after laser in situ keratomileusis. *J Cataract Refract Surg.* 2003;29:788-791.

41. Randleman JB, Banning CS, Stulting RD. Corneal ectasia after hyperopic LASIK. *J Refract Surg.* 2007;23:98-102.

42. Amoils SP, Deist MB, Gous P, Amoils PM. Iatrogenic keratectasia after laser in situ keratomileusis for less than -4.0 to -7.0 diopters of myopia. *J Cataract Refract Surg.* 2000;26:967-977.

43. Klein SR, Epstein RJ, Randleman JB, Stulting RD. Corneal ectasia after laser in situ keratomileusis in patients without apparent preoperative risk factors. *Cornea.* 2006;25:388-403.

44. Zadnik K, Barr JT, Gordon MO, Edrington TB. Biomicroscopic signs and disease severity in keratoconus. Collaborative Longitudinal Evaluation of Keratoconus (CLEK) Study Group. *Cornea.* 1996;15:139-146.

45. Garcia-Lledo M, Feinbaum C, Alio JL. Contact lens fitting in keratoconus. *Compr Ophthalmol Update.* 2006;7:47-52.

46. Edrington TB, Szczotka LB, Barr JT, et al. Rigid contact lens fitting relationships in keratoconus. Collaborative Longitudinal Evaluation of Keratoconus (CLEK) Study Group. *Optom Vis Sci.* 1999;76:692-699.

47. Lim N, Vogt U. Characteristics and functional outcomes of 130 patients with keratoconus attending a specialist contact lens clinic. *Eye.* 2002;16:54-59.

48. Zadnik K, Barr JT, Steger-May K, et al. Comparison of flat and steep rigid contact lens fitting methods in keratoconus. *Optom Vis Sci.* 2005;82:1014-1021.

49. O'Donnell C, Maldonado-Codina C. A hyper-Dk piggyback contact lens system for keratoconus. *Eye Contact Lens.* 2004;30:44-48.

50. Rubinstein MP, Sud S. The use of hybrid lenses in management of the irregular cornea. *Contact Lens Anterior Eye.* 1999;22:87-90.

51. Visser ES, Visser R, van Lier HJ, Otten HM. Modern scleral lenses part I: clinical features. *Eye Contact Lens.* 2007;33:13-20.

52. Betts AM, Mitchell GL, Zadnik K. Visual performance and comfort with the Rose K lens for keratoconus. *Optom Vis Sci.* 2002;79:493-501.

53. Pramanik S, Musch DC, Sutphin JE, Farjo AA. Extended long-term outcomes of penetrating keratoplasty for keratoconus. *Ophthalmology.* 2006;113:1633-1638.

54. Boxer Wachler BS, Christie JP, Chandra NS, et al. Intacs for keratoconus. *Ophthalmology.* 2003;110:1031-1040.

55. Colin J, Cochener B, Savary G, et al. INTACS inserts for treating keratoconus: one-year results. *Ophthalmology.* 2001;108:1409-1414.

56. Siganos CS, Kymionis GD, Kartakis N, et al. Management of keratoconus with Intacs. *Am J Ophthalmol.* 2003;135:64-70.

57. Kymionis GD, Aslanides IM, Siganos CS, Pallikaris IG. Intacs for early pellucid marginal degeneration. *J Cataract Refract Surg.* 2004;30:230-233.

58. Ertan A, Bahadir M. Intrastromal ring segment insertion using a femtosecond laser to correct pellucid marginal corneal degeneration. *J Cataract Refract Surg.* 2006;32:1710-1716.

59. Ertan A, Bahadir M. Management of superior pellucid marginal degeneration with a single intracorneal ring segment using femtosecond laser. *J Refract Surg.* 2007;23:205-208.

60. Mularoni A, Torreggiani A, di Biase A, et al. Conservative treatment of early and moderate pellucid marginal degeneration: a new refractive approach with intracorneal rings. *Ophthalmology.* 2005;112:660-666.

61. Alio JL, Shabayek MH. Intracorneal asymmetrical rings for keratoconus: where should the thicker segment be implanted? *J Refract Surg.* 2006;22:307-309.

62. Alio JL, Shabayek MH, Artola A. Intracorneal ring segments for keratoconus correction: long-term follow-up. *J Cataract Refract Surg.* 2006;32:978-985.

63. Rabinowitz YS. INTACS for keratoconus. *Int Ophthalmol Clin.* 2006;46:91-103.

64. Hofling-Lima AL, Branco BC, Romano AC, et al. Corneal infections after implantation of intracorneal ring segments. *Cornea.* 2004;23:547-549.

65. Rabinowitz YS, Li X, Ignacio TS, Maguen E. INTACS inserts using the femtosecond laser compared to the mechanical spreader in the treatment of keratoconus. *J Refract Surg.* 2006;22:764-771.

66. Alio J, Salem T, Artola A, Osman A. Intracorneal rings to correct corneal ectasia after laser in situ keratomileusis. *J Cataract Refract Surg.* 2002;28:1568-1574.

67. Lovisolo CF, Fleming JF. Intracorneal ring segments for iatrogenic keratectasia after laser in situ keratomileusis or photorefractive keratectomy. *J Refract Surg.* 2002;18:535-541.

68. Siganos CS, Kymionis GD, Astyrakakis N, Pallikaris IG. Management of corneal ectasia after laser in situ keratomileusis with INTACS. *J Refract Surg.* 2002;18:43-46.

69. Chan CC, Wachler BS. Reduced best spectacle-corrected visual acuity from inserting a thicker Intacs above and thinner Intacs below in keratoconus. *J Refract Surg.* 2007;23:93-95.

70. Siganos D, Ferrara P, Chatzinikolas K, et al. Ferrara intrastromal corneal rings for the correction of keratoconus. *J Cataract Refract Surg.* 2002;28:1947-1951.

71. Wollensak G. Crosslinking treatment of progressive keratoconus: new hope. *Curr Opin Ophthalmol.* 2006;17:356-360.

72. Wollensak G, Spoerl E, Seiler T. Riboflavin/ultraviolet-a-induced collagen crosslinking for the treatment of keratoconus. *Am J Ophthalmol.* 2003;135:620-627.

73. Sady C, Khosrof S, Nagaraj R. Advanced Maillard reaction and crosslinking of corneal collagen in diabetes. *Biochem Biophys Res Commun.* 1995;214:793-797.

74. Seiler T, Huhle S, Spoerl E, Kunath H. Manifest diabetes and keratoconus: a retrospective case-control study. *Graefes Arch Clin Exp Ophthalmol.* 2000;238:822-825.

75. Chan CC, Sharma M, Wachler BS. Effect of inferior-segment Intacs with and without C3-R on keratoconus. *J Cataract Refract Surg.* 2007;33:75-80.

76. Geerards AJ, Vreugdenhil W, Khazen A. Incidence of rigid gas-permeable contact lens wear after keratoplasty for keratoconus. *Eye Contact Lens.* 2006;32:207-210.

77. Gordon MO, Steger-May K, Szczotka-Flynn L, et al. Baseline factors predictive of incident penetrating keratoplasty in keratoconus. *Am J Ophthalmol.* 2006;142:923-930.

78. Javadi MA, Motlagh BF, Jafarinasab MR, et al. Outcomes of penetrating keratoplasty in keratoconus. *Cornea.* 2005;24:941-96.

79. Fogla R, Padmanabhan P. Results of deep lamellar keratoplasty using the big-bubble technique in patients with keratoconus. *Am J Ophthalmol.* 2006;141:254-259.

80. Fontana L, Parente G, Tassinari G. Clinical outcomes after deep anterior lamellar keratoplasty using the big-bubble technique in patients with keratoconus. *Am J Ophthalmol.* 2007;143:117-124.

8

SYSTEMIC AND IMMUNOLOGIC CONDITIONS OF THE CORNEA

Howard A. Lane, MD, FACS and Jodi I. Luchs, MD, FACS

The cornea is a unique structure whose clarity makes deposition of materials relatively easy to identify. Though it has no inherent blood supply, it is affected by immunologic and systemic disease processes that affect their pathology in the cornea via the nearby limbal vasculature. The disease spectrum can vary in severity from benign, asymptomatic corneal deposits to severe corneal destruction.

SYSTEMIC IMMUNOLOGIC DISEASES AFFECTING THE CORNEA

Rheumatoid Arthritis

Rheumatoid arthritis is a common, chronic, systemic autoimmune disease characterized by a symmetric, erosive, and deforming polyarthritis. It is more common in women and affects approximately 1% of the population.[1] The metacarpophalangeal and interphalangeal joints are most commonly involved, although any joint may be affected. Ligamentous changes associated with later stage arthritis may result in joint subluxation and angulation. This is associated with the characteristic "swan neck" deformity of the digits. Numerous extraarticular inflammatory manifestations involving multiple organ systems may affect up to 25% of rheumatoid arthritis patients.

Ocular manifestations most frequently involve the anterior segment. These include episcleritis, scleritis, keratoconjunctivitis sicca, sclerosing keratitis, stromal keratitis, paracentral keratolysis, peripheral ulcerative keratitis (PUK), and limbal furrowing. Posterior segment findings are less common and include posterior scleritis, retinal vasculitis, and choroidal effusion.

Keratoconjunctivitis sicca, which may affect up to 25% of rheumatoid patients,[2] is the most common ocular manifestation of rheumatoid arthritis (Figure 8-1). The triad of keratoconjunctivitis sicca, xerostomia, and an autoimmune disease such as rheumatoid arthritis is referred to as *secondary Sjögren's syndrome*. An aqueous tear deficiency resulting in a dry eye syndrome occurs due to autoimmune

Trattler WB, Majmudar PA, Luchs JI, Swartz TS, eds.
Cornea Handbook (pp. 123-140)
© 2010 SLACK Incorporated

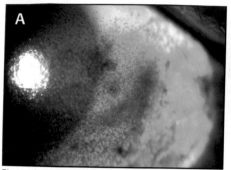
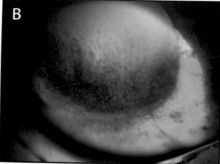

Figure 8-1. (A) Severe keratoconjunctivitis sicca as seen using Lissamine green stain. (B) The inferior portion of the cornea stains heavily with Lissamine green in cases of exposure, particularly at night.

Figure 8-2. Episcleritis may be simple, seen here, or nodular. Published with permission from Rapuano CJ, Luchs JI, Kim T, eds. *Anterior Segment: The Requisites in Ophthalmology.* New York, NY: Mosby Publishing; 2000. (Courtesy of Jodi I. Luchs, MD.)

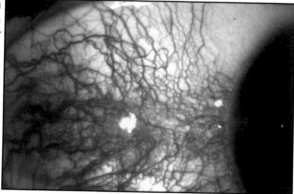

involvement of the lacrimal glands. Dry eye syndrome and aqueous tear deficiency states are discussed in further detail in Chapter 12.

Episcleritis either alone or associated with an underlying scleritis may occur in patients with rheumatoid arthritis (Figure 8-2). Simple or nodular forms may occur, with injection of the radial episcleral vasculature. Patients typically complain of mild pain and tenderness, although there may be no pain associated with it. The injection tends to blanch after the application of topical phenylephrine, distinguishing it from scleritis.

Scleritis is the second most common ocular manifestation of rheumatoid arthritis after keratoconjunctivitis sicca (Figure 8-3). Its presence may have serious implications regarding the systemic stage of disease. Scleritis has been reported in approximately 6% of rheumatoid arthritis patients and may present in an anterior or posterior form.[3] Anterior scleritis most commonly presents as a diffuse form (most common), but nodular or necrotizing forms may also occur. Though other etiologies for scleritis exist, rheumatoid arthritis is the most common underlying cause. Patients present with a deep, boring pain typically radiating through the orbit, temple, and jaw. Diffuse scleral injection and swelling upon biomicroscopy are associated with the diffuse form. Localized tender nodules of scleral inflammation are characteristic of the nodular form. The involved areas have a violaceous hue best seen using gross inspection in natural light. There is associated conjunctival and episcleral injection. Distinguishing between episcleri-

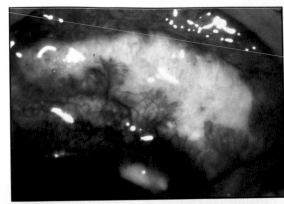

Figure 8-3. Surgically induced necrotizing scleritis. A large area of necrotizing scleritis is seen at the superior limbus, where extracapsular cataract surgery was performed several months earlier. Published with permission from Rapuano CJ, Luchs JI, Kim T, eds. *Anterior Segment: The Requisites in Ophthalmology.* New York, NY: Mosby Publishing; 2000. (Courtesy of Jodi I. Luchs, MD.)

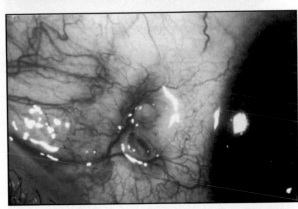

Figure 8-4. Necrotizing scleritis. An area of necrotizing scleritis with an overlying conjunctival epithelial defect and visible uveal pigment. Published with permission from Rapuano CJ, Luchs JI, Kim T, eds. *Anterior Segment: The Requisites in Ophthalmology.* New York, NY: Mosby Publishing; 2000. (Courtesy of Jodi I. Luchs, MD.)

tis and scleritis is often difficult. Scleritis is associated with more severe pain and less blanching with topical phenylephrine.

The least common form seen clinically is necrotizing anterior scleritis, which may occur either with or without inflammation. Necrotizing anterior scleritis with inflammation is associated with intense scleritis and severe pain (Figure 8-4). Involved areas show signs of scleral necrosis, often with a conjunctival epithelial defect. As the sclera thins, choroidal pigment may be visible. Necrotizing anterior scleritis with inflammation is an ominous sign because 40% to 60% of these patients may lose best corrected vision, and it indicates life-threatening systemic complications.[4] Adequate systemic immunosuppression is required because 30% to 50% of these patients may die within 5 to 10 years of the onset of scleritis from complications related to severe systemic vasculitis.[4]

Necrotizing anterior scleritis without inflammation, or scleromalacia perforans, is found in patients with long-standing, severe rheumatoid arthritis (Figure 8-5). Patients present with painless necrotic scleral lesions in a relatively quiet eye. Active lesions generally produce no significant ocular inflammation or pain, yet result in extensive scleral thinning with visible underlying choroid. Despite thinning, perforation rarely occurs. Patients may present complaining of a recently noted discoloration on the eye or reduced vision secondary to induced astigmatism.

Corneal manifestations of rheumatoid arthritis may be associated with scleritis or episcleritis or occur alone. Nonulcerative corneal manifestations include

Figure 8-5. Scleromalacia perforans. A large area of superior scleral thinning, protrusion, and uveal show is seen. Published with permission from Rapuano CJ, Luchs JI, Kim T, eds. *Anterior Segment: The Requisites in Ophthalmology.* New York, NY: Mosby Publishing; 2000. (Courtesy of Jodi I. Luchs, MD.)

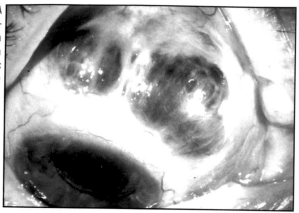

Figure 8-6. Peripheral ulcerative keratitis in a patient with rheumatoid arthritis.

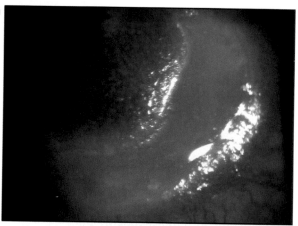

Figure 8-7. Paracentral keratolysis with a descemetocele.

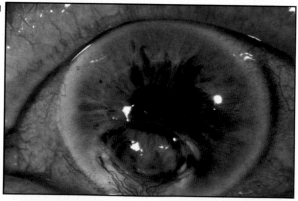

sclerosing keratitis and acute stromal keratitis. Ulcerative manifestations include PUK (also called marginal keratolysis; Figure 8-6), paracentral keratolysis (Figure 8-7), and limbal guttering. Sclerosing keratitis is frequently associated with scleritis and presents as a thickening of the corneal periphery and opacification adjacent to an area of active scleritis. It may progress to include the central cornea and become vascularized. Untreated cases may result in corneal scarring and lipid deposition. Stromal keratitis presents with edema and peripheral stromal infiltrates with an intact epithelium, usually associated with scleritis. Untreated, the infiltrates may coalesce, producing vascularization, scarring, and stromal melting similar to PUK.

PUK is corneal ulceration in isolation or associated with necrotizing scleritis. The ulcer appears as an area of peripheral infiltration and thinning, with an epithelial defect. There is usually associated limbal and conjunctival injection. It may extend circumferentially and progress centrally. Untreated, lesions may thin progressively and form a descemetocele or perforate. Limbal guttering may also occur, with variable peripheral corneal thinning associated with an intact epithelium.

Paracentral keratolysis is characterized by a severe, acute corneal ulceration often without a significant infiltrate and melting. This typically occurs with necrotizing scleritis or keratoconjunctivitis sicca. The lesion may rapidly progress to descemetocele formation and perforation in a previously clear cornea.

All of these findings are not unique to rheumatoid arthritis and may be found in patients with other collagen vascular diseases. Their presence should alert the clinician to the possibility of underlying systemic autoimmune disease and, if not previously performed, a systemic workup should be ordered.

Treatment of ocular manifestations of rheumatoid arthritis varies according to the specific condition. The treatment of keratoconjunctivitis sicca is described in detail in Chapter 12.

Episcleritis may respond to topical or systemic corticosteroids, or topical or systemic nonsteroidal anti-inflammatory medications. The treatment of scleritis, however, is more complicated. Topical therapy is typically ineffective for scleritis, and systemic therapy is necessary. Oral nonsteroidal anti-inflammatory medications such as ibuprofen, naproxen, or indomethacin may be effective in mild or moderate cases, and systemic corticosteroids or other immunosuppressive agents are often required for more severe cases. Therapy must be continued for weeks or months, with gradual tapering of anti-inflammatories.[5-8] Periocular corticosteroids are generally contraindicated because they increase the risk of scleral melting or perforation.[6] Necrotizing scleritis should be considered both an ocular and a medical emergency because it represents an ocular manifestation of systemic vasculitis. These patients require prompt evaluation by a rheumatologist and the initiation of systemic immunosuppression to reduce ocular and systemic morbidity. Though systemic corticosteroids provide a rapid immunosuppressive effect, side effects of long-term therapy are problematic. Systemic methotrexate, azathioprine, cyclophosphamide, and cyclosporine are potent immunosuppressive agents that may be effective in the treatment of necrotizing scleritis, as well as severe nonnecrotizing scleritis that fails to respond to other treatments.[7-10] The goal is to reduce inflammation, limit tissue destruction, and promote healing. Aggressive treatment of dry eye is also essential. The integrity of the globe may be compromised by severe tissue loss, requiring surgical procedures such as scleral, pericardial, or fascia-lata patch grafts. Secondary bacterial, fungal, or atypical mycobacterial infections may occur, and suspicious lesions should be cultured and aggressively treated prior to high-dose immunosuppression, when possible.

Sclerosing keratitis and stromal keratitis are usually associated with scleritis and generally respond to topical corticosteroid treatment. The treatment of associated scleritis is also necessary.

PUK and paracentral keratolysis are thought to be partly related to the increased collagenase activity. Promotion of epithelial healing using aggressive lubrication with preservative-free tears and tear ointments is the initial goal. Corneal melting should cease when the epithelial defect has healed. Punctal occlusion or a lateral tarsorrhaphy may be helpful. Topical corticosteroids, which may enhance collagenase activity, should be used cautiously because they may hasten tissue loss and increase risk of perforation. When used, the minimal effective dose should be prescribed, with frequent follow-up visits. Patients presenting taking topical corticosteroids should be tapered gradually.

Periocular use of corticosteroids is controversial because of the inability to withdraw the drug should progressive melting occur. Topical cyclosporine may offer local immunosuppression without enhancement of collagenase activity.[11] Other anticollagenase agents may be helpful in selected cases and include tetracyclines, N-acetylcysteine, and medroxyprogesterone. Tumor necrosis factor alpha (TNF-alpha) antagonists have been shown to be effective for the treatment of PUK not responsive to conventional immunosuppressive therapy.[12] When required, conjunctival resection or recession adjacent to the involved cornea to keep the conjunctival collagenases away from the cornea may be beneficial. Amniotic membrane transplantation for persistent epithelial defects may be beneficial as well, but its utility is limited due to underlying severe ischemia.[13] Lamellar patch grafting may be required to avoid perforation. Cyanoacrylate glue with a bandage hydrogel lens may be useful for small perforations,[14] although larger perforations may require PK.

Systemic Lupus Erythematosis

Systemic lupus erythematosis (SLE) is a collagen vascular disease affecting multiple organ systems. Associated conditions include arthralgia, skin rashes, glomerulonephritis, and central nervous system manifestations. The diagnosis can be made by the presence of antinuclear antibodies, anti-double-stranded DNA antibodies, and other autoantibodies.

Ocular manifestations of SLE involve both the anterior and posterior segment. Lid manifestations include chronic blepharitis and the typical lupus rash on the eyelids. Conjunctival injection and symblepharon are rare. A secondary Sjögren's syndrome occurs in 25% of patients.[15] Corneal involvement, though uncommon, may include stromal keratitis and neovascularization. Episcleritis and scleritis have also been reported.[16] Similar to rheumatoid arthritis, the presence of scleritis may indicate the severity of the systemic disease or occasionally be the initial manifestation of SLE. Posterior segment findings usually related to vasculitis include cotton wool spots and retinal hemorrhages.

Wegener's Granulomatosis

Wegener's granulomatosis (WG) is an autoimmune disease characterized by a systemic vasculitis. Upper and lower respiratory tracts, as well as the kidneys, are typically affected, although other organs may become involved. Sinusitis, pulmonary infiltrates, hemoptysis, and glomerulonephritis may occur. Rapidly progressive orbital inflammation is commonly associated with Wegener's. Anterior segment ocular findings result from focal vasculitis and include localized or diffuse conjunctival and episcleral injection, peripheral subepithelial and anterior stromal infiltrates, scleritis, and PUK. WG should be ruled out in all patients with necrotiz-

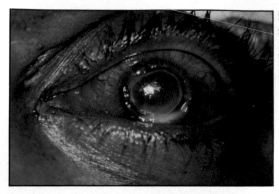

Figure 8-8. Mooren's ulcer. Published with permission from Rapuano CJ, Luchs JI, Kim T, eds. *Anterior Segment: The Requisites in Ophthalmology.* New York, NY: Mosby Publishing; 2000. (Courtesy of Jodi I. Luchs, MD.)

ing sclerokeratitis. Necrotizing scleritis may produce severe tissue loss, and PUK may progress circumferentially and centrally, resembling a Mooren's ulcer. Secondary Sjögren's syndrome producing keratoconjunctivitis sicca is also common.

Ocular manifestations of WG are managed by addressing the systemic disease using corticosteroids and other immunosuppressive agents, most commonly cyclophosphamide. Keratoconjunctivitis sicca should be aggressively treated using lubricating ointments and tears, punctal occlusion, and lateral tarsorrhaphy when necessary. Conjunctivitis and episcleritis may respond to topical corticosteroids, but use should be minimized in the presence of ulcerative keratitis to avoid corneal melting.

Other autoimmune diseases such as polyarteritis nodosa, scleroderma, relapsing polychondritis, and dermatomyositis may also produce anterior segment findings similar to the above conditions. This wide variety of systemic autoimmune conditions demonstrates the importance of a complete systemic autoimmune workup in patients who present with these conditions. An initial workup is often unrevealing. When recurrent, a workup should be repeated 6 to 12 months later. This second workup is often more revealing.

Mooren's Ulceration

Mooren's ulceration is a painful ulceration of the cornea that is not related to infection or trauma (Figure 8-8). It starts as a peripheral infiltrate, which progresses to an epithelial defect, and then to an ulcer. This painful peripheral ulceration progresses circumferentially, with a classic grey "overhanging ledge," which is undermined. The ulceration in Mooren's is purely corneal; scleral involvement is usually associated with PUK.[17]

Two types of Mooren's ulcer have been identified.[18] Type 1 is a unilateral, slowly progressive, milder type that usually occurs in older patients. Type 2 is a more painful, bilateral variant that occurs in younger patients, most commonly of African descent.[19] This variant responds poorly to medical or surgical interventions, and perforation is common.[20]

The true cause of Mooren's ulcer is not known. Autoimmunity is believed to play a crucial role in disease development. Some suggest an autoreactivity to a cornea-specific antigen as the catalyst; humoral and cell-mediated mechanisms may perpetuate the corneal destruction.[21] Patients with Mooren's ulcer have a deficiency of T suppressor cells and an increased concentration of plasma cells and lymphocytes in the conjunctiva adjacent to the ulcerated areas. Resection of the limbal conjunctiva has proven to be beneficial in Mooren's patients.[22]

Accidental trauma, surgery, exposure to parasites, and hepatitis C infection[23] may be predisposing factors for Mooren's ulcer. Some hypothesize that inflammation from these factors alters the expression of corneal antigens, thereby causing autoantibodies to be produced.[24]

Due to the clinical similarity to PUK, one must rule out autoimmune diseases before defining a case of Mooren's. If a history of a collagen vascular disorder is not already present, serologic testing for rheumatoid factor (RF), antinuclear antibodies (ANA), antineutrophil cytoplasmic antibody (ANCA), and a medical consult is indicated.

Unilateral, mild type of Mooren's (type 1) may respond well to topical steroids, in conjunction with topical antibiotic coverage. Conjunctival recession extending 3 to 4 mm from the limbus may also be helpful if topical steroids alone do not work. Topical cyclosporine has been utilized with some success.[25]

Type 2 Mooren's is usually resistant to topical therapy and requires systemic immunosuppression. Oral corticosteroids, cyclosporine, cyclophosphamide, methotrexate, and azathioprine may be required. Mooren's ulcer associated with hepatitis C have been responsive to interferon treatment.[26] Even with these aggressive systemic measures, conjunctival recession, cyanoacrylate glue, patch grafts, or full-thickness PK may be required for impending corneal perforation.[22]

SYSTEMIC DISEASES WITH CORNEAL MANIFESTATIONS

Multiple Myeloma

Multiple myeloma is a malignant neoplasm of plasma cells that causes monoclonal proliferation and secretion of excessive immunoglobulin. Ophthalmic manifestations may involve the conjunctiva, cornea, uveal tract, retina, optic nerve, and orbit and are usually secondary to immunoglobulin deposition or hyperviscosity. Hyperviscosity and a crystalline deposition may manifest as a sludging of red blood cells in the conjunctival vasculature. Deposition of immunoglobulins in the cornea may appear as fine crystals throughout the stroma. Peripheral deposition is usually heaviest because the immunoglobulins gain access through the limbal blood vessels.[27] Multiple myeloma crystalline deposits may be the first manifestation of the disease process. Associated hypercalcemia may produce band keratopathy. Copper deposition in Descemet's membrane and crystalline deposits in the lens may also occur.

Vernal and Atopic Conjunctivitis

Vernal keratoconjunctivitis (VKC) is a chronic, bilateral inflammatory condition of the conjunctiva and cornea. It occurs more commonly in males and typically presents in the spring or summer months, though some patients have symptoms year round. A family history of atopy is present in about 50% of cases.[28]

Clinical findings are confined to the conjunctiva and cornea, in comparison to atopic keratoconjunctivitis (AKC), which is often associated with atopic dermatitis. VKC patients complain of severe itching and photophobia. A thick mucous discharge (often stringy) may be present. The conjunctiva shows a heavy papillary response, primarily on the upper limbus or tarsus. When the tarsal papillae become large, with diameters greater than 1.0 mm and with flattened tops, they take on the appearance of the classic "cobblestone" papillae (Figure 8-9).

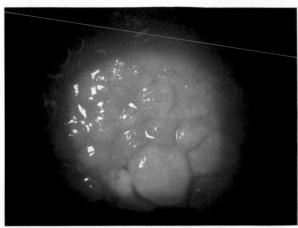

Figure 8-9. Cobblestone papillae in a patient with VKC.

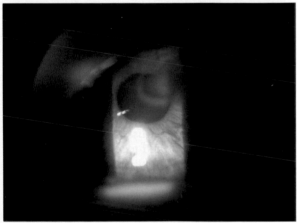

Figure 8-10. Shield ulcer in a patient with VKC.

The condition manifests in 2 clinical forms: palpebral and limbal. In the palpebral form, patients have diffuse giant papillae that are most prominent on the upper rather than the lower palpebral conjunctiva. This form is often associated with corneal changes, ranging from punctuate erosions to a sight-threatening shield ulcer. The limbal variant of VKC occurs primarily in boys of African and Asian descent. In this form, giant papillae develop along the limbal border, producing thick, gelatinous nodules. White Horner-Trantas dots—collections of eosinophils and epithelial cells—may appear amid the limbal papillae.

Corneal findings in VKC range from minimal to extensive. Mediators from the inflamed tarsal conjunctiva may cause punctate keratitis in VKC patients. If the areas coalesce, they may create a full epithelial erosion; a plaque with mucus and fibrin may then form over the defect, impairing the healing process. This sterile corneal ulceration is known as a *shield ulcer*. (Figure 8-10). It is usually within the upper half of the visual axis. After resolution, it may leave a subepithelial scar that has the potential to affect vision.

The immunopathogenesis of VKC most likely involves both type I and type IV hypersensitivity reactions.[29] The conjunctival epithelium of VKC patients contains large numbers of mast cells and eosinophils, which are not found in normal individuals.

In addition to supportive therapy, treatment includes suppressing the inflammatory process. Topical corticosteroids, including fluorometholone, prednisolone acetate 1%, or loteprednol QID, are effective in treating the acute inflammation until topical mast-cell stabilizers, such as olopatadine, ketotifen, epinastine, azelastine, nedocromil, pemirolast BID, become effective. Topical and systemic antihistamines may also alleviate symptoms. The initiation and duration of these medications should be based upon the individual patient's history of disease. Those with regular seasonal exacerbations can be started on topical mast cell stabilizers 2 weeks before the anticipated onset of symptoms, and those with continuous disease can be maintained on this therapy all year long. Literature has also shown topical cyclosporine to be effective in the management of severe or refractory cases of vernal and AKC.

Atopic Keratoconjunctivitis

AKC is a bilateral, chronic inflammation of the eyelids and conjunctiva that usually affects people 20 to 50 years old. AKC does not feature any racial or sex predilection, and is a perennial rather than seasonal disease. Approximately 3% of the population has atopic dermatitis,[30] and almost one third of patients with atopic dermatitis develop keratoconjunctivitis.

Clinically, AKC patients often complain of severe itching. There may be ocular discharge, but this is usually more watery than in VKC. Signs include skin, lid margin, conjunctival, and corneal changes. AKC has similar clinical findings to VKC, with some clear distinguishing features. Patients usually have extensive lid changes. The periocular skin manifests a scaly dermatitis, often associated with loss of cilia and meibomianitis (Figure 8-11). The eyelid may become cicatricial, resulting in lagophthalmos. In contrast to VKC, the papillae in AKC are smaller than those found in VKC, and they are more prominent in the inferior conjunctival fornix. Subepithelial fibrosis and subsequent symblepharon formation, similar to ocular cicatricial pemphigoid, may occur.

Punctate epithelial erosions are the most commonly seen corneal finding in AKC.[31] However, extensive corneal neovascularization secondary to chronic epithelial disease may be present, possibly due to limbal stem cell dysfunction. Vision loss in AKC patients results from corneal vascularization with scarring and secondary infections. Characteristic anterior and posterior subcapsular cataract changes may occasionally occur.[32]

Though atopic individuals demonstrate type I hypersensitivity with large numbers of mast cells and extensive mast cell activation, they also demonstrate a depressed cell-mediated immunity.[33] Consequently, AKC patients are more susceptible to *Staphylococcus aureus* infection as well as herpes simplex keratitis.[34]

Treatment of both vernal and AKC is complex and involves environmental controls in addition to topical and systemic therapies. Environmental irritants should be avoided as much as possible in patients with AKC and VKC. Cool compresses and utilization of home air filtration is helpful.

Mild cases of AKC and VKC may respond to topical mast cell stabilizers, as outlined above. Cromolyn sodium has repeatedly shown to be effective in treating VKC.[35] Dual-acting mast cell stabilizing and antihistamine medications are often effective perennial therapies, and a steroid pulse may be given at a time of exacerbation. The risks of long-term topical steroid abuse should be thoroughly discussed with these patients, who may need relief year-round.

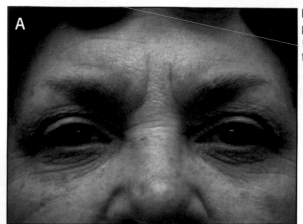

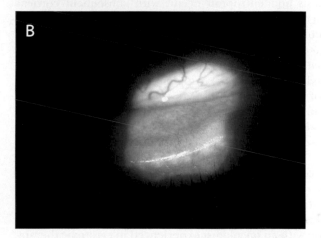

Figure 8-11. (A) Atopic patients typically present with dermatitis and meibomianitis. (B) Lid changes associated with atopic keratoconjunctivitis.

Topical CsA has shown promise in the treatment of VKC. CsA diminishes the release of interleukin-2, thereby reducing T-cell expansion. There are a number of studies showing reduction of inflammation and symptoms after use of CsA for VKC.[36] Oral therapies for AKC and VKC include antihistamines, steroids, and nonsteroidal anti-inflammatory agents. For vision-threatening corneal disease, oral steroids may be necessary along with aggressive topical modalities. Corneal shield ulcers may be treated with antibiotic–steroid combination drops or ointments, as well as bandage contact lenses or patching. Some physicians have had success with a superficial scraping of the mucous plaque in order to promote healing. Recent reports have shown amniotic membrane placement to be effective in treating shield ulcers.[37] Systemic immunosuppression may be required for cicatrizing sequelae of AKC.

Ocular Cicatricial Pemphigoid

Ocular cicatricial pemphigoid (OCP) is an autoimmune-related chronic cicatrizing conjunctivitis that may have severe ocular implications. It affects women more frequently than men. Patients are typically older than 50 when OCP is diagnosed, though early forms of the disease are likely present before the patient presents with symptoms. Though OCP primarily affects the conjunctiva, it frequently affects other mucous membranes, including the mouth, oropharynx, anus, and genitalia. Skin involvement occurs in about one quarter of cases and usually takes the form of a scarring dermatitis.[38]

OCP patients usually present with nonspecific unilateral conjunctival inflammation. Close inspection of the conjunctival fornices in early stages of the disease may reveal subepithelial fibrosis, which forms when transient bullae of the conjunctiva rupture (stage 1). Another early sign might be trichiasis. Stage 2 is classically associated with fornix foreshortening, and symblepharon formation is typically known as stage 3. Rarely, adhesions may form between the lid and the globe, leading to reduced ocular motility (stage 4).[39]

Conjunctival (Figures 8-12 to 8-14) inflammation from OCP may lead to goblet cell destruction, resultant loss of mucin from the tear film, and obstruction of the lacrimal gland ductules, producing a secondary aqueous deficiency.[40] Lack of aqueous and mucous in the tear film leads to keratinization and conjunctival thickening. In turn, trichiasis and entropion occur, with subsequent corneal abnormalities. The corneal changes in OCP include abrasions to neovascularization, corneal ulceration, and scarring.[41]

The typical clinical course of OCP is slow progression, with variable periods of remission. If OCP is suspected by ophthalmic exam, referral to a dermatologist and internist should be considered. Characteristic skin and mucous membrane changes may help in the diagnosis of pemphigoid. Even with a high clinical suspicion of OCP, pathologic confirmation is necessary before the institution of a therapy, which may be effective but potentially toxic. Biopsy specimens should be obtained from actively affected areas of the conjunctiva and sent for immunofluorescent or immunoperoxidase staining (PIC). The diagnosis of OCP is confirmed by staining of C3, IgG, IgM, and/or IgA in the conjunctival basement membrane zone (BMZ).[42]

It is important to remember that OCP is a systemic disorder that usually requires a systemic approach to treatment. Although systemic steroids may be used for short-term pulse therapy, they are often not useful as a sole medical therapy in advancing OCP. Consultation with an oncologist experienced in cytotoxic therapy is recommended before beginning immunosuppressive therapy. With correct treatment, these modalities can bring about remission.

Dapsone is currently the drug of choice in mild OCP. Caution must be taken in patients with G6PD deficiency or sulfa allergy. Hemolytic anemia is a serious side effect of dapsone in patients with or without G6PD deficiency.

Cyclophosphamide is a helpful modality in severe cases of OCP. The therapeutic target, when treating with cyclophosphamide, is a reduction of the white blood count to 2000 to 3000 cells per microliter. Azathioprine, methotrexate, mycophenolate mofetil, daclizumab, or intravenous immunoglobulin therapy[43] have been useful as alternative agents when cyclophosphamide can not be tolerated.

Controlling the stability of the ocular surface is often difficult in OCP patients. Depending on the stage of OCP, nonpreserved artificial tears and ointments, punctal occlusion, and tarsorrhaphy may be necessary. Ocular surgery should be delayed until disease activity is under control. Hard palate and buccal mucosal grafting may be used in fornix reconstruction. PK has a low success rate in moderate to severe OCP patients due to the poor ocular surface environment.[44] Permanent keratoprosthesis placement has been shown to have some success in end-stage patients.[45]

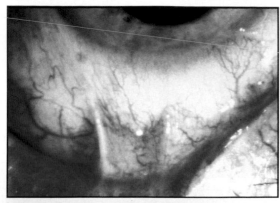

Figure 8-12. Ocular cicatricial pemphigoid stage 2. Shortening of the conjunctival fornix is evident with early symblepharon formation. Published with permission from Rapuano CJ, Luchs JI, Kim T, eds. *Anterior Segment: The Requisites in Ophthalmology.* New York, NY: Mosby Publishing; 2000. (Courtesy of Jodi I. Luchs, MD.)

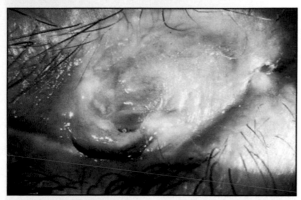

Figure 8-13. Ocular cicatricial pemphigoid stage 4.

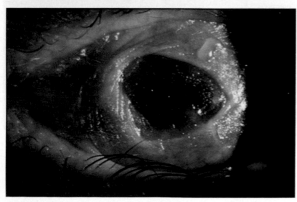

Figure 8-14. Ocular cicatricial pemphigoid stage 4 is associated with extensive symblepharon formation between the eyelid and the ocular surface. Extensive ocular surface keratinization is also present. Published with permission from Rapuano CJ, Luchs JI, Kim T, eds. *Anterior Segment: The Requisites in Ophthalmology.* New York, NY: Mosby Publishing; 2000. (Courtesy of Jodi I. Luchs, MD.)

Stevens-Johnson Syndrome (Erythema Multiforme Major)

Stevens-Johnson syndrome (SJS) is an acute inflammatory bullous disorder of the mucous membranes and skin characterized by immune complex deposition in the skin and conjunctiva (Figures 8-15 to 8-17). Causative agents include drugs such as penicillin, ampicillin, isoniazid, sulfonamides, salicylates, cardiovascular medications, and anticonvulsants.[46] Infections such as HSV, adenovirus, and streptococci have also been implicated.[47]

When the skin alone is involved, the term *erythema multiforme minor* is used; erythema multiforme major or SJS involves skin and mucous membranes.

Figure 8-15. Stevens-Johnson syndrome. Stevens-Johnson syndrome developed 1 month earlier in this patient as a result of amoxicillin treatment. The eyelid and skin lesions are beginning to resolve. Published with permission from Rapuano CJ, Luchs JI, Kim T, eds. *Anterior Segment: The Requisites in Ophthalmology.* New York, NY: Mosby Publishing; 2000. (Courtesy of Jodi I. Luchs, MD.)

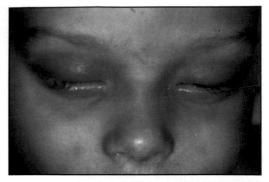

Figure 8-16. Stevens-Johnson syndrome. The left eye of this patient shows severe membranous conjunctivitis. Published with permission from Rapuano CJ, Luchs JI, Kim T, eds. *Anterior Segment: The Requisites in Ophthalmology.* New York, NY: Mosby Publishing; 2000. (Courtesy of Jodi I. Luchs, MD.)

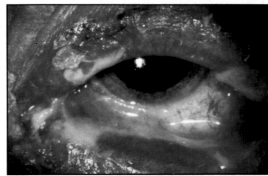

Figure 8-17. Stevens-Johnson syndrome. Extensive symblepharon formation and corneal scarring with ocular surface keratinization have developed after an episode of Stevens-Johnson syndrome. Published with permission from Rapuano CJ, Luchs JI, Kim T, eds. *Anterior Segment: The Requisites in Ophthalmology.* New York, NY: Mosby Publishing; 2000. (Courtesy of Jodi I. Luchs, MD.)

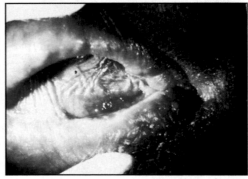

Sudden onset of malaise, fever, and upper respiratory congestion is the typical presentation. A few days later, skin manifestations take place; erythematous macules and papules, "bull's eye" lesions, and vesicular lesions are found on the arms, hands, legs, and feet (but not the trunk).[48] The mucous membranes of the eyes, mouth, and genitalia can be affected with vesicular changes that may progress to scarring and necrosis.

Early ocular findings in SJS are mucopurulent conjunctivitis and episcleritis. Bullae formation later leads to membrane formation. With continued inflammation, diffuse conjunctival scarring and symblepharon formation occurs. Cicatrization then leads to entropion/ectropion, trichiasis, and tear deficiency.

SJS is rare, with about 5 cases per million per year, and it occurs most commonly in young adults and children. AIDS patients are at a higher risk of developing SJS.[49] Patients with SJS are usually admitted to the hospital and care is coordinated by a team of infectious disease specialists, dermatologists, and ophthalmologists. If a causative agent is a medication, it is discontinued; if the cause is a microorganism, proper antimicrobial therapy is critical. Supportive therapy and close observation for secondary infections is important; studies have shown that patients admitted to the hospital burn unit have a better prognosis than those who are not. Treatment with systemic steroids still remains controversial; most authorities will treat severe cases of SJS with oral steroids, watching carefully for any serious complications, including infection.[50]

Ocular management in SJS surrounds the maintenance of the health of the ocular surface, particularly the cornea. Frequent ocular lubrication with artificial tears and ointments is the mainstay of treatment. Many physicians will use topical antibiotics as prophylaxis in these debilitated patients. Topical steroid use is controversial. Though surface inflammation is controlled with topical steroids, there is a higher risk of corneal thinning and infection.

Lysis of symblephara and use of symblepharon rings have been advocated as useful in SJS patients, but they are usually ineffective in ultimately preventing symblepharon formation.[51] Once the disease quiets, surgical correction of trichiasis, entropion, ectropion, and forniceal shortening can be attempted. Treatment of trichiasis and liberal use of tarsorrhaphy are crucial in protecting the ocular surface. The use of limbal allografts, with or without amniotic membrane placement, has been shown to be useful in corneal surface reconstruction in SJS patients with limbal stem cell failure.[52] PK has a poor prognosis in these severe SJS patients and may require simultaneous limbal stem cell transplantation. Permanent keratoprosthesis placement has had limited success in certain end-stage SJS cases, but long-term outcomes are still very poor.[53]

Graft-Versus-Host Disease

Graft-versus-host disease is a systemic condition resulting from allogenic bone marrow transplantation. In this disease, the grafted cells attack the patient's tissues, including the skin, lungs, liver, gastrointestinal system, and eyes. Most likely, graft-versus-host disease is a result of systemic sensitization of the donor cells, which recognize the recipient as foreign.

The most frequent ocular manifestation of this process is severe keratoconjunctivitis sicca. Lacrimal gland infiltration by T-lymphocytes and conjunctival inflammation with subepithelial fibrosis are causes of severe ocular surface dryness in these patients.[54] Intense conjunctival inflammation in graft-versus-host disease leads to limbal stem cell deficiency and subsequent corneal scarring.

Maintenance of the ocular surface with punctual occlusion and frequent lubrication is critical. Filamentary keratitis can be managed with 10% acetylcysteine. For severe cases of graft-versus-host disease, increased immunosuppression with tacrolimus (FK506)[55] or cyclosporine[56] may be required.

REFERENCES

1. Wilder RL. Rheumatoid arthritis: epidemiology, pathology and pathogenesis. In: *Primer on the Rheumatic Diseases*. 10th ed. Atlanta, GA: Arthritis Foundation; 1993.
2. Talal N. Sjogren's syndrome. In: Samter M, ed. *Immunologic Diseases*. 4th ed. Boston, MA: Little, Brown; 1988.
3. Jayson MI, Jones, DE. Scleritis and rheumatoid arthritis. *Ann Rheum Dis*. 1971;30:343-347.

4. Foster CS, Forstot SL, Wilson LA. Mortality rate in rheumatoid arthritis patients developing necrotizing scleritis or peripheral ulcerative keratits. *Ophthalmology.* 1984;91:1253-1263.

5. Watson PG. The diagnosis and management of scleritis. *Ophthalmology.* 1980;87:716-720.

6. Tuft SJ, Watson PG. Progression of scleral disease. *Ophthalmology.* 1991;98:467-471.

7. Foster CS. Immunosuppressive therapy for external ocular inflammatory disease. *Ophthalmology.* 1980;87:140-150.

8. Foster CS, Forstot SL, Wilson LA. Mortality rate in rheumatoid arthritis patients developing necrotizing scleritis or peripheral ulcerative keratitis: effects of systemic immunosuppression. *Ophthalmology.* 1984;91:1253-1263.

9. McCarthy JM, Dubord PJ, Chalmers A, Kassen BO, Rangno KK. Cyclosporine A for the treatment of necrotizing scleritis and corneal melting in patients with rheumatoid arthritis. *J Rheumatol.* 1992;19:1358-1361.

10. Jabs DA, Rosenbaum JT, Foster CS, et al. Guidelines for the use of immunosuppressive drugs in patients with ocular inflammatory disorders: recommendations of an expert panel. *Am J Ophthalmol.* 2000;130:492-513.

11. Liegner JT, Yee RW, Wild JH. Topical cyclosporine therapy for ulcerative keratitis associated with rheumatoid arthritis. *Am J Ophthalmol.* 1990;109:610-612.

12. Thomas JW, Pflugfelder SC. Therapy of progressive rheumatoid arthritis-associated corneal ulceration with infliximab. *Cornea.* 2005;24:742-744.

13. Tseng SC. Amniotic membrane transplantation for persistent corneal epithelial defect. *Br J Ophthalmol.* 2001;85:1400-1401.

14. Eiferman RA, Carothers DJ, Yankeelov JA Jr. Peripheral rheumatoid ulceration and evidence for conjunctival collagenase production. *Am J Ophthalmol.* 1979;87:703-709.

15. Hochberg MC, Boyd RE, Ahearn JM, et al. Systemic lupus erythematosis: a review of clinico-laboratory features and immunologic markers in 150 patients with emphasis on demographic subsets. *Medicine.* 1985;64:285-295.

16. Frith P, Burge SM, Millard PR, Wojnarowska F. External ocular findings in lupus erythematosis: a clinical and immunopathological study. *Br J Ophthalmol.* 1990;74:163-167.

17. Sangwan VS, Zafirakis P, Foster CS. Mooren's ulcer: current concepts in management. *Indian J Ophthalmol.* 1997;45:7-17.

18. Wood TO, Kaufman HE. Mooren's ulcer. *Am J Ophthalmol.* 1971;71:417-422.

19. Kietzman B. Mooren's ulcer in Nigeria. *Am J Ophthalmol.* 1968;65:679-685.

20. Young RD, Watson PG. Light and electron microscopy of corneal melting syndrome (Mooren's ulcer). *Br J Ophthalmol.* 1982;66:341-356.

21. Gottsch JD, Liu SH, Minkovitz JB, Goodman DF, Srinivasan M, Stark WJ. Autoimmunity to a cornea-associated stromal antigen in patients with Mooren's ulcer. *Invest Ophthalmol Vis Sci.* 1995;36:1541-1547.

22. Brown SI, Mondino BJ. Therapy of Mooren's ulcer. *Am J Ophthalmol.* 1984;98:1-6.

23. Wilson SE, Lee WM, Murakami C, et al. Mooren-type hepatitis C virus associated corneal ulceration. *Ophthalmology.* 1994;101:736-745.

24. Foster CS. Systemic immunosuppressive therapy for progressive bilateral Mooren's ulcer. *Ophthalmology.* 1985;92:1436-1439.

25. Wakefield D, Robinson LP. Cyclosporine therapy in Mooren's ulcer. *Br J Ophthalmol.* 1987;71:415-417.

26. Mozami G, Auran JD, Florakis GJ, et al. Interferon treatment of Mooren's ulcers associated with hepatitis C. *Am J Ophthalmol.* 1995;119:365-366.

27. Miller KH, Green WR, Stark WJ, Wells HA, Mendelsohn G, Kanhofer H. Immunoprotein deposition in the cornea. *Ophthalmology.* 1980;87:944-950.

28. Neumann E, Gutmann MJ, Blumenkrantz N, Michaelson IC. A review of 400 cases of vernal conjunctivitis. *Am J Ophthalmol.* 1959;74:166-172.

29. Allansmith MR. Vernal conjunctivitis. In: Duane T, ed. *Clinical Ophthalmology.* Vol 4. New York, NY: Harper and Row; 1978.

30. Garrity JA, Liesegang TJ. Ocular complications of atopic dermatitis. *Can J Ophthalmol.* 1984;19:21-24.

31. Tuft SJ, Kemeny DM, Dart JK, Buckley RJ. Clinical features of atopic keratoconjunctivitis. *Ophthalmology.* 1991;98:150-158.

32. Rich LF, Hanifin JM. Ocular complications of atopic dermatitis and other eczemas. *Int Ophthalmol Clin.* 1985;25:61-76.

33. McGeady SJ, Buckley RH. Depression of cell-mediated immunity in atopic eczema. *J Allergy Clin Immunol.* 1975;56:393-406.

34. Prabriputaloong T, Margolis TP, Lietman TM, Wong IG, Mather R, Gritz DC. Atopic disease and herpes simplex eye disease: a population-based case-control study. *Am J Ophthalmol.* 2006;142:745-749.

35. Foster CS. Evaluation of topical cromolyn sodium in the treatment of vernal keratoconjunctivitis. *Ophthalmology.* 1988;95:194-201.

36. BenEzra D, Pe'er J, Brodsky M, Cohen E. Cyclosporine eyedrops for the treatment of severe vernal keratoconjunctivitis. *Am J Ophthalmol.* 1986;101:278-282.

37. Rouher N, Pilon F, Dalens H, et al. Implantation of preserved human amniotic membrane for the treatment of shield ulcers and persistent corneal epithelial defects in chronic allergic keratoconjunctivitis. *J Fr Ophthalmol.* 2004;7:1091-1097.

38. Brusting LA, Perry HO. Benign pemphigoid? *Arch Dermatol.* 1957;75:489-501.

39. Foster CS, Wilson LA, Ekins MB. Immunosuppressive therapy for progressive ocular cicatricial pemphigoid. *Ophthalmology.* 1982;89(4):340-353.

40. Leonard JN, Wright P, Haffenden GP, Williams DM, Griffiths CE, Fry L. Skin diseases and the dry eye. *Trans Ophthalmol Soc UK.* 1985;104:467-476.

41. Mondino BJ, Brown SI. Ocular cicatricial pemphigoid. *Ophthalmology.* 1981;88:95-100.

42. Leonard JN, Hobday CM, Haffenden GP, et al. Immunofluorescent studies in ocular cicatricial pemphigoid. *Br J Dermatol.* 1988;118:209-217.

43. Foster CS, Sainz De La Maza M. Ocular cicatricial pemphigoid review. *Curr Opin Allergy Clin Immunol.* 2004;4:435-439.

44. Tugal-Tutkun I, Akova Y, Foster CS. Penetrating keratoplasty in cicatrizing conjunctival diseases. *Ophthalmology.* 1995;102:576-585.

45. Khan B, Dudenhoefer E, Dohlman C. Keratoprosthesis: an update. *Curr Opin Ophthalmol.* 2001;12:282-287.

46. Yetiv JZ, Bianchine JR, Owen JA. Etiologic factors of the Stevens-Johnson syndrome. *South Med J.* 1980;73:599-602.

47. Foerster DW, Scott LV. Isolation of herpes simplex virus from a patient with erythema multiforme exudativum. *N Engl J Med.* 1958;259:473-475.

48. Mondino BJ. Cicatricial pemphigoid and erythema multiforme. *Ophthalmology.* 1990;97:939-952.

49. Fagot JP, Mockenhaupt M, Bouwes-Bavinck JN, et al. Nevirapine and the risk of Stevens-Johnson syndrome or toxic epidermal necrolysis. *AIDS.* 2001;15:1843-1848.

50. Hynes AY, Kafkala C, Daoud YJ, Foster CS. Controversy in the use of high-dose systemic steroids in the acute care of patients with Stevens-Johnson syndrome. *Int Ophthalmol Clin.* 2005;45:25-48.

51. Yip LW, Thong BY, Lim J, et al. Ocular manifestations and complications of Stevens-Johnson syndrome and toxic epidermal necrolysis: an Asian series. *Allergy.* 2007;62:527-531.

52. Tsubota K, Toda I, Saito H, Shinozaki N, Shimazaki J. Reconstruction of the corneal epithelium by limbal allograft transplantation for severe ocular surface disorders. *Ophthalmology.* 1995;102:1486-1496.

53. Sayegh RR, Ang LP, Foster CS, Dohlman CH. The Boston keratoprosthesis in Stevens-Johnson syndrome. *Am J Ophthalmol.* 2008;145:438-444.

54. Bahn AK, Fujikawa LS, Foster CS. T-cell subsets and Langerhans cells in normal and diseased conjunctiva. *Am J Ophthalmol.* 1882;94:205-212.

55. Miyakoshi S, Kami M, Tanimoto T. Tacrolimus as prophylaxis for acute graft-versus-host disease in reduced intensity cord blood transplantation for adult patients with advanced hematologic diseases. *Transplantation*. 2007;84:316-322.

56. HJ Deeg, R Storb, ED Thomas, et al. Cyclosporine as prophylaxis for graft-versus-host disease: a randomized study in patients undergoing marrow transplantation for acute nonlymphoblastic leukemia. *Blood*. 1985;65:1325-1334.

9
METABOLIC AND CONGENITAL DISORDERS

Tracy S. Swartz, OD, MS; Michael D. Duplessie, MD; and Jodi I. Luchs, MD, FACS

Corneal manifestations of systemic disease related to metabolic disorders are frequent and may be the first indication of disease. Conditions are typically rare due to recessive inheritance, bilateral, and result in loss of corneal clarity due to deposition of various substances in the different layers of the cornea.

LIPID METABOLISM DISORDERS

Hyperlipoproteinemias

Ocular manifestations of hyperlipoproteinemias result from extracellular deposits of cholesterol, cholesterol esters, phospholipids, and triglycerides. They are common and often manifest as xanthelasma and arcus. Though arcus is common in older patients, presentation in a patient 35 to 40 years old or asymmetric presentation warrants investigation to rule out a lipid abnormality. Arcus may be associated with hypercholesterolemia, xanthelasma, alcohol, elevated blood pressure, cigarette smoking, diabetes, increasing age, and coronary heart disease. It remains unclear whether corneal arcus is an independent risk factor for coronary heart disease.[1]

Schnyder crystalline corneal dystrophy (crystalline stromal dystrophy) is thought to be a localized defect of lipid metabolism, which is covered in detail in Chapter 6.

Hypolipoproteinemias

Lecithin-cholesterol acyltransferase (LCAT) facilitates removal of cholesterol from the liver. Its deficiency leads to accumulation of unesterified cholesterol in the tissues, causing atherosclerosis, renal insufficiency, arcus, and nebular corneal clouding due to focal lipid deposition. Five disorders are related to abnormally low serum lipoprotein levels: LCAT deficiency, Tangier disease, fish eye disease, familial hypobetalipoproteinemia, and Bassen-Kornzweig syndrome.

Trattler WB, Majmudar PA, Luchs JI, Swartz TS, eds.
Cornea Handbook (pp. 141-162)
© 2010 SLACK Incorporated

Familial hypobetalipoproteinemia and Bassen-Kornzweig syndrome are not associated with corneal findings. The remaining disorders in the group are autosomal recessive conditions, and serum lipid profiles confirm characteristically low levels of high-density lipoprotein (HDL). LCAT deficiency and fish eye disease share the same genetic locus on chromosome 16q22.1. However, fish eye disease has normal levels of LCAT that fail to aid HDL in esterifying cholesterol. LCAT deficiency manifests with arcus and nebular stromal haze due to lipid deposition and rarely interferes with visual acuity.

Fish eye disease manifests with obvious clouding, which progresses toward the central cornea possibly reducing vision. Corneal opacities develop at the end of the second decade of life and consist of numerous minute grayish dots throughout the corneal stroma, giving the cornea its classic misty appearance.[2]

Tangier disease is associated with enlarged liver, spleen, and lymph nodes; hypocholesterolemia; abnormal chylomicron remnants; and low HDL in plasma, in addition to large, orange tonsils. Diffuse clouding of the cornea with stromal opacities may be noted. Confocal microscopy has suggested that pathologic corneal changes are limited to the stroma. The same study reported that reduced corneal sensation and lid abnormalities, previously described in Tangier disease, may not be present in all patients.[3] Tangier disease maps to chromosome 9q22-q31, and patients with the disease suffer from a complete absence of serum high-density α-lipoproteins.

Sphingolipidoses

Sphingolipidoses are disorders of complex lipids: gangliosides and sphingomyelin. They are rare, autosomal recessive (except for Fabry's disease), associated with retinal and optic nerve abnormalities, and may progress to central nervous system dysfunction. Three conditions involve the cornea: Fabry's disease, multiple sulfatase deficiency, and generalized gangliosidosis.

Fabry's disease is X-linked recessive. It is caused by an α-galactosidase A deficiency, resulting in accumulation of glycosphingolipids in the renal and cardiovascular systems. Systemic manifestations include skin lesions, renal failure, and peripheral neuropathy in the lower extremities. Ocular findings include cornea verticillata (Figure 9-1), conjunctival and retinal vessel tortuosity, and anterior and posterior cataracts.[4] Vessel tortuosity may indicate severity of the disease because it was found in those with more severe disease.[5] Women who are heterozygous for the gene may transmit the condition but are usually symptom-free, although they may have cornea verticillata.[6]

Multiple sulfatase deficiency is similar to metachromatic leukodystrophy and mucopolysaccharidoses. Corneal opacities, macular changes and optic nerve atrophy, and psychomotor delay are often seen in children, who typically die within the first decade of life. Enzyme replacement therapy studies may prove to be beneficial.[7]

Generalized gangliosidosis results from deficiencies of β-galactosidase and accumulation of gangliosides within the central nervous system and keratan sulfate in somatic tissues. Early infantile GM1 is the most severe subtype. It typically manifests shortly after birth and may include neurodegeneration, seizures, liver and spleen enlargement, skeletal irregularities, joint stiffness, distended abdomen, muscle weakness, deafness, and gait problems. Onset of late infantile GM1

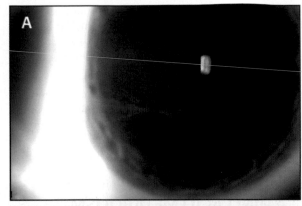

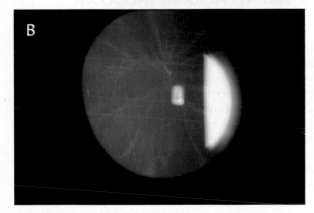

Figure 9-1. (A) Corneal verticillata associated with Fabry's disease. (Courtesy of University of Iowa Department of Ophthalmology and Visual Sciences.) (B) Verticillata associated with Fabry's disease seen in retroillumination. (Courtesy of University of Iowa Department of Ophthalmology and Visual Sciences.)

is typically between ages 1 and 3 years. Symptoms include ataxia, seizures, dementia, and speech difficulties. Adult GM1 manifests between ages 3 and 30, is less severe, and is associated with muscle atrophy, corneal clouding, and dystonia.[8] Cherry-red spot, optic atrophy, and corneal clouding have been reported,[9] as well as marked degeneration of the retinal ganglion cell and nerve fiber layers.[10]

Impaired elastic-fiber assembly may result in the corneal manifestations typically seen with these disorders. Corneal verticillata within the basal layers of the epithelium are typical. History rules out chloroquine or amiodarone treatment as the cause of the corneal changes. When vision is affected, PK is not recommended due to poor prognosis. Enzyme replacements with infusion of α-galactosidase A have been found to be beneficial.

Mucolipidoses

These conditions are similar to mucopolysaccharidoses and lipidoses due to the etiology and inherited defects of carbohydrate and lipid metabolism. They are due to a defect in lysosomal acid hydrolase enzymes. Mucopolysaccharides accumulate in the cornea, whereas sphingolipids deposit in the retina and central nervous system. These conditions are all autosomal recessive and include mucolipidosis I (dysmorphic sialidosis), II (inclusion cell disease), III (pseudo-Hurler polydystrophy), and IV (Goldberg syndrome; mannosidoses; and fucosidosis).

Retinal degeneration and a cherry-red spot are often found with many of these conditions. The epithelium is abnormal, making penetrating and lamellar keratoplasty in severe cases risky, in addition to the guarded visual prognosis.

Bietti Crystalline Corneoretinal Dystrophy

This disorder is autosomal recessive chorioretinal dystrophy characterized by progressive night blindness, tiny yellowish glistening retinal crystals, choroidal sclerosis, and crystalline deposits in the peripheral cornea. The CYP4V2 gene, which encodes a CYP450 family protein, is the causative gene of the disease.[11] Crystalline deposits are seen in the skin and lymphocytes rather than cholesterol or cholesterol esters.

DISORDERS OF AMINO ACID METABOLISM

Cystinosis

Cystinosis is caused by a defect in transport across lysosomal membranes that leads to accumulation of cystine within lysosomes. It has been mapped to chromosome 17p13 and is autosomal recessive. Typical presentation occurs at 1 year of age but it could occur much later. The infantile form (also called *nephropathic*) features dwarfism, renal dysfunction, deposits of fine crystals in the conjunctiva, corneal stroma, and other ocular structures.[12] This deposition results in photophobia, corneal erosions, and keratopathy.[13] Without renal transplant, these patients typically die within the first year.

The intermediate or adolescent form typically has less severe renal involvement, and these patients may live to the second or third decade. Life expectancy is normal in the adult form. Photophobia and glaucoma may result from crystals in the stroma and in the trabecular meshwork.[14]

Topical cysteamine reacts with intracellular cystine forming a cysteine-cysteamine disulfide resembling lysine. This is transported by the lysine transport system through the lysosomes. Cysteamine used topically reduces the crystalline deposits and improves pain associated with recurrent corneal erosions.[15]

Tyrosinemia

Tyrosinemia (II) is an autosomal recessive disorder caused by a defect in the hepatic tyrosine aminotransferase gene responsible for converting tyrosine to 4-hydroxyphenylpyruvate. The condition typically presents with herpetiform corneal ulcers, photophobia, conjunctival injection, hyperkeratotic skin lesions, and mental retardation.

A special diet restricting phenylalanine and tyrosine may improve the eye condition as well as other manifestations. Maintaining tyrosine levels below 800μmol/L appears to be protective against pathology, including neurological sequelae. 2-(2-Nitro-4-trifluoromethylbenzoyl)-1,3-cyclohexanedione (NTBC) for tyrosinemia type I treatment has been found to be beneficial.[16]

Alkaptonuria

Alkaptonuria is an autosomal recessive disorder due to defective tyrosine metabolism mapping to gene locus 3q21-q23. Patients lack the enzyme homogentisate 1,2-dioxygenase (HGO) required to fully metabolize tyrosine and phenylalanine. This deficiency results in accumulation of homogentisic acid, which is rapidly cleared in the kidney and excreted. Pigmentation of the eye, nose, and earlobes (ochronosis) is an early finding. Ocular involvement may be seen in up to 70% of patients who may present with a blue/black deposition in the sclera, just anterior to the insertion of the rectus muscles. Deposits may also be found in the corneal epithelium or Bowman's layer as a dark pigment. The hallmark sign of the disorder is urine that turns black upon standing.[17]

DISORDERS OF PROTEIN METABOLISM

Amyloidosis

Amyloidosis is a multisystem disease that can be classified as primary or secondary, local or systemic, or according to which type of amyloid is deposited. The presentation and prognosis will vary according to the etiology. Precurser protein mutations will cause inherited flaws.[18] Systemic primary amyloidosis arises from immunocyte dyscrasias.[19] Secondary amyloidosis results from chronic inflammation.[20] Many different proteins are associated with amyloid in humans. Most are constituents of the plasma.[21]

Neurological diseases such as Alzheimer's disease,[22] bovine spongiform encephalopathy,[23] Creutzfeldt-Jakob disease,[15] Huntington's disease,[24] kuru,[25] and Parkinson's disease[26] all show amyloid deposition.

The amyloid is deposited in a fibril formed by the stacking of beta-pleated sheets.[27] Amyloid is the core of the fibril.[28] The secondary structure of the protein is altered, resulting in a relatively insoluble protein. Histologically, amyloid will stain orange/red with Congo red stain and exhibit a distinctive apple green birefringence and dichroism when viewed under polarized light (Figure 9-2). It will also exhibit metochromasia when stained with crystal violet and yellow-green ultraviolet fluorescence when stained with thioflavin T. Biopsies should be taken where possible from affected organs such as the kidney, conjunctiva, rectum, or anterior adipose tissue. A circulating protein called *serum amyloid* P component (SAP) is also found in amyloid.[29] Radionuclide SAP scans can locate amyloid deposits.[30]

Ocular manifestations of amyloid are varied and may be found in primary or secondary localized or systemic amyloid (Figures 9-3 and 9-4). The classifications and ocular manifestations of amyloid are summarized in Table 9-1.

DISORDERS OF CARBOHYDRATE METABOLISM

Mucopolysaccharidoses

These disorders are rare, inherited diseases resulting from absence of lysosomal acid hydrolases, enzymes that catabolize the GAGs, dermatan sulfate, heparin sulfate, and keratan sulfate. The lack of the enzymes causes accumulation of metabolites that cause changes in the cornea. All syndromes are autosomal recessive with the exception of Hunter syndrome, which is X-linked recessive. They affect multiple organs and physiologic systems and have variable ages of onset and variable rates of progression.[31]

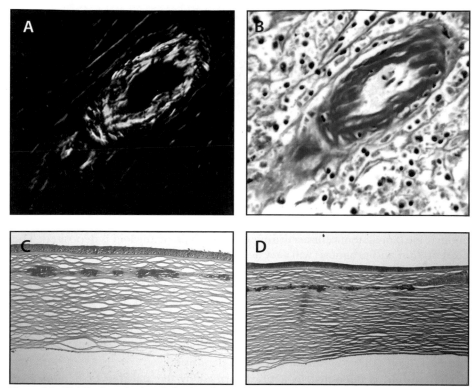

Figure 9-2. (A) A blood vessel with amyloid in the wall, stained by Congo red. This appears red in unpolarized light. (Courtesy of Professor Alec J. Howie.) (B) The blood vessel in Figure 9-2A, examined between crossed polarizer and analyzer. This shows a bright green anomalous color. (Courtesy of Professor Alec J. Howie.) (C) Low-magnification histopathological corneal button section depicting Congo red staining of amyloid deposits in Avellino corneal dystrophy. (Courtesy of W. Barry Lee, MD.) (D) Low-magnification histopathological corneal button section depicting Masson's trichrome staining of hyaline deposits in Avellino dystrophy. (Courtesy of W. Barry Lee, MD.)

Figure 9-3. A slit-lamp photograph depicting Avellino corneal dystrophy with a combination of amyloid and hyaline deposition in the anterior stroma. (Courtesy of W. Barry Lee, MD.)

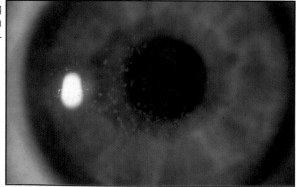

GAGs normally constitute the ground substance of the cornea. In these disorders, microscopic mucopolysaccharide deposits are found in the stroma and, in some cases, the endothelium and epithelium. Specific diagnosis requires biochemical assays for enzymes in tears, amniotic cells, and leukocytes and testing for elevated urinary GAG levels. Treatment may include enzyme replacement

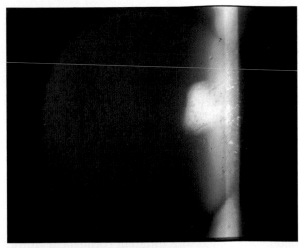

Figure 9-4. A slit-lamp photograph demonstrating polymorphic amyloid degeneration with amyloid deposits seen on retroillumination. (Courtesy of W. Barry Lee, MD.)

Table 9-1

OCULAR MANIFESTATIONS OF AMYLOIDOSIS

Primary systemic amyloidosis	Amyloid deposition in eyelids, extraocular muscles, orbit and vitreous
Primary localized amyloidosis	Amyloid deposition in conjunctiva and cornea (gelatinous drop-like dystrophy) May be associated with systemic lymphoma
Secondary systemic amyloidosis	Associated with rheumatoid arthritis, leprosy, Mediterranean fever, and bronchiectasis Eyelids less commonly affected than in primary systemic amyloidosis
Secondary localized amyloidosis	Secondary to chronic ocular inflammation (ie, trachoma, interstitial keratitis) Conjunctival and corneal deposition

Adapted from Rapuano CJ, Luchs JI, Kim T, eds. *Anterior Segment: The Requisites in Ophthalmology.* New York, NY: Mosby Publishing; 2000.

therapy with recombinant human iduronate-2-sulphatase (idursulfase). Weekly intravenous infusions of idursulfase have been shown to improve many of the clinical manifestations in patients with MPS II.[32]

These syndromes as a group are characterized by corneal clouding, retinopathy, and optic neuropathy. Hunter syndrome and Sanfilippo rarely show corneal changes. The quantity of GAGs that accumulates is directly related to the amount of corneal clouding, which typically affects the entire cornea and may be present at birth. These patients may have severe physical impairments and shorter life expectancies. Though the risk for corneal graft failure is significant, the improvement of vision for a short time may allow these patients to function better during their short lifetimes.[33]

Diabetes

Diabetes is the most common carbohydrate metabolism disorder and is associated with nonspecific corneal findings. These may include dry eye, punctuate epithelial keratitis, basement membrane irregularities (Figure 9-5), decreased corneal sensation, folds in Descemet's membrane, and microbial keratitis.[34] Corneal abnormalities typically result from structural abnormalities in the basement membrane complex. Problems which affect epithelial-stromal adhesion include thickened basement membranes and reduced hemidesmosomes, resulting in recurrent corneal erosions. Diabetic patients have been found to have a significantly reduced Schirmer's test result and corneal sensitivity, suggesting reduced basal tear production due to a peripheral neuropathy affecting corneal sensation and lacrimal gland function.[5]

The peripheral neuropathy can now be directly imaged using noninvasive corneal confocal microscopy, which enables direct visualization of the peripheral nerve in vivo.[35] This has been suggested as a method to evaluate the severity of diabetes. The advances in technology have led to further classification of diabetes to include prediabetic neuropathy or neuropathy of impaired glucose tolerance.[36] This technology may also be used to monitor treatment.[37,38]

Though diabetes is not commonly associated with different corneal curvature, one study found that the optical power of the posterior corneal surface of the patients with diabetes differed significantly from that of the healthy subjects. Corneal thickness, anterior radius and asphericity, and overall corneal power were similar to those of healthy subjects.[39]

DISORDERS OF IMMUNOGLOBULIN SYNTHESIS: NONINFLAMMATORY DISORDERS OF THE CONNECTIVE TISSUE

Ehlers-Danlos Syndrome

Ehlers-Danlos syndrome represents a group of inherited disorders that affect connective tissues.[40] The inheritance pattern and prevalence of Ehlers-Danlos syndrome (EDS) varies by type (Table 9-2). The most common form of inheritance pattern is autosomal dominant. Mutations in the ADAMTS2, COL1A1, COL1A2, COL3A1, COL5A1, COL5A2, PLOD1, and TNXB genes cause Ehlers-Danlos syndrome.[41] These mutations affect proteins that involve collagen, disrupting its formation.

Features vary by type, with the joints and skin commonly affected. Loose joints have a greater incidence of complications such as arthritis, chronic pain, joint instability, and dislocation. The shoulders, hips, and knees are frequently involved.

Skin has increased elasticity but tends to be delicate, with a tendency for bruising and poor wound healing. Small blood vessels are fragile. Scarring tends to be more pronounced. Chronic recurrent headaches may be the neurologic presentation of EDS.[42]

Myopia, occasionally extreme, is a typical presentation of Ehlers-Danlos syndrome.[43] Blue sclera can be seen with an increased susceptibility to traumatic injury,[44] as well as spontaneous perforation.[45] Abnormal retinal blood vessels have been noted with type VI.[46] Type VI Ehlers-Danlos syndrome is associated with deficient activity of lysyl hydroxylase.[47] Ectopia lentis is also seen.[48]

The cornea is often abnormally thin with limbus-to-limbus corneal thinning. Steep corneas often manifest astigmatism, but no increase in the incidence of

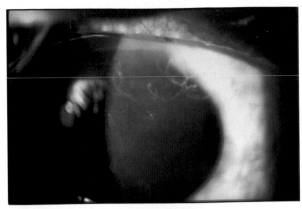

Figure 9-5. Irregular epithelium in a diabetic patient.

Table 9-2

TYPES OF EHLERS-DANLOS SYNDROME[134]

Hypermobility type[135]	1 in 10 000
Classic type	1 in 30 000
Vascular type[136]	1 in 250 000
Dermatosparaxis type[137]	Rare
Arthrochalasia type[138]	Rare
Kyphoscoliosis type	Rare

keratoconus has been reported.[49] The eyelids can be floppy.[50] All types of Ehlers-Danlos remain a contraindication to laser refractive surgery.[51]

Marfan Syndrome

Marfan syndrome is an autosomal dominant disorder of the connective tissue. Those with Marfan's tend to be tall, slender individuals. The signs and symptoms vary widely in timing of initial presentation, rate of progression, and severity. The incidence of Marfan syndrome is 1 in 5000.[52] Most Marfan patients have mutations in the FBN1 gene.[53] The FBN1 gene is responsible for the protein fibrillin-1,[54] which forms microfibrils[55] that are essential elements in elastic and nonelastic tissues. They account for the flexibility and strength of connective tissue. A small percentage of Marfan syndrome cases are caused by mutations in the TGFBR2 gene[56] (Marfan type II). A significant percentage is due to de novo genetic mutations.

Aside from being typically tall and slender, individuals tend to have an arm span that exceeds their body height.[57] There is often arachnodactyl of the fingers with joint laxity.[58] The chest bony structure is often abnormal, and scoliosis, pectus excavatum, and pectus carinatum are often seen.[59] There is an increased risk of pneumothorax.[60] The palate is high and arched.[61] Abnormalities of the heart and the aorta are not uncommon. Mitral valve prolapse, aortic aneurysm, aortic incompetence, and aortic dissection[62] can be life threatening.

Subluxation of the lens[63] may occur in up to 70% of patients and is generally bilateral, superotemporal, or upward (Figure 9-6). Glaucoma occurs more frequently in people with Marfan syndrome, and angle closure glaucoma has also been reported.[64] There was a significant difference in keratometry values between Marfan and control patients,[65] as well as an increased incidence of keratoconus[66] and hypoplasia of the dilator papillae. Increased axial myopia in these patients is associated with a corresponding increase in rates sf retinal detachment.[67]

Eye surgery can be safely performed on Marfan's patients.[68] Primary anterior chamber intraocular lens (ACIOL) placement in children with Marfan syndrome has shown promise.[69] Reports also suggest that iris fixation of foldable intraocular lenses (IOLs) for ectopia lentis in children can lead to good results.[70] Endocapsular ring implantation has also been used to aid cataract surgery in Marfan syndrome.[71]

NUCLEOTIDE METABOLISM DISORDERS

Gout

Gout is a metabolic disorder that results from an excess of uric acid in the blood and tissues; it is typically associated with acute inflammatory attacks of arthritis.[72] It is the most common cause of inflammatory joint disease in men over 40 years of age. The joints of the foot, knee, ankle, and hand are commonly affected; the big toe is affected in 70% of cases.[75] Gout can affect the eyelids, cornea,[74] conjunctiva, iris,[73] and muscles. It has been also known to cause uveitis.[76]

The Egyptians first described gout in 2640 BC.[77] It typically affects men between the ages of 40 and 60, particularly those who are overweight.[78] It can occur from excess consumption of protein or alcohol, and its prevalence is increasing.[79]

Gout is usually diagnosed on the basis of its classic signs and symptoms. Elevated serum uric acid levels are usually found in these patients,[80] and joint aspirations will show the needle-like uric acid crystals.[81] Ocular manifestations vary and are listed in Table 9-3.

Nonsteroidal anti-inflammatory drugs are used as first-line therapy. Lifestyle modification is vital[82]; patients should avoid foods rich in purines. Patients with recurrent gout will require long-term drug treatment. Allopurinol reduces production of uric acid[83] but is associated with an increased risk of cataract formation.[84] Probenecid also increases the excretion of uric acid.[85]

Porphyria

Porphyrias are a group of disorders caused by abnormalities in the production of hemoglobin.[86] Enzyme abnormalities cause the accumulation of the precursor products called *porphyrin*.[87] The failure of porphyrin precursors to be excreted causes an accumulation in the skin or central nervous system. They are inherited in both an autosomal dominant and autosomal recessive fashion.[88] Descriptions of porphyria date from the time of Hippocrates.[89] Porphyria is a derivative of the Greek word for *purple*; darkening of urine is seen in some types of porphyria.[41]

The clinical manifestations and treatments for each porphyria are different.[90,91] Active symptoms can be triggered by drugs, infections, stress, menstruation, and exposure to the sun.[91] Early diagnosis with initiation of therapy is beneficial.[92] Porphyria is diagnosed through blood,[93] urine,[94] and stool tests.

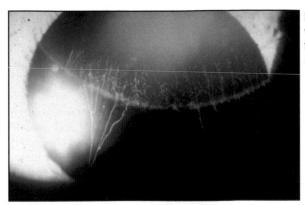

Figure 9-6. Marfan syndrome is associated with crystalline lens dislocation. Reprinted from Barkana et al.[64] (Courtesy of Robert Ritch, MD.)

Table 9-3

DEPOSITION OF URATE CRYSTALS IN OCULAR TISSUE CAN RESULT IN A VARIETY OF OCULAR COMPLICATIONS[139]

- Conjunctival nodules containing needle-like crystals[140]
- Anterior uveitis[141]
- Band keratopathy with crystals deposited in the epithelium[142] and Bowman's membrane. There was no increased incidence of dry eye[143]
- Crystals deposit in the sclera and the tendons of the muscles[139]
- Increased incidence of cataracts[144] as a result of allopurinol[145,146]
- Epithelial breakdown resulting in keratitis[147]
- Eyelid tophi[148]
- Increased retinal venule diameter[149] and retinal aneurysms[150]
- Macular changes[151]

The incidence of age-related macular degeneration (ARMD) is higher in patients with gout. No relationship to asteroid hyalosis.[152]

Ocular complications can include decreased vision,[95,96] scleromalacia,[97] cicatricial conjunctivitis,[98] scleritis,[99] and optic atrophy.[100]

MINERAL METABOLISM DISORDERS

Wilson's Disease

Wilson's disease is a rare autosomal recessive disorder in which excessive amounts of copper accumulate in the body.[101] There is a mutation in the copper-transporting gene ATP7B[102] such that copper is not released properly into bile.[103] Excessive copper in the liver causes hepatitis and an increased concentration of copper in the bloodstream, leading to damage of the liver, brain, eyes, and kidneys.[61] Failure to properly treat Wilson's disease can result in liver failure, brain damage, and death.[104] One in 30 000 people have Wilson's disease; most patients have no family history of Wilson's disease.[105]

Symptoms can appear in late childhood or early adolescence.[106] Acute or chronic hepatitis, liver failure, and progressive liver disease[107] can be early presentations. Copper deposition in the central nervous system, specifically the basal ganglia,[108] can cause psychiatric problems,[109] tremors, dysarthria, dystonia, bradykinesia, dysphagia, and spasticity.[110]

The diagnosis can be made by slit-lamp examination (Figure 9-7) of Kayser-Fleischer rings, low serum ceruloplasmin, normal total serum copper levels, high urine copper, liver biopsy for histology, and copper quantification,[111] and genetic testing, haplotype analysis for siblings, and mutation analysis. The most characteristic sign is the Kayser-Fleisher ring, in which copper deposits in Descemet's membrane produce a brownish yellow limbal ring. It appears first in the superior cornea and then becomes circumferential. Early deposits may only be visible gonioscopically. Almost all patients with central nervous system disease will have rings, whereas slightly more than half of patients with hepatic disease will have a Kayser-Fleischer ring.[112] Copper chelating will cause a disappearance of the Kayser-Fleischer ring. A green sunflower cataract can be also seen in some patients.[113] There are some reports of an increased difficulty with accommodation,[114,115] and one case of rapid vision loss from Wilson's disease has been reported.[116]

Hypercalcemia

Hypercalcemia is a blood disease caused by elevated levels of blood calcium. Parathyroid gland hyperactivity is the most common reason. Calcium balance is controlled by the parathyroid hormone, calcitonin, and vitamin D3.[117] Band keratopathy may be seen in patients with elevated calcium levels (Figure 9-8).

Osteogenesis Imperfecta

Osteogenesis imperfecta is a genetic disorder characterized by fragile bones that break easily. Its prevalence in the United States is 20 000 to 50 000 individuals. It is inherited in an autosomal dominant and autosomal recessive manner. It is possible to diagnose based on clinical features but collagen biopsies and DNA testing will detect 90% of all type I collagen mutations.

Clinical characteristic features vary greatly. The majority of cases are caused by a dominant mutation in a gene coding for type I collagen. There are as many as 8 different types of osteogenesis imperfecta. Bones fracture easily. Stature can vary. Facial and other bony deformities are not uncommon.

Sclera usually have a blue,[118,119] purple, or gray[120] tint.[121] Central corneal thickness is lower in osteogenesis imperfecta and negatively correlates with the presence of blue sclera.[122]

CONGENITAL DISORDERS

Mesodermal Dysgenesis

Mesodermal dysgenesis is a group of congenital disorders that can affect the iris, cornea, and lens and are frequently associated with congenital glaucoma. These congenital corneal abnormalities typically involve incomplete migration of mesodermal or neural crest tissues. Ocular abnormalities may be evident during the newborn examination or, for the milder variants, may present during routine

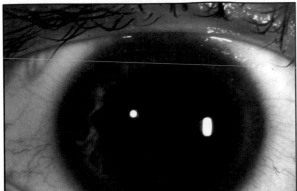

Figure 9-7. Ocular copper deposition associated with monoclonal gammopathy. (Courtesy of Patrick Tzelikis, MD, and Peter Laibson, MD.)

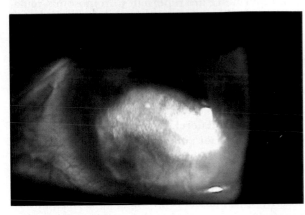

Figure 9-8. Band keratopathy may be noted in patients with hypercalcemia.

examination. This group includes posterior embryotoxon, Axenfield's, Rieger's, and Peter's anomalies.

Posterior Embryotoxon

The typical anterior segment findings including a prominent, thickened anteriorly displaced Schwalbe's line.[123] This typically presents as a white arc central to the limbus. It may be found in 15% to 30% of normal individuals. Systemic associations are rare. No treatment is necessary if it is an isolated finding. Posterior embryotoxon is not a precursor to forme fruste of Axenfeld-Rieger's syndrome.[124] It is typically autosomal dominantly inherited.

Axenfeld's Anomaly and Axenfeld's Syndrome

An autosomal dominant condition, Axenfeld's anomaly manifests on slit-lamp examination with posterior embryotoxon and prominent iris processes attached to Schwalbe's line. It may be associated with hypertelorism and Down syndrome.[125]

Axenfeld's syndrome is the Axenfeld's anomaly plus glaucoma. Skeletal, auditory, and cardiac anomalies, including tetralogy of Fallot, have been reported.[126] The etiology of both Axenfeld's and Reiger's is a developmental arrest of neural crest cells leaving primordial endothelial changes, causing the resultant iris changes. Secondary glaucoma results from an incomplete maturation of the trabecular meshwork and Schlemm's canal and a high insertion of the iris,[127] and is difficult to control.[128]

Reiger's Anomaly and Reiger's Syndrome

Also autosomal dominant by inheritance, this anomaly includes posterior embryotoxon, prominent iris processes, and atrophy of the iris stroma. It results in anterior iris stromal hypoplasia and pupillary abnormalities, including peripheral anterior synechiae, corectopia, and pseudopolycoria. The syndrome has all the characteristics of Reiger's anomaly with associated systemic problems. Microdontia, maxillary hypoplasia, and other bony malformations have been described. Cardiac anomalies have been reported[129] and a careful cardiac workup is suggested in these patients.

Peter's Anomaly

Peter's anomaly shows a more sporadic genetic pattern, but both autosomal recessive and dominant modes of inheritance are reported. Chromosomal mutations at chromosome 11 and 13 have been proposed. Pax6 3' deletion has been associated with Peter's anomaly.[130] The anomaly has been reported as a feature of fetal alcohol syndrome.[131] There is an absence of posterior corneal tissue with a central corneal leukoma. The absence of corneal endothelium and Descemet's membrane in the area of the defect produces an overlying corneal opacity due to chronic corneal edema and stromal scarring. There often are iridocorneal adhesions to the leukoma, adhesions with a cataract, corectopia, and scleralization of the cornea. Eighty percent of the cases are bilateral. Fifty percent of the patients have glaucoma. The lens usually has an anterior polar cataract. Associated ocular abnormalities include microphthalmos, persistent hyperplastic primary vitreous, optic nerve hypoplasia, and retinal dysplasia.

Systemic abnormalities associated with Peter's anomaly include mental retardation, urogenital malformations, craniofacial and skeletal abnormalities, hydrocephalus, pulmonary hypoplasia, cleft and palate deformities, and cardiac complications.

Early PK is often performed to correct the leukoma in bilateral cases to reduce the risk of amblyopia; however, there is a high risk of failure in Peter's anomaly.[132] The long-term probability of maintaining a clear graft after initial PK for Peter's anomaly is 35%, with subsequent grafts rarely surviving.[133]

Megalocornea and Microcornea

These corneal abnormalities are due to growth abnormalities of the optic cup during development.

Megalocornea

X-linked, nonprogressive enlargement of anterior segment. The patients are typically myopic. Corneal size is between 13 and 18 mm. The finding is associated with Marfan syndrome, craniosynostosis and ichthyosis, and Alport and Down syndromes.

Microcornea

Microcornea is defined as corneal size less than 10 mm. It is generally autosomal dominant, and patients are typically hyperopic. It may be complicated by glaucoma and is associated with Weill-Markesan, Ehlers-Danlos, Reiger's syndrome, and Norrie's disease.

CORNEAL HYPOSTHESIA

This disorder can be either physiological, due to increasing aging of the peripheral cornea, or pathological, due to congenital maldevelopment, Riley-Day syndrome, congenital corneal hyposthesia proper, or corneal dystrophies such as Reis Buckler's dystrophy or lattice dystrophy. It can be acquired in cases of herpes simplex, diabetes mellitus, and leprosy, or iatrogenic in cases of contact lens wear, use of certain topical eye drops (timolol, atropine, sulphur drugs), and due to corneal surgery (ECCE, PK, LASIK, epikeratophakia).

REFERENCES

1. Fernandez A, Sorokin A, Thompson PD. Corneal arcus as coronary artery disease risk factor. *Atherosclerosis.* 2007;193:235-240.

2. Clerc M, Dumon MF, Sess D, Freneix-Clerc M, Mackness M, Conri C. A "Fish-eye disease" familial condition with massive corneal opacities and hypoalphalipoproteinaemia: clinical, biochemical and genetic features. *Eur J Clin Invest.* 1991;21:616-624.

3. Herrmann WA, von Mohrenfels CW, Lohmann CP. Confocal microscopy and corneal sensitivity in a patient with corneal manifestations of Tangier disease. *Cornea.* 2004;23:825-827.

4. Nguyen TT, Gin T, Nicholls K, Low M, Galanos J, Crawford A. Ophthalmological manifestations of Fabry disease: a survey of patients at the Royal Melbourne Fabry Disease Treatment Centre. *Clin Exp Ophthalmol.* 2005;33:164-168.

5. Sodi A, Ioannidis AS, Mehta A, Davey C, Beck M, Pitz S. Ocular manifestations of Fabry's disease: data from the Fabry Outcome Survey. *Br J Ophthalmol.* 2007;91:210-214.

6. Masson C, Cissé I, Simon V, Insalaco P, Audran M. Fabry disease: a review. *Joint Bone Spine.* 2004;71:381-383.

7. Tomatsu S, Gutierrez M, Nishioka T, et al. Development of MPS IVA mouse (Galnstm(hC79S. mC76S)slu) tolerant to human N-acetylgalactosamine-6-sulfate sulfatase. *Hum Mol Genet.* 2005;14:3321-3335.

8. NINDS gangliosidoses information page. National Institute of Neurological Disorders and Stroke Web site. http://www.ninds.nih.gov/disorders/gangliosidoses/Gangliosidoses. htm. Accessed April 8, 2008.

9. Sorcinelli R, Sitzia A, Loi M. Cherry-red spot, optic atrophy and corneal cloudings in a patient suffering from GM1 gangliosidosis type I. *Metab Pediatr Syst Ophthalmol,* 1987;10(3):62-63.

10. Cairns LJ, Green WR, Singer HS. GM1 gangliosidosis, type 2: ocular clinicopathologic correlation. *Graefes Arch Clin Exp Ophthalmol.* 1984;222(2):51-62.

11. Nakamura M, Lin J, Nishiguchi K, Kondo M, Sugita J, Miyake Y. Bietti crystalline corneoretinal dystrophy associated with CYP4V2 gene mutations. *Adv Exp Med Biol.* 2006;572:49-53.

12. Fung AT, Fraser-Bell S, Ojaimi E, Sutton G. In vivo confocal microscopy and polarizing microscopy of the cornea in a patient with nephropathic cystinosis. *Clin Exp Ophthalmol.* 2007;35:292-293.

13. Gahl WA, Kuehl EM, Iwata F, et al. Corneal crystals in nephropathic cystinosis: natural history and treatment with cysteamine eyedrops. *Mol Genet Metab.* 2000;71:100-120.

14. Mungan N, Nischal KK, Héon E, MacKeen L, Balfe JW, Levin AV. Ultrasound biomicroscopy of the eye in cystinosis. *Arch Ophthalmol.* 2000;118:1329-1333.

15. Debatin L, Streffer J, Geissen M, Matschke J, Aguzzi A, Glatzel M. Association between deposition of beta-amyloid and pathological prion protein in sporadic Creutzfeldt-Jakob disease. *Neurodegener Dis.* 2008;5:347-354.

16. Masurel-Paulet A, Poggi-Bach J, Rolland MO, et al. NTBC treatment in tyrosinaemia type I: long-term outcome in French patients. *J Inherit Metab Dis.* 2008;31:81-87.

17. Cheskes J, Buettner H. Ocular manifestations of alkaptonuric ochronosis. *Arch Opthalmol.* 2000;118:724-725.

18. Ahn KW, Joo Y, Choi Y, et al. Swedish amyloid precursor protein mutation increases cell cycle-related proteins in vitro and in vivo. *J Neurosci Res.* 2008;86:2476-2487.

19. Tanasilovi S, Zivanovi D, Nikoli M, Tomovi M, Elezovi I, Medenica L. Primary systemic amyloidosis. *Vojnosanit Pregl.* 2007;64:859-862.

20. Nakamura T, Higashi S, Tomoda K, Tsukano M, Baba S. Efficacy of etanercept in patients with AA amyloidosis secondary to rheumatoid arthritis. *Clin Exp Rheumatol.* 2007;25:518-522.

21. Ando Y, Jono H. Pathogenesis and therapy for transthyretin related amyloidosis. *Rinsho Byori.* 2008;56:114-120.

22. Fein JA, Sokolow S, Miller CA, et al. Co-localization of amyloid beta and tau pathology in Alzheimer's disease synaptosomes. *Am J Pathol.* 2008;172:1683-1692.

23. Bishop MT, Kovacs GG, Sanchez-Juan P, Knight RS. Cathepsin D SNP associated with increased risk of variant Creutzfeldt-Jakob disease. *BMC Med Genet.* 2008;9:31.

24. Calingasan NY, Ho DJ, Wille EJ, et al. Influence of mitochondrial enzyme deficiency on adult neurogenesis in mouse models of neurodegenerative diseases. *Neuroscience.* 2008; 153:986-996.

25. Liberski PP. Amyloid plaques in transmissible spongiform encephalopathies (prion diseases). *Folia Neuropathol.* 2004;42(suppl B):109-119.

26. Jellinger KA. Striatal beta-amyloid deposition in Parkinson disease with dementia. *J Neuropathol Exp Neurol.* 2008;67:484.

27. Xu S. Aggregation drives "misfolding" in protein amyloid fiber formation. *Amyloid.* 2007; 14:119-131.

28. Lin MS, Chen LY, Tsai HT, et al. Investigation of the mechanism of beta-amyloid fibril formation by kinetic and thermodynamic analyses. *Langmuir.* 2008;24:5802-5808.

29. Voss A, Nielsen EH, Svehag SE, Junker P. Serum amyloid P component-DNA complexes are decreased in systemic lupus erythematosus. Inverse association with anti-dsDNA antibodies. *J Rheumatol.* 2008;35:625-630.

30. Hawkins PN, Lavender JP, Pepys MB. Evaluation of systemic amyloidosis by scintigraphy with 123I-labeled serum amyloid P component. *N Engl J Med.* 1990;323:508-513.

31. Martin R, Beck M, Eng C, et al. Recognition and diagnosis of mucopolysaccharidosis II (Hunter syndrome). *Pediatrics.* 2008;121:e377-e386.

32. Wraith JE, Scarpa M, Beck M, et al. Mucopolysaccharidosis type II (Hunter syndrome): a clinical review and recommendations for treatment in the era of enzyme replacement therapy. *Eur J Pediatr.* 2008;167:267-277.

33. Käsmann-Kellner B, Weindler J, Pfau B, Ruprecht KW. Ocular changes in mucopolysaccharidosis IV A (Morquio A syndrome) and long-term results of perforating keratoplasty. *Ophthalmologica.* 1999;213:200-205.

34. Cousen P, Cackett P, Bennett H, Swa K, Dhillon B. Tear production and corneal sensitivity in diabetes. *J Diabetes Complicat.* 2007;21:371-373.

35. Ruggeri A, Scarpa F, Grisan E. Analysis of corneal images for the recognition of nerve structures. *Conf Proc IEEE Eng Med Biol Soc.* 2006;1:4739-4742.

36. Boulton AJ. Diabetic neuropathy: classification, measurement and treatment. *Curr Opin Endocrinol Diabetes Obes.* 2007;14:141-145.

37. Mehra S, Tavakoli M, Kallinikos PA, et al. Corneal confocal microscopy detects early nerve regeneration after pancreas transplantation in patients with type 1 diabetes. *Diabetes Care.* 2007;30:2608-2612.

38. Babu K, Narasimha Murthy K, Ramachandra Murthy K. Wavelike epitheliopathy after phacoemulsification: role of in vivo confocal microscopy. *Cornea.* 2007;26:747-748.

39. Wiemer NG, Dubbelman M, Kostense PJ, Ringens PJ, Polak BC. The influence of chronic diabetes mellitus on the thickness and the shape of the anterior and posterior surface of the cornea. *Cornea.* 2007;26:1165-1170.

40. Parapia LA, Jackson C. Ehlers-Danlos syndrome—a historical review. *Br J Haematol.* 2008;141:32-35.

41. A 27-year-old woman with abdominal pain, vomiting, dark urine and hyponatremia. *Rev Clin Esp.* 1995;195:726-736.

42. Jacome DE. Headache in Ehlers-Danlos syndrome. *Cephalalgia.* 1999;19:791-796.

43. Paluru P, Ronan SM, Heon E, et al. New locus for autosomal dominant high myopia maps to the long arm of chromosome 17. *Invest Ophthalmol Vis Sci.* 2003;44:1830-1836.

44. Cosar CB, Ceyhan N, Sevim S, et al. Corneal perforation with minor trauma: Ehlers-Danlos syndrome type VI. *Ophthalmic Surg Laser Imaging.* 2005;36:350-351.

45. Puri P, Gupta M, Chan J. Spontaneous perforation of the globe in Ehlers Danlos syndrome. *Eye.* 2001;15(pt 4):553-554.

46. Chikamoto N, Teranishi S, Chikama T, Nishida T, Ohshima K, Hatsukawa Y. Abnormal retinal blood vessels in Ehlers-Danlos syndrome type VI. *Jpn J Ophthalmol.* 2007;51:453-455.

47. Walker LC, Overstreet MA, Siddiqui A, et al. A novel mutation in the lysyl hydroxylase 1 gene causes decreased lysyl hydroxylase activity in an Ehlers-Danlos VIA patient. *J Invest Dermatol.* 2005;124:914-918.

48. Sharma Y, Sudan R, Gaur A. Post traumatic subconjunctival dislocation of lens in Ehlers-Danlos syndrome. *Indian J Ophthalmol.* 2003;51:185-186.

49. McDermott ML, Holladay J, Liu D, Puklin JE, Shin DH, Cowden JW. Corneal topography in Ehlers-Danlos syndrome. *J Cataract Refract Surg.* 1998;24:1212-1215.

50. Segev F, Héon E, Cole WG, et al. Structural abnormalities of the cornea and lid resulting from collagen V mutations. *Invest Ophthalmol Vis Sci.* 2006;47:565-573.

51. Pesudovs K. Orbscan mapping in Ehlers-Danlos syndrome. *J Cataract Refract Surg.* 2004; 30:1795-1798.

52. Matt P, Habashi J, Carrel T, Cameron DE, Van Eyk JE, Dietz HC. Recent advances in understanding Marfan syndrome: should we now treat surgical patients with losartan? *J Thorac Cardiovasc Surg.* 2008;135:389-394.

53. Blyth M, Foulds N, Turner C, Bunyan D. Severe Marfan syndrome due to FBN1 exon deletions. *Am J Med Genet A.* 2008;146:1320-1324.

54. Faivre L, Collod-Beroud G, Loeys BL, et al. Effect of mutation type and location on clinical outcome in 1,013 probands with Marfan syndrome or related phenotypes and FBN1 mutations: an international study. *Am J Hum Genet.* 2007;81:454-466.

55. Chaudhry SS, Cain SA, Morgan A, Dallas SL, Shuttleworth CA, Kielty CM. Fibrillin-1 regulates the bioavailability of TGFbeta1. *J Cell Biol.* 2007;176:355-367.

56. Zangwill SD, Brown MD, Bryke CR, Cava JR, Segura AD. Marfan syndrome type II: there is more to Marfan syndrome than fibrillin 1. *Congenit Heart Dis.* 2006;1:229-232.

57. Ramirez F, Dietz HC. Marfan syndrome: from molecular pathogenesis to clinical treatment. *Curr Opin Genet Dev.* 2007;17:252-258.

58. Louis DS, Tsai E. Congenital hand and forearm anomalies. *Curr Opin Pediatr.* 1996;8:61-64.

59. Baran S, Igny A, Igny I. Respiratory dysfunction in patients with Marfan syndrome. *J Physiol Pharmacol.* 2007;58(suppl 5, pt 1):37-41.

60. Kouerinis IA, Hountis PA, Loutsidis AK, Bellenis IP. Spontaneous pneumothorax: are we missing something? *Interact Cardiovasc Thorac Surg.* 2004;3:272-273.

61. Ozçakar ZB, Ekim M, Ensari A, et al. Membranoproliferative glomerulonephritis in a patient with Wilson's disease. *J Nephrol.* 2006;19:831-833.

62. Gandhi SD, Iqbal Z, Markan S, Almassi GH, Pagel PS. Massive retrograde acute type B aortic dissection in a postpartum woman with a family history of Marfan syndrome. *J Clin Anesth.* 2008;20:50-53.

63. Li D, Yu J, Gu F, et al. The roles of two novel FBN1 gene mutations in the genotype-phenotype correlations of Marfan syndrome and ectopia lentis patients with marfanoid habitus. *Genet Test.* 2008.

64. Barkana Y, Shihadeh W, Oliveira C, Tello C, Liebmann JM, Ritch R. Angle closure in highly myopic eyes. *Ophthalmology.* 2006;113:247-254.

65. Heur M, Costin B, Crowe S, et al. The value of keratometry and central corneal thickness measurements in the clinical diagnosis of Marfan syndrome. *Am J Ophthalmol.* 2008;145:997-1001.

66. Grünauer-Kloevekorn C, Duncker GI. Keratoconus: epidemiology, risk factors and diagnosis. *Klin Monatsbl Augenheilkd.* 2006;223:493-502.

67. Siganos DS, Siganos CS, Popescu CN, Margaritis VN. Clear lens extraction and intraocular lens implantation in Marfan's syndrome. *J Cataract Refract Surg.* 2000;26:781-784.

68. Ladewig MS, Robinson PN, Neumann LM, Holz FG, Foerster MH. Ocular manifestations and surgical results in patients with Marfan syndrome [in German]. *Ophthalmologe*. 2006; 103:777-782.

69. Morrison D, Sternberg P, Donahue S. Anterior chamber intraocular lens (ACIOL) placement after pars plana lensectomy in pediatric Marfan syndrome. *J AAPOS*. 2005;9:240-242.

70. Dureau P, de Laage de Meux P, Edelson C, Caputo G. Iris fixation of foldable intraocular lenses for ectopia lentis in children. *J Cataract Refract Surg*. 2006;32:1109-1114.

71. Bahar I, Kaiserman I, Rootman D. Cionni endocapsular ring implantation in Marfan's Syndrome. *Br J Ophthalmol*. 2007;91:1477-1480.

72. Berman EL. Clues in the eye: ocular signs of metabolic and nutritional disorders. *Geriatrics*. 1995;50:34-36, 43-44.

73. Joseph J, McGrath H. Gout or "pseudogout": how to differentiate crystal-induced arthropathies. *Geriatrics*. 1995;50:33-39.

74. Bernad B, Narvaez J, Diaz-Torné C, Diez-Garcia M, Valverde J. Clinical image: corneal tophus deposition in gout. *Arthritis Rheum*. 2006;54:1025.

75. Coassin M, Piovanetti O, Stark WJ, Green WR. Urate deposition in the iris and anterior chamber. *Ophthalmology*. 2006;113:462-465.

76. Lo WR, Broocker G, Grossniklaus HE. Histopathologic examination of conjunctival tophi in gouty arthritis. *Am J Ophthalmol*. 2005;140:1152-1154.

77. Nuki G, Simkin PA. A concise history of gout and hyperuricemia and their treatment. *Arthritis Res Ther*. 2006;8(suppl 1).

78. Lange RK. The varying picture in gout. *Med Clin North Am*. 1967;51:1035-1040.

79. Hakoda M. Epidemiology of hyperuricemia and gout in Japan. *Nippon Rinsho*. 2008;66:647-652.

80. Fels E, Sundy JS. Refractory gout: what is it and what to do about it? *Curr Opin Rheumatol*. 2008;20:198-202.

81. Pascual E, Doherty M. Aspiration of normal or asymptomatic pathological joints for diagnosis and research: indications, technique and success rate. *Ann Rheum Dis*. 2009;68:3-7.

82. Mineo I, Kamiya H, Tsukuda A. Practical strategies for lifestyle modification in people with hyperuricemia and gout treatment through diet, physical activity, and reduced alcohol consumption. *Nippon Rinsho*. 2008;66:736-741.

83. Stocker SL, Williams KM, McLachlan AJ, Graham GG, Day RO. Pharmacokinetic and pharmacodynamic interaction between allopurinol and probenecid in healthy subjects. *Clin Pharmacokinet*. 2008;47:111-118.

84. Garbe E, Suissa S, LeLorier J. Exposure to allopurinol and the risk of cataract extraction in elderly patients. *Arch Ophthalmol*. 1998;116:1652-1656.

85. Jelley MJ, Wortmann R. Practical steps in the diagnosis and management of gout. *BioDrugs*. 2000;14:99-107.

86. Sarkany RP. Making sense of the porphyrias. *Photodermatol Photoimmunol Photomed*. 2008;24:102-108.

87. Richard E, Robert-Richard E, Ged C, Moreau-Gaudry F, de Verneuil H. Erythropoietic porphyrias: animal models and update in gene-based therapies. *Curr Gene Ther*. 2008;8:176-186.

88. Bulat V, Lugovi L, Situm M, Buljan M, Bradi L. Porphyria cutanea tarda as the most common porphyria. *Acta Dermatovenerol Croat*. 2007;15:254-263.

89. Rimington C. Was Hippocrates the first to describe a case of acute porphyria? *Int J Biochem*. 1993;25:1351-1352.

90. Harper P, Wahlin S. Treatment options in acute porphyria, porphyria cutanea tarda, and erythropoietic protoporphyria. *Curr Treat Options Gastroenterol*. 2007;10:444-455.

91. Sheerani M, Urfy MZ, Hassan A, Islam Z, Baig S. Acute porphyrias: clinical spectrum of hospitalized patients. *J Coll Physicians Surg Pak*. 2007;17:662-665.

92. Karpova IV, Pustovoit IaS, Luchinina IuA, et al. Acute porphyrias: problem of primary diagnosis in Russia and CIS countries. *Ter Arkh*. 2007;79(8):52-56.

93. Poblete-Gutiérrez P, Wiederholt T, Merk HF, Frank J. Laboratory tests and therapeutic strategies for the porphyrias [in German]. *Hautarzt*. 2006;16:230-240.

94. Roshal M, Turgeon J, Rainey PM. Rapid quantitative method using spin columns to measure porphobilinogen in urine. *Clin Chem.* 2008;54:429-431.

95. Tsuboi H, Yonemoto K, Katsuoka K. Erythropoietic protoporphyria with eye complications. *J Dermatol.* 2007;34:790-794.

96. Gürses C, Durukan A, Sencer S, Akça S, Baykan B, Gökyiqit A. A severe neurological sequela in acute intermittent porphyria: presentation of a case from encephalopathy to quadriparesis. *Br J Radiol.* 2008;81(965):e135-e140.

97. Bandyopadhyay R, Bhaduri G, Banerjee A, et al. Bilateral scleromalacia in a case of congenital erythropoietic porphyria. *J Indian Med Assoc.* 2006;104:406-407.

98. Park AJ, Webster GF, Penne RB, Raber IM. Porphyria cutanea tarda presenting as cicatricial conjunctivitis. *Am J Ophthalmol.* 2002;134:619-621.

99. Veenashree MP, Sangwan VS, Vemuganti GK, Parthasaradhi A. Acute scleritis as a manifestation of congenital erythropoietic porphyria. *Cornea.* 2002;21:530-531.

100. DeFrancisco M, Savino PJ, Schatz NJ. Optic atrophy in acute intermittent porphyria. *Am J Ophthalmol.* 1979;87:221-224.

101. Gupta A, Aikath D, Neogi R, et al. Molecular pathogenesis of Wilson disease: haplotype analysis, detection of prevalent mutations and genotype-phenotype correlation in Indian patients. *Hum Genet.* 2005;118:49-57.

102. Park S, Park JY, Kim GH, et al. Identification of novel ATP7B gene mutations and their functional roles in Korean patients with Wilson disease. *Hum Mutat.* 2007;28:1108-1113.

103. Günther P, Hermann W, Kühn HJ, Wagner A. Wilson's disease. *Ther Umsch.* 2007;64:57-61.

104. Pfeil SA, Lynn DJ. Wilson's disease: copper unfettered. *J Clin Gastroenterol.* 1999;29:22-31.

105. Brewer GJ. Neurologically presenting Wilson's disease: epidemiology, pathophysiology and treatment. *CNS Drugs.* 2005;19:185-192.

106. Chakravarty A, Mukherjee A, Sen A. Familial pediatric rapidly progressive extrapyramidal syndrome: is it Hallervorden-Spatz disease? *Pediatr Neurol.* 2003;29:170-172.

107. Maier KP. Rare, but important chronic liver diseases. *Schweiz Rundsch Med Prax.* 2002;91:2077-2085.

108. Mueller A, Reuner U, Landis B, Kitzler H, Reichmann H, Hummel T. Extrapyramidal symptoms in Wilson's disease are associated with olfactory dysfunction. *Mov Disord.* 2006;21:1311-1316.

109. Müller J, Landgraf F, Trabert W. Schizophrenia-like symptoms in the Westphal-Strümpell variation of Wilson disease. *Nervenarzt.* 1998;69:264-268.

110. Chilcott-Lauber C, Burkhard PR, Giostra E. Wilson's disease: clinical presentations [in French]. *Rev Med Suisse.* 2005;1:2018, 2020-2022.

111. Siordia-Reyes AG, Ferman-Cano F, García GR, Rodríguez-Velasco A. Wilson disease. Report of a case of autopsy with copper tissue quantification and electronic microscopy. *Rev Gastroenterol Mex.* 2001;66:38-41.

112. Tankanow RM. Pathophysiology and treatment of Wilson's disease. *Clin Pharm.* 1991;10:839-849.

113. Deguti MM, Tietge UJ, Barbosa ER, Cancado EL. The eye in Wilson's disease: sunflower cataract associated with Kayser-Fleischer ring. *J Hepatol.* 2002;37:700.

114. Klingele TG, Newman SA, Burde RM. Accommodation defect in Wilson's disease. *Am J Ophthalmol.* 1980;90:22-24.

115. Curran RE, Hedges TR 3rd, Boger WP III. Loss of accommodation and the near response in Wilson's disease. *J Pediatr Ophthalmol Strabismus.* 1982;19:157-160.

116. Gow PJ, Peacock SE, Chapman RW. Wilson's disease presenting with rapidly progressive visual loss: another neurologic manifestation of Wilson's disease? *J Gastroenterol Hepatol.* 2001;16:699-701.

117. Mazzaglia PJ, Berber E, Kovach A, Milas M, Esselstyn C, Siperstein AE. The changing presentation of hyperparathyroidism over 3 decades. *Arch Surg.* 2008;143:260-266.

118. Lang NK, Schalhorn A, Hiddemann W. Pronounced osteoporosis, shrunken stature and blue coloration of sclerae in a 47-year old patient. *Internist (Berl).* 2001;42:1151-1155.

119. Sillence D, Butler B, Latham M, Barlow K. Natural history of blue sclerae in osteogenesis imperfecta. *Am J Med Genet.* 1993;45:183-186.

120. Wilcox RA, McDonald FS. Gray-blue sclerae and osteopenia secondary to osteogenesis imperfecta. *Mayo Clin Proc.* 2007;82:265.

121. Alikadic-Husovic A, Merhemc Z. The blue sclera syndrome (Van der Heave syndrome). *Med Arh.* 2000;54:325-326.

122. Evereklioglu C, Madenci E, Bayazit YA, Yilmaz K, Balat A, Bekir NA. Central corneal thickness is lower in osteogenesis imperfecta and negatively correlates with the presence of blue sclera. *Ophthalmic Physiol Opt.* 2002;22:511-515.

123. Waring GO III, Rodrigues MM, Laibson PR. Anterior chamber cleavage syndrome. A stepladder classification. *Surv Ophthalmol.* 1975;20:3-27.

124. Sim KT, Karri B, Kaye SB. Posterior embryotoxon may not be a forme fruste of Axenfeld-Rieger's syndrome. *AAPOS.* 2004;8:504-506.

125. Stokes DW, Parrish CM. Axenfeld's anomaly associated with Down's syndrome. *Cornea.* 1992;11:163-164.

126. Brear DR, Insler MS. Axenfeld's syndrome associated with systemic abnormalities. *Ann Ophthalmol.* 1985;17:291-294.

127. Shields MB. Axenfeld-Rieger syndrome: a theory of mechanism and distinctions from the iridocorneal endothelial syndrome. *Trans Am Ophthalmol Soc.* 1983;81:736-784.

128. Shields MB, Buckley E, Klintworth GK, Thresher R. Axenfeld-Rieger syndrome. A spectrum of developmental disorders. *Surv Ophthalmol.* 1985;29:387-409.

129. Mammi I, De Giorgio P, Clementi M, Tenconi R. Cardiovascular anomaly in Rieger syndrome: heterogeneity or contiguity? *Acta Ophthalmol Scand.* 1998;76:509-512.

130. Davis LK, Meyer KJ, Rudd DS, et al. Pax6 3' deletion results in aniridia, autism and mental retardation. *Hum Genet.* 2008;123:371-378.

131. Miller MT, Epstein RJ, Sugar J, et al. Anterior segment anomalies associated with the fetal alcohol syndrome. *J Pediatr Ophthalmol Strabismus.* 1984;21:8-18.

132. Comer RM, Daya SM, O'Keefe M. Penetrating keratoplasty in infants. *J AAPOS.* 2001;5:285-290.

133. Yang LL, Lambert SR, Lynn MJ, Stulting RD. Long-term results of corneal graft survival in infants and children with Peters anomaly. *Ophthalmology.* 1999;106:833-848.

134. Gawthrop F, Mould R, Sperritt A, Neale F. Ehlers-Danlos syndrome. *Br Med J.* 2007;335(7617):448-450.

135. Milhorat TH, Bolognese PA, Nishikawa M, McDonnell NB, Francomano CA. Syndrome of occipitoatlantoaxial hypermobility, cranial settling, and chiari malformation type I in patients with hereditary disorders of connective tissue. *J Neurosurg Spine.* 2007;7:601-609.

136. Perdu J, Boutouyrie P, Lahlou-Laforêt K, et al. Vascular Ehlers-Danlos syndrome. *Presse Med.* 2006;35(pt 2):1864-1875.

137. De Coster PJ, Malfait F, Martens LC, De Paepe A. Unusual oral findings in dermatosparaxis (Ehlers-Danlos syndrome type VIIC). *J Oral Pathol Med.* 2003;32:568-570.

138. Giunta C, Chambaz C, Pedemonte M, Scapolan S, Steinmann B. The arthrochalasia type of Ehlers-Danlos syndrome (EDS VIIA and VIIB): the diagnostic value of collagen fibril ultrastructure. *Am J Med Genet A.* 2008;146:1341-1346.

139. Ferry AP, Safir A, Melikian HE. Ocular abnormalities in patients with gout. *Ann Ophthalmol.* 1985;17:632-635.

140. Lo WR, Broocker G, Grossniklaus HE. Histopathological examination of conjunctival tophi in gouty arthritis. *Am J Ophthalmol.* 2005;140:1152-1154.

141. Wood DJ. Inflammatory disease in the eye caused by gout. *Br J Ophthalmol.* 1936;20:510-519.

142. Slansky HH, Kubara T. Intranuclear urate crystals in corneal epithelium. *Arch Ophthalmol.* 1968;80:338-344.

143. Moss SE, Klein R, Klein BE. Incidence of dry eye in an older population. *Arch Ophthalmol.* 2004;122:369-373.

144. Lerman S, Megaw J, Fraunfelder FT. Further studies on allopurinol therapy and human cataractogenesis. *Am J Ophthalmol.* 1984;97:205-209.

145. Liu CS, Brown NA, Leonard TJ, Bull PW, Scott JT. The prevalence and morphology of cataract in patients on allopurinol treatment. *Eye.* 1988;2(pt 6):600-606.

146. Fraunfelder FT, Hanna C, Dreis MW, Cosgrove KW Jr. Cataracts associated with allopurinol therapy. *Am J Ophthalmol.* 1982;94:137-140.

147. Bernad B, Narvaez J, Diaz-Torné C, Diez-Garcia M, Valverde J. Clinical image: corneal tophus deposition in gout. *Arthritis Rheum.* 2006;54:1025.

148. Martínez-Cordero E, Barreira-Mercado E, Katona G. Eye tophi deposition in gout. *J Rheumatol.* 1986;13:471-473.

149. Klein R, Klein BE, Knudtson MD, Wong TY, Tsai MY. Are inflammatory factors related to retinal vessel caliber? The Beaver Dam Eye Study. *Arch Ophthalmol.* 2006;124:87-94.

150. Fichte C, Streeten BW, Friedman AH. A histopathologic study of retinal arterial aneurysms. *Am J Ophthalmol.* 1978;85:509-518.

151. Laval J. Allopurinol and macular lesions. *Arch Ophthalmol.* 1968;80:415.

152. Mitchell P, Wang MY, Wang JJ. Asteroid hyalosis in an older population: the Blue Mountains Eye Study. *Ophthalmic Epidemiol.* 2003;10:331-335.

10

ANTERIOR SEGMENT NEOPLASIA

David A. Hollander, MD, MBA

Neoplasia, which literally means "new growth" in Greek, represents an abnormal proliferation of cells that is uncoordinated with the growth of normal tissues. Neoplasias of the conjunctiva and cornea range in severity from benign lesions to highly invasive tumors with metastatic potential. These tumors of the ocular surface are often categorized into subtypes based upon the cells of origin, such as epithelial, melanocytic, lymphoid, vascular, and histiocytic.[1] Metastatic tumors to the conjunctiva are rare but may include breast carcinoma, bronchogenic carcinoma, and cutaneous melanoma.[2] Though there may be overlap in the clinical characteristics between tumors of different cellular origins, as well as between benign and malignant conditions, a detailed examination and understanding of pertinent history and clinical findings may aid in the diagnosis and treatment planning for patients presenting with masses of the ocular surface.

Understanding key features of ocular surface anatomy provides the basis for appreciating the common clinical characteristics and behaviors of particular conjunctival and corneal tumors. The corneoscleral limbus, the primary site of many ocular surface tumors, is a site rich in melanocytes and, perhaps more importantly, the region of mitotically active epithelial cells. The conjunctival epithelium is contiguous with the corneal epithelium, thereby allowing for tumors of the conjunctival epithelium to easily extend directly onto the corneal surface. Epithelial tumors, however, rarely invade the corneal stroma secondary to the presence of the dense connective tissue of Bowman's layer, a direct contrast to the lack of any significant barrier separating the conjunctival epithelium from the underlying substantia propria. A wide array of neoplasms may arise from the caruncle, located in the medial canthus, because this specialized region contains both conjunctival and cutaneous structures.[3,4]

Unlike tumors of the posterior segment, tumors of the ocular surface and anterior segment often present at a relatively early stage. In evaluating a patient with an ocular surface mass, a detailed history is required regarding the onset and growth pattern of the lesion as well as any history of systemic diseases, immunosuppression, or ocular trauma. Careful slit-lamp examination with lid eversion is critical, with attention to color and pigmentation, layer of involvement (epithelial

Trattler WB, Majmudar PA, Luchs JI, Swartz TS, eds.
Cornea Handbook (pp. 163-190)
© 2010 SLACK Incorporated

or subepithelial), internal tumor vasculature and associated feeder vessels, evidence of intraocular invasion, adherence to underlying tissues, and associated ocular inflammation. Examination should also include palpation of the orbit and regional lymph nodes, as well as detailed drawings and/or photographs for both possible surgical planning and follow-up. Systemic evaluation is also necessary, particularly in cases of suspected lymphoma or melanoma. The degree of clinical suspicion, the size of a lesion, and the patient's symptoms all play key roles in dictating the course of treatment and the need for surgery. In selected cases, the use of impression cytology,[5-7] ultrasound,[8,9] and anterior segment optical coherence tomography[9] may prove useful prior to any surgical intervention.

EPITHELIAL NEOPLASMS

Conjunctival Squamous Papilloma

Conjunctival squamous papillomas are benign epithelial tumors, often with multiple finger-like projections, composed of acanthotic squamous epithelium overlying a central fibrovascular core.[10] The surface of these tumors is typically transparent, with a glistening appearance, through which the central capillary fronds are easily visualized. Focal areas of pigmentation may be present.[11] Conjunctival papillomas are most commonly found inferiorly and nasally, though they may occur anywhere on the conjunctival surface.[12] These tumors may present as single or multiple unilateral as well as bilateral lesions.[13-15] Conjunctival papillomas may arise in both children and adults, occurring most commonly between 20 and 39 years of age.[12]

Conjunctival papillomas typically grow in an exophytic manner and may be categorized as either sessile (flat) or pedunculated (from a stalk; Figures 10-1 and 10-2).[12] More rarely, conjunctival papillomas may be inverted (endophytic).[16] There is a strong association with HPV, most commonly types 6 and 11,[10,17,18] with rare reports secondary to types 13,[19] 16,[20] 33,[21] and 45.[10] In several large series, HPV has been detected using polymerase chain reaction (PCR) in 58% to 92% of conjunctival papillomas.[10,17,22,23] Transmission of HPV infection is via direct contact. In children, the HPV infection is likely acquired by vertical transmission during delivery.[22]

Conjunctival papillomas are unlikely to undergo malignant transformation.[12,24] In a histopathologic study of 245 papillomas, evidence of dysplasia was found in only 6% of samples, none of which were classified as severe dysplasia.[12] This may be due to the low oncogenic potential of the HPV types 6 and 11 most commonly identified in papillomas. In contrast, HPV types 16 and 18, which are considered high-risk for oncogenic potential, are commonly associated with conjunctival neoplasia.[25,26]

No treatment is recommended for asymptomatic lesions because conjunctival papillomas may resolve spontaneously over months to years. The size, location, and associated inflammation, however, may warrant surgical intervention. Recurrence rates range from 6% to 27%,[12] and the use of a number of adjuvant therapies has been reported, including intraoperative and postoperative mitomycin C (MMC),[27,28] topical and intralesional interferon-alpha (IFN-α),[13,29] cryotherapy,[30] carbon dioxide laser,[31] dinitrochlorobenzene immunotherapy,[32] and oral cimetidine.[14]

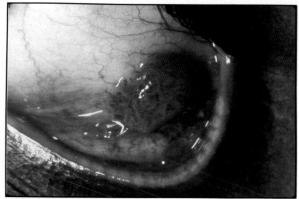

Figure 10-1. Conjunctival papilloma. Slit-lamp photograph of a sessile inferior bulbar conjunctival papilloma. The central fibrovascular core is visible below the transparent epithelial surface. (Courtesy of Peter J. McDonnell, MD.)

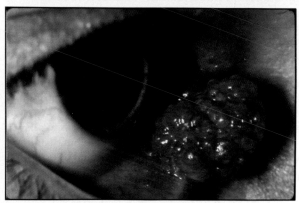

Figure 10-2. Conjunctival papilloma. Slit-lamp photograph of a pedunculated papilloma of the inferior palpebral conjunctiva. (Courtesy of Peter J. McDonnell, MD.)

Keratoacanthoma

Keratoacanthoma is a benign squamous epithelial lesion that commonly occurs on the skin and only rarely presents on the conjunctiva. Keratoacanthoma may develop at the limbus in the interpalpebral fissure and is characterized by rapid growth (~4 to 8 weeks).[33] The pathogenesis of keratoacanthoma has yet to be determined, though both ultraviolet exposure and trauma may play a role.[34,35] Keratoacanthoma typically appears as a white nodule with rounded edges and a central hyperkeratotic area.[36,37] Histologically, acanthotic epithelium surrounds a keratin-filled crater.[33,35,36,38,39] Complete excision is required based on the significant clinical and histological overlap between squamous cell carcinoma and keratoacanthoma. Though invasive features have been reported with keratoacanthoma,[40] it remains unclear whether such cases simply represented highly differentiated squamous cell carcinomas.

Hereditary Benign Intraepithelial Dyskeratosis

Hereditary benign intraepithelial dyskeratosis (HBID) is an autosomal dominant disorder of the oral and ocular mucosa that primarily affects descendents of the Haliwa Indians in North Carolina. In early childhood, patients develop bilateral elevated fleshy plaques on the nasal and/or temporal perilimbal conjunctiva.[41-44] Histopathological analysis reveals dyskeratosis, acanthosis, parakeratosis, and chronic inflammation.[41-44] Patients may experience chronic relapsing

Figure 10-3. Conjunctival intraepithelial neoplasia. A raised, vascularized gelatinous conjunctival mass with an inferior feeder vessel is seen at the temporal limbus.

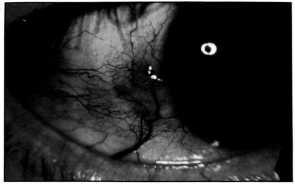

courses of conjunctival inflammation and photophobia.[41] Though recurrence is common following local excision, there is no malignant potential. Recently, the HBID gene has been located to chromosome 4q35.[45]

Conjunctival and Corneal Intraepithelial Neoplasia

Conjunctival and corneal intraepithelial neoplasia (CIN), the most common neoplasm of the ocular surface, is a slowly progressive lesion with low malignant potential.[46,47] By definition, CIN consists of dysplastic epithelial cells that have not invaded either the substantia propria of the conjunctiva or Bowman's layer of the cornea. Previously referred to as Bowen's disease, CIN typically occurs in middle-aged and elderly individuals, with a greater incidence in males.[47-49] Risk factors include ultraviolet exposure,[50] HPV (types 16 and 18),[51-53] HIV,[54] smoking,[55] lightly pigmented irides,[50] and xeroderma pigmentosa.[56,57]

CIN is most commonly found on the bulbar conjunctiva at the limbus within the interpalpebral fissure. Clinically, this lesion often appears as an elevated gelatinous mass that is highly vascularized, with fine superficial vessels (Figure 10-3).[46,58,59] The dysplastic conjunctival epithelium may extend onto the corneal surface above Bowman's layer, resulting in thickened and opaque epithelium, often with scalloped edges (Figures 10-4 and 10-5). Leukoplakia (white keratinized plaques) and feeder vessels are common. Lesions of CIN may also be present at the caruncle as well as the palpebral conjunctiva.[60] In addition, CIN may appear in isolation without any associated conjunctival abnormalities.[59,61] Vital stains such as fluorescein, rose bengal, and toluidine blue can be used at the slit lamp or intraoperatively to identify the extent of dysplastic epithelium.[62]

Surgical treatment of CIN typically involves complete excision with wide margins and adjuvant cryotherapy. Reports of adjuvant therapies have also included the use of radiation,[63] PTK,[64] photodynamic therapy,[65] topical retinoic acid,[66] MMC,[67-71] 5-fluorouracil (5-FU),[72] cidofovir,[73] and interferon alfa-2b (IFNα2b).[49,74,75] Though reports of local recurrence rates following complete excision are as low as 5%, these rates may rise to 56% when the tumor extends to the surgical margins.[47,58,76-79] Topical MMC and IFNα2b offer alternatives to excision in cases of recurrent disease, because repeat excision and extensive cryotherapy may result in limbal stem cell deficiency and cicatricial changes. The use of topical MMC may achieve faster tumor regression than topical IFNα2b but typically requires medication cycling to minimize pain and ocular surface side effects such as punctate keratopathy and conjunctival hyperemia.[49,70,71,74,75,80]

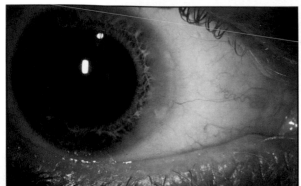

Figure 10-4. Conjunctival intraepithelial neoplasia. A gelatinous limbal mass with leukoplakia and peripheral corneal neovascularization is seen on slit-lamp examination.

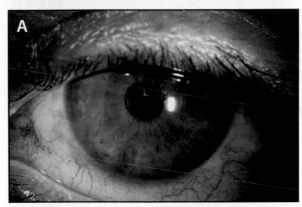

Figure 10-5. Conjunctival intraepithelial neoplasia. (A) Slit-lamp photograph demonstrates mild vascular tortuosity on the nasal conjunctiva in a patient who presented with complaints of reduced visual acuity. (B) High-power magnification reveals scalloped opaque dysplastic epithelium that had encroached on the visual axis.

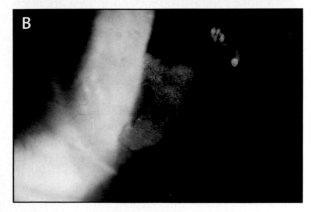

Adverse ocular events secondary to topical IFNα2b are typically mild but include conjunctival hyperemia, follicular conjunctivitis, and the development of epithelial microcysts.[49,81] Though CIN rarely progresses to squamous cell carcinoma, close follow-up is necessary because local recurrences have been reported more than 10 years following initial treatment.[78]

Squamous Cell Carcinoma

CIN is often a precursor of squamous cell carcinoma. Squamous cell carcinoma is defined by the invasion of neoplastic cells through the underlying basement membrane to the substantia propria of the conjunctiva. Similar to CIN, squamous cell carcinoma typically presents as an elevated gelatinous lesion at the limbus in the interpalpebral region. Intraocular involvement is rare because both Bowman's layer and the sclera serve as barriers to extension. Clinical findings suggestive of invasion include tumor immobility, anterior chamber inflammation, synechiae, glaucoma, and scleritis.[82,83] Ultrasound may aid in assessing the depth of tumor involvement.[84,85]

Treatment of squamous cell carcinoma typically involves wide local excision with cryotherapy, corneal alcohol epitheliectomy for corneal involvement, and partial scleral resections in areas with tumor adherence to the globe. Extensive and recurrent disease may be treated with topical MMC or IFNα2b.[70,71,86] Intraocular or orbital involvement typically requires enucleation or exenteration, respectively. Squamous cell carcinoma is only rarely associated with regional or distant metastases.[87] More aggressive behavior may be seen in the setting of immunosuppression, such as organ transplant patients or individuals with HIV.[88-90] Mucoepidermoid carcinoma, adenoid squamous carcinoma, and spindle cell carcinoma represent aggressive variants of squamous cell carcinoma with a greater risk for intraocular invasion and metastases.[91-93]

PIGMENTED NEOPLASMS

Conjunctival Nevus

Conjunctival nevi are benign tumors typically seen in Caucasian patients between 10 and 40 years of age.[94,95] They are most commonly found on the bulbar conjunctiva and caruncle.[95-97] Unlike conjunctival melanosis, nevi are often elevated and rarely extend into the corneal epithelium. Conjunctival nevi are categorized histologically as junctional (intraepithelial), subepithelial, compound (intraepithelial plus subepithelial), and blue nevi. Most conjunctival nevi are compound or subepithelial, though a high percentage of junctional nevi are present in patients younger than 20 years.[95,98]

The diagnosis of a conjunctival nevus is often made clinically based on the presence of intralesional cysts, which are rarely observed in conjunctival melanoma (Figure 10-6).[95] Nevi are most commonly brown but may appear tan or nonpigmented. Both feeder vessels and intrinsic vessels, prominent features of conjunctival melanoma, may also be observed in approximately one third of conjunctival nevi.[95] Changes in the appearance of conjunctival nevi may be observed, especially during puberty, secondary to inflammation, enlargement of cysts, and melanocytic proliferation.[95,99] In a series of 149 nevi treated with observation alone (mean time of 11 years), Shields and colleagues reported a change in size in 8% and a change in color in 13% of cases.[95] Though excision is recommended for suspicious lesions to obtain a histological diagnosis, the use of argon green laser therapy has been reported as an alternative treatment option in select patients with stable, benign-appearing lesions.[100]

Racial Melanosis

Racial melanosis is flat, conjunctival pigmentation that usually appears bilaterally in darkly pigmented patients. The pigmentation is typically found in the

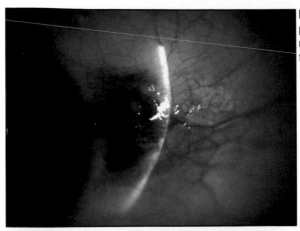

Figure 10-6. High-magnification slit-lamp photograph reveals pigmented conjunctival nevus at the limbus with multiple cystic structures. (Courtesy of Anthony J. Aldave, MD.)

perilimbal region and may extend onto the peripheral cornea. The pigmented cells are benign melanocytes located in the basal epithelium.

Ocular Melanocytosis

Ocular melanocytosis is a congenital increase in pigmentation of the sclera and episclera. The condition most commonly occurs unilaterally but may be found bilaterally.[101] Clinically, clusters of melanocytes produce gray-brown areas deep to the overlying conjunctiva, which typically remains free of pigmentation. A corresponding increase in the size and number of uveal melanocytes may result in heterochromia iridis.[102] Ocular melanocytosis may also be associated with pigmentation of the orbital tissues, meninges, and the periocular dermis (Nevus of Ota) in the distribution of the ophthalmic and maxillary divisions of the trigeminal nerve. Both ocular and oculodermal melanocytosis are most commonly seen in the Asian population.[103] In patients with ocular melanocytosis, there is a 1 in 400 risk of developing uveal melanoma.[104]

Primary Acquired Melanosis

Primary acquired melanosis (PAM) is a flat, patchy acquired pigmentation of the conjunctiva that may undergo malignant transformation to melanoma. Primary acquired melanosis most commonly presents in middle-aged and elderly Caucasians as a unilateral area of superficial pigmentation in the bulbar conjunctiva (Figure 10-7).[105,106] When the canthus or palpebral conjunctiva is affected, the adjacent skin may also be involved.[105] Corneal involvement has been reported in up to 23% of cases.[106] Simple inspection may not reveal the full extent of PAM as areas may be amelanotic (PAM *sine pigmento*).[107,108] In addition, the areas of pigmentation have also been described to "wax and wane" over time.[105,109]

Primary acquired melanosis is categorized histologically into PAM with and without atypia with critical implications on prognosis. Primary acquired melanosis without atypia and PAM with only mild atypia (atypical melanocytes confined to the basal layer of epithelium) are unlikely to progress to melanoma.[106,110] In contrast, the risk for progression to melanoma with severe atypia ranges from 13% to 90%.[106,110] Histological signs of severe atypia include the presence of epithelioid cells as well as pagetoid spread within the epithelium beyond the basilar

Figure 10-7. (A) Slit-lamp photograph of a Caucasian male with PAM inferiorly and temporally on the bulbar conjunctiva. (B) PAM seen diffusely on the temporal bulbar conjunctiva. (C) PAM extends onto the inferior palpebral conjunctiva.

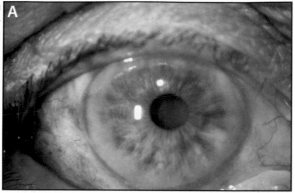

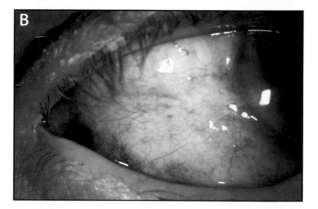

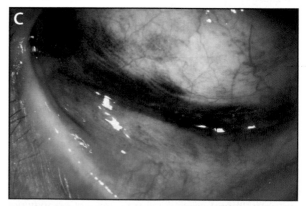

layer.[106,110] Shields and colleagues have demonstrated that the most significant risk factor for recurrence following treatment and progression to melanoma is the extent of PAM (in clock hours).[106] The development of any areas of elevation is often a sign of malignancy.[105]

Treatment recommendations for PAM vary based upon the extent of melanosis. Though small foci of PAM (less than 1 clock hour) may be observed initially, larger lesions should be treated with complete excision and cryotherapy. In cases of diffuse PAM, map biopsies can be performed with cryotherapy to all pigmented

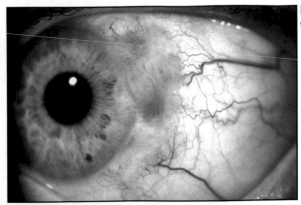

Figure 10-8. Recurrent limbal conjunctival melanoma with multiple feeder vessels. (Courtesy of Gary N. Holland, MD.)

areas.[106,111] Regions of corneal PAM can be treated with alcohol epitheliectomy. Courses of topical MMC drops have been recommended in cases of recurrence, incomplete excision, or as an alternative to cryotherapy.[112-115]

Conjunctival Melanoma

Conjunctival melanoma is a rare malignant tumor of atypical melanocytes, which accounts for approximately 2% of all ocular malignancies.[116] This invasive neoplasm predominantly affects middle-aged and elderly Caucasian individuals and is exceedingly rare in non-Caucasian populations.[117-119] Conjunctival melanoma most commonly presents as an elevated mass on the bulbar conjunctival surface in the perilimbal region. Limbal tumors often extend into the corneal epithelium yet rarely invade the corneal stroma.[120,121] Melanomas detected in the fornix, palpebral conjunctiva, plica semilunaris, and caruncle are associated with a worse prognosis.[121,122]

Conjunctival melanoma may arise from regions of PAM (36% to 75%), a pre-existing conjunctival nevus (4% to 16%), or de novo (12% to 47%).[110,121,123,124] Histologically, conjunctival melanomas are classified by cell type as spindle, mixed, or epithelioid. Conjunctival melanomas may be unifocal or multicentric, and prominent feeder vessels are often present.[111,121,125] On examination, conjunctival melanomas may appear brown, yellow, or red in color, with rare reports of amelanotic melanoma arising from areas of PAM sine pigmento (Figure 10-8).[121,126-128] In contrast to initial presentations, recurrent melanomas of the conjunctiva are typically amelanotic (Figure 10-9).[121]

The behavior of conjunctival melanomas more closely resembles that of cutaneous than uveal melanomas.[129] Unlike uveal melanoma, which spreads hematogenously, conjunctival and cutaneous melanomas spread predominantly via the lymphatics. Following invasion of the underlying substantia propria, tumor cells often first metastasize to the regional preauricular and submandibular lymph nodes.[130] Distant metastases, most commonly to the lung, brain, liver, skin, bone, and gastrointestinal tract, may occur without evidence of prior or concurrent lymph node involvement.[130,131]

Conjunctival melanoma is associated with frequent local recurrences as well as high mortality rates secondary to metastatic disease. At 5 years, rates of local recurrence range from 26% to 61%.[121,132,133] Estimates of melanoma-related mortality rates are 7% to 23% at 5 years and 27% to 38% at 10 years.[121,123-125,127,129,134]

Figure 10-9. Slit-lamp photograph of superior amelanotic melanoma seen on lid eversion. (Courtesy of M. Reza Vagefi, MD.)

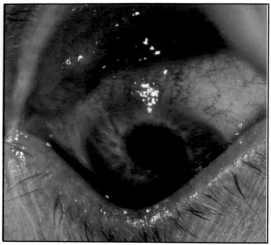

The clinical features consistently observed to have the greatest impact on survival are tumor thickness[121,125,129,132,134] and extralimbal location.[121,125,129,132]

Though randomized studies evaluating surgical treatment options have not been conducted, current evidence suggests that the ideal management of conjunctival melanoma includes partial lamellar scleroconjunctivectomy using a "no touch" technique, adjuvant cryotherapy to the conjunctival margins, and alcohol corneal epitheliectomy as described by Shields and colleagues.[121,135] Wide margins (~3-4 mm) are recommended, and any positive margin necessitates repeat excision with cryotherapy.[121,135] Both incisional biopsy as well excision without adjuvant cryotherapy may increase the risk of local recurrences.[111,121,127] In select cases, additional treatment options include plaque brachytherapy,[125,132,134,136] proton beam radiotherapy,[137,138] as well as postoperative topical MMC[139,140] or IFNα2b.[141] Orbital exenteration has not been shown to lead to improved survival rates and is currently recommended only as palliative therapy.[142] The role of sentinel lymph node biopsy in the treatment of conjunctival melanoma remains under investigation.[131,143]

Similar to trends observed in cutaneous melanoma, recent studies in the United States and Finland have demonstrated an increasing incidence of conjunctival melanoma.[129,144-146] However, the impact of increased exposure to ultraviolet radiation on the development of conjunctival melanoma has yet to be determined.[120]

SUBEPITHELIAL NEOPLASIA

Kaposi's Sarcoma

Kaposi's sarcoma, originally described as a sarcoma of the skin, is a multifocal vascular tumor that may also affect the mucous membranes, gastrointestinal tract, liver, spleen, and lymph nodes. Though Kaposi's sarcoma was a rare ocular tumor prior to the acquired immune deficiency syndrome (AIDS) epidemic, Kaposi's sarcoma of the ocular adnexa (eyelids and conjunctiva) may occur in up to 20% of patients infected with HIV.[147-149] In addition, Kaposi's sarcoma may

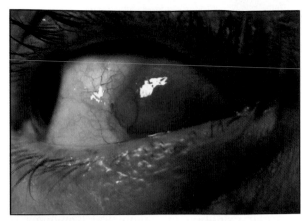

Figure 10-10. Conjunctival lymphoma: slit-lamp photograph of a patient with a sub-epithelial, salmon-colored diffuse mass of the midbulbar conjunctiva diagnosed histologically as a lymphoma. (Courtesy of M. Reza Vagefi, MD.)

be the first clinical sign arising in patients with HIV infection.[150,151] Kaposi's sarcomas of the conjunctiva are most commonly found in the inferior fornix as deep reddish blue elevated masses that may be either nodular or diffuse.[147,148,152] Kaposi's sarcomas are typically painless but may cause local irritation, ptosis, conjunctival edema, trichiasis, and visual obstruction. Kaposi's sarcoma has been attributed to infection of the human herpes virus 8.[153-155] Disseminated disease requires systemic chemotherapy, yet localized conjunctival disease may be treated by observation, surgical excision,[156,157] radiation,[147,158,159] cryotherapy,[156,157] or local injections of chemotherapy/immunotherapy (interferon alpha-2a, vinblastine, human chorionic gonadotropin).[160,161] Suppression of viral replication and immune reconstitution with highly active antiretroviral therapy (HAART) have reduced the incidence and improved the prognosis of HIV-related Kaposi's sarcoma.[149,162-164]

Lymphoid Tumors

Lymphoproliferative tumors of the conjunctiva, which most commonly develop in the elderly, encompass a spectrum of neoplastic disorders ranging from benign lymphoid hyperplasia to malignant lymphoma.[165,166] Clinically, patients typically present with unilateral or bilateral elevated salmon-colored diffuse masses located in the conjunctival stroma or deep to Tenon's fascia (Figure 10-10).[167] The lesions are usually painless, though they may cause irritation, and the surrounding conjunctival tissue is rarely inflamed. Unlike most conjunctival tumors, which tend to arise at the limbus, lymphoid tumors of the conjunctiva are typically found on the midbulbar conjunctiva superiorly beneath the eyelid or inferiorly in the fornix.[167] Conjunctival lymphoid tumors may be associated with additional sites of ocular involvement (orbit, eyelid, vitreous, choroid) as well as with systemic disease.[167]

Benign and malignant lymphoid tumors are often difficult to differentiate based on clinical characteristics, thereby necessitating tissue biopsy and complete workup in every patient to evaluate for systemic disease. In addition to conventional light microscopy, newer techniques such as flow cytometry, immunohistochemistry, and PCR may be critical in differentiating reactive lymphoid hyperplasia from low-grade lymphomas.[166,168] The majority of conjunctival lymphoid tumors in adults are categorized as low-grade B cell lymphomas of the mucosa-associated lymphoid tissue lymphoma (MALT) subtype, followed by follicular lymphoma, with rare reports of diffuse large B-cell, T-cell lymphoma, and other more aggressive subtypes.[166,168-172] Most lymphoid tumors in children represent benign lymphoid hyperplasia.[173]

Among patients with lymphoid tumors of the ocular adnexa, individuals with lymphomas confined to the conjunctiva tend to have a better prognosis and lower likelihood of developing systemic lymphoma than those with eyelid or orbital involvement.[165] Patients with conjunctival infiltration have an approximately 20% to 37% risk of presenting with or eventually developing systemic lymphoma.[165,167,174] The presence of bilateral conjunctival involvement and extralimbal tumor location may be associated with higher rates of systemic disease.[167]

In the absence of systemic disease, treatment options for localized conjunctival infiltration include radiotherapy, excisional biopsy and cryotherapy, or intralesional injections of IFNα2b.[135,167,175,176] If systemic lymphoma is present, incisional or excisional biopsy may be performed in conjunction with systemic chemotherapy.[167] Overall, intraocular extension of conjunctival lymphoma is rare,[177-179] and most cases of conjunctival lymphomas are associated with good prognoses.[167,180,181] However, close follow-up is necessary because systemic disease may arise many years following initial conjunctival involvement.[167]

Fibrous Histiocytoma

Fibrous histiocytoma is a mesenchymal tumor that may originate in the orbit and, more rarely, the conjunctiva, eyelids, and sclera. Conjunctival fibrous histiocytoma often arises near the limbus and appears as a yellow or tan-colored subepithelial mass with prominent superficial vessels.[182-184] The neoplasm consists of 2 different populations of cells, namely, fibroblasts and histiocytes, and may demonstrate either benign or malignant histopathologic features.[183-185] Treatment requires complete surgical excision with wide margins.[184] Close follow-up is necessary because recurrent lesions may exhibit more aggressive clinical and histological features.[183,186]

SEBACEOUS GLAND CARCINOMA

Sebaceous gland carcinoma is a rare ocular tumor that may originate from the meibomian glands in the tarsus, the glands of Zeiss in the eyelid margin, and the sebaceous glands in the caruncle.[187-189] The tumor most often occurs in elderly individuals with a slight increased prevalence in females.[187,188] Sebaceous gland carcinoma may arise from a single or multiple (multicentric) glands, and the diagnosis is often delayed due to variable clinical findings. The tumor may present as a nodular mass, potentially mistaken for a chalazion, or as diffuse infiltrative disease, often misdiagnosed as a unilateral chronic blepharoconjuctivitis or superior limbic keratitis (Figure 10-11).[187,188,190] Intraepithelial invasion and pagetoid spread occurs in 40% to 80% of cases, though the extent of invasion is often not evident on clinical examination.[190,191]

Treatment of sebaceous gland carcinoma requires excision with wide margins. Map biopsies may be necessary in cases of diffuse disease for surgical planning.[192,193] Treatment options in cases with significant pagetoid spread include adjuvant cryotherapy, topical MMC, and exenteration.[188,194-196] Radiotherapy may be best reserved for palliative treatment.[197] Despite surgical excision, local recurrence ranges between 6% and 36% at 5 years[198] and mortality rates have been reported as high as 45%.[191]

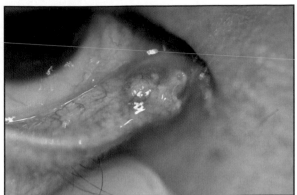

Figure 10-11. Sebaceous cell carcinoma diagnosed on excisional biopsy following repeat treatments for recurrent chalazion. (Courtesy of M. Reza Vagefi, MD.)

IRIS MASSES AND NEOPLASMS

Iris masses often can be diagnosed based on history (growth pattern) and clinical features. Overall, most iris tumors are of melanocytic or pigment epithelial origin. In addition to assessing clinical features, the use of ultrasound biomicroscopy (UBM),[199,200] fine-needle aspiration,[201] and minimally invasive incisional biopsy techniques[202,203] may all aid in establishing a diagnosis prior to devising a definitive treatment plan.

In selected cases, a constellation of ocular and systemic findings may aid in determining the underlying diagnosis of an iris mass. Iris nodules may arise in cases of infectious as well as noninfectious uveitis. Iris lesions are common early features of neurofibromatosis (Lisch nodules; multiple tan-brown neurofibromas of the iris surface) and juvenile xanthogranuloma (iris xanthogranulomas; vascularized grey-yellow masses associated with spontaneous hyphema and secondary glaucoma). White iris nodules and infiltrates may also develop secondary to retinoblastoma, leukemia, and metastases.

Iris Freckle and Iris Nevus

Iris freckles, commonly found in the adult population, are quiescent lesions produced by clusters of melanocytes in the anterior border layer of the iris.[204,205] Iris freckles appear as areas of hyperpigmentation on the anterior iris surface without any alteration in the normal stromal architecture of the iris.

An iris nevus is a benign tumor composed of atypical melanocytes that may be classified histologically into spindle, epithelioid, and polyhedral cell types. Clinical features of iris nevi may overlap with findings more commonly associated with iris melanoma, including ectropion iridis, intrinsic vessels, sectoral cataract, and glaucoma.[206,207] Ultrasound biomicroscopy may aid in differentiating iris nevi from melanoma because the posterior iris plane is typically maintained with iris nevi, yet becomes irregular and distorted in the setting of melanoma.[199,200] The majority of iris nevi remain stable over time, though iris nevi have the potential to grow and undergo malignant transformation.[207] Close observation of iris nevi is recommended because growth is often a sign of malignancy.[208] Controversy persists over whether iris nevi pose an increase in the risk of developing posterior uveal melanomas.[209-211]

Iris Melanocytoma

Iris melanocytoma is a rare variant of an iris nevus that may simulate a melanoma. Unlike iris melanomas, which rarely present in non-Caucasians, melanocytomas may occur in people of diverse racial and ethnic backgrounds.[212] Though typically diagnosed in adults, melanocytomas most likely represent a congenital lesion.[213] Histologically, the tumor consists of deeply pigmented plump melanocytes with abundant cytoplasm and small nuclei.[212,213] On clinical examination, iris melanocytomas are dark brown or black nodular tumors, which are most commonly located inferiorly at the iris root.[212] The tumor may be elevated, with a corrugated surface. Focal areas of necrosis may lead to seeding on the iris surface and anterior chamber angle.[212,214] Tumor necrosis may induce pigment dispersion and a secondary glaucoma.[212,214-216] Risk factors for elevated IOP include anterior chamber inflammation and pigmented keratic precipitates. Ectropion irides, intrinsic tumor vascularization, and sentinel vessels, common findings with iris melanoma, are rarely seen with melanocytomas.[212]

Initially, melanocytomas are usually treated by observation alone. Both fine-needle aspiration and localized resection may be performed for diagnostic purposes.[201,212] In cases of secondary glaucoma, localized tumor resection may facilitate IOP control.[217] Histopathologic diagnosis is warranted prior to any glaucoma filtering surgery. Though melanocytomas are benign, these tumors may undergo malignant transformation.[218] Growth alone, however, does not necessarily imply malignancy.[212,213]

Iris Cysts

Iris cysts may arise either spontaneously (primary) or following penetrating trauma, intraocular surgery, or prolonged use of topical miotics (secondary). Primary iris cysts are further categorized as epithelial (pigmented) and stromal (nonpigmented) subtypes. Epithelial cysts may be detected in both children and adults, whereas stromal cysts are usually identified in young children.[219-221] Epithelial cysts are more common than stromal cysts and originate from a separation in the 2 epithelial layers lining the posterior iris. The origin of stromal cysts, in contrast, remains controversial, though a surface ectodermal etiology is supported by the presence of goblet cells and other histopathological findings.[221-223] Familial cases of primary epithelial cysts have been reported.[224,225]

Primary epithelial cysts of the iris may be located peripherally, in the midzonal regions, at the pupillary margin, or be found as free-floating cysts in the anterior chamber or vitreous cavity.[219,226] The majority of epithelial cysts are located peripherally and temporally. The iris stroma overlying a pigment epithelial cyst is typically intact without any structural abnormalities (Figure 10-12). Though central cysts may be detected upon dilated examination, the diagnosis of peripheral cysts often requires the use of gonioscopy (localized peripheral anterior iris displacement) or UBM (low internal reflectivity).[199,219,227,228]

Most epithelial iris cysts are asymptomatic, rarely increase in size, and typically do not require treatment. Stromal cysts, however, tend to increase in size and may lead to reduced visual acuity, anterior chamber inflammation, corneal endothelial decompensation, and secondary glaucoma.[223,229,230] The treatment options for symptomatic iris cysts include aspiration, surgical excision, diathermy, and laser application (argon, Nd:YAG).[219,226,230-233] Rarely, multiple peripheral primary

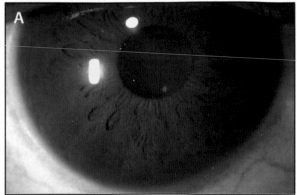

Figures 10-12. Pigment epithelial iris cyst. (A) Normal iris stromal architecture observed on slit-lamp examination. (B) High magnification demonstrates anterior bowing of iris and shallowing of anterior chamber inferotemporally.

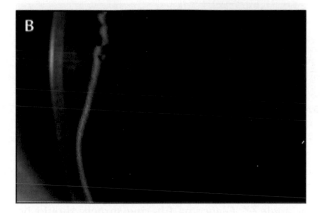

epithelial cysts of the iris or ciliary body may produce a plateau iris configuration, which may be treated by laser iridoplasty[234] or direct endoscopic laser photocoagulation (J. Alvarado, personal communication, 2003) of the individual cysts.

Iris Melanoma

Iris melanomas account for 2% to 3% of all cases of uveal melanomas.[235,236] Iris melanomas most commonly occur in Caucasian patients with blue irides[236-238] and may be categorized as either circumscribed (distinct margins) or diffuse (poorly defined margins with confluence or multifocality). Common findings on examination include inferior location, corectopia, ectropion irides, iris feeder vessels, intrinsic tumor vascularity, prominent episcleral vessels, and elevated IOP (Figure 10-13). Additionally, anterior chamber inflammation, secondary cataract, and hyphema may also be present.

Though most circumscribed iris melanomas are low-grade, spindle cell tumors, the vast majority of diffuse iris melanomas consist of epithelioid cells.[236,238-240] Epithelioid cells are less cohesive than spindle cells and are more likely to produce seeding of the angle and iris surface, resulting in elevated IOP and iris heterochromia.[238] Overall, 5-year and 10-year rates of metastases with iris melanomas are approximately 1% to 3% and 5% to 6%, respectively.[236,241] Diffuse melanoma has a worse prognosis than circumscribed tumors, with a 13% metastatic rate at 5 years.[238] Factors that increase the likelihood of metastases secondary to iris melanoma include increasing patient age at diagnosis, elevated IOP, and tumor

Figures 10-13. Iris melanoma. (A) Slit-lamp photograph reveals inferior iris melanoma. (B) Goniophotograph demonstrates mild ectropion iridis with angle structures obscured.

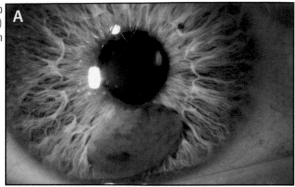

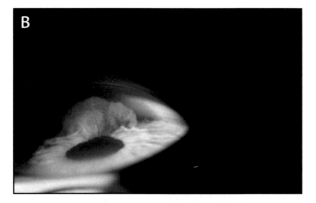

involvement of the iris root or angle.[236] Glaucoma filtering surgery should be avoided due to risk of metastases.

Diagnosis of iris melanoma is typically based upon clinical features. In addition, UBM has become a useful tool in diagnosing iris melanoma (masses of medium to high internal reflectivity with irregularity and convex bowing of posterior iris plane), documenting tumor growth, as well as assessing invasion of surrounding tissues.[199,200] In select cases, fine-needle aspiration[201] and minimally invasive incisional biopsy techniques[202,203] implementing a vitreous cutter may be necessary to establish a diagnosis. The tumor margins are critical in designing a treatment regimen for iris melanoma. For circumscribed tumors, local resection with a "no-touch" technique and 1 to 2 mm tumor-free margins is recommended. Iris root involvement or angle involvement necessitates either an iridocyclectomy or an iridogoniocyclectomy, respectively, with tumor removed ideally as a single specimen. Plaque radiotherapy may be performed as primary therapy for diffuse tumors or following resection of high-grade tumors. Enucleation is typically reserved for diffuse iris melanomas or tumors with significant seeding of the anterior chamber structures.[236,238]

Financial disclosure: Dr. Hollander is an employee of Allergan, Inc.

REFERENCES

1.   Shields CL, Demirci H, Karatza E, Shields JA. Clinical survey of 1643 melanocytic and nonmelanocytic conjunctival tumors. *Ophthalmology.* 2004;111:1747-1754.

2. Kiratli H, Shields CL, Shields JA, De Potter P. Metastatic tumours to the conjunctiva; report of 10 cases. *Br J Ophthalmol.* 1996;80:5-8.

3. Luthra CL, Doxanas MT, Green WR. Lesions of the caruncle: a clinicohistopathologic study. *Surv Ophthalmol.* 1978;23:183-195.

4. Kaeser PF, Uffer S, Zografos L, Hamedani M. Tumors of the caruncle: a clinicopathologic correlation. *Am J Ophthalmol.* 2006;142:448-455.

5. Paridaens AD, McCartney AC, Curling OM, Lyons CJ, Hungerford JL. Impression cytology of conjunctival melanosis and melanoma. *Br J Ophthalmol.* 1992;76:198-201.

6. Tole DM, McKelvie PA, Daniell M. Reliability of impression cytology for the diagnosis of ocular surface squamous neoplasia employing the Biopore membrane. *Br J Ophthalmol.* 2001;85:154-158.

7. Keijser S, Missotten GS, De Wolff-Rouendaal D, et al. Impression cytology of melanocytic conjunctival tumours using the Biopore membrane. *Eur J Ophthalmol.* 2007;17:501-506.

8. Lin HC, Shen SC, Huang SF, Tsai RJ. Ultrasound biomicroscopy in pigmented conjunctival cystic nevi. *Cornea.* 2004;23:97-99.

9. Buchwald HJ, MullerA, Kampmeier J, Lang GK. Optical coherence tomography versus ultrasound biomicroscopy of conjunctival and eyelid lesions [in German]. *Klin Monatsbl Augenheilkd.* 2003;220:822-829.

10. Sjö NC, von Buchwald C, Cassonnet P, et al. Human papillomavirus in normal conjunctival tissue and in conjunctival papilloma: types and frequencies in a large series. *Br J Ophthalmol.* 2007;91:1014-1015.

11. Kremer I, Sandbank J, Weinberger D, Rotem A, Shapiro A. Pigmented epithelial tumours of the conjunctiva. *Br J Ophthalmol.* 1992;76:294-296.

12. Sjö N, Heegaard S, Prause JU. Conjunctival papilloma. A histopathologically based retrospective study. *Acta Ophthalmol Scand.* 2000;78:663-666.

13. Lass JH, Foster CS, Grove AS, et al. Interferon-alpha therapy of recurrent conjunctival papillomas. *Am J Ophthalmol.* 1987;103(pt 1):294-301.

14. Chang SW, Huang ZL. Oral cimetidine adjuvant therapy for recalcitrant, diffuse conjunctival papillomatosis. *Cornea.* 2006;25:687-690.

15. Tritten JJ, Beati D, Sahli R, Uffer S. Bilateral conjunctivo-palpebral tumor in an immunocompetent man cause by human papilloma virus [in German]. *Klin Monatsbl Augenheilkd.* 1994;204:453-455.

16. Streeten BW, Carrillo R, Jamison R, Brownstein S, Font RL, Zimmerman LE. Inverted papilloma of the conjunctiva. *Am J Ophthalmol.* 1979;88:1062-1066.

17. Sjö NC, Heegaard S, Prause JU, von Buchwald C, Lindeberg H. Human papillomavirus in conjunctival papilloma. *Br J Ophthalmol.* 2001;85:785-787.

18. Minchiotti S, Masucci L, Serapiao Dos Santos M, et al. Conjunctival papilloma and human papillomavirus: identification of HPV types by PCR. *Eur J Ophthalmol.* 2006;16:473-477.

19. Benevides dos Santos PJ, Borborema dos Santos CM, Rufino Mendonça R, Vieira do Carmo MA, Astofi-Filho S. Human papillomavirus type 13 infecting the conjunctiva. *Diagn Microbiol Infect Dis.* 2005;53:71-73.

20. Saegusa M, Takano Y, Hashimura M, Okayasu I, Shiga J. HPV type 16 in conjunctival and junctional papilloma, dysplasia, and squamous cell carcinoma. *J Clin Pathol.* 1995;48:1106-1110.

21. Buggage RR, Smith JA, Shen D, Chan CC. Conjunctival papillomas caused by human papillomavirus type 33. *Arch Ophthalmol.* 2002;120:202-204.

22. McDonnell PJ, McDonnell JM, Kessis T, Green WR, Shah KV. Detection of human papillomavirus type 6/11 DNA in conjunctival papillomas by in situ hybridization with radioactive probes. *Hum Pathol.* 1987;18:1115-1119.

23. Eng HL, Lin TM, Chen SY, Chen WJ. Failure to detect human papillomavirus DNA in malignant epithelial neoplasms of conjunctiva by polymerase chain reaction. *Am J Clin Pathol.* 2002;117:429-436.

24. Heuring AH, Hütz WW, Eckhardt HB, Bohle RM. Inverted transitional cell papilloma of the conjunctiva with peripheral carcinomatous transformation [in German]. *Klin Monatsbl Augenheilkd.* 1998;212:61-63.

25. McDonnell JM, McDonnell PJ, Sun YY. Human papillomavirus DNA in tissues and ocular surface swabs of patients with conjunctival epithelial neoplasia. *Invest Ophthalmol Vis Sci.* 1992;33:184-189.

26. Scott IU, Karp CL, Nuovo GJ. Human papillomavirus 16 and 18 expression in conjunctival intraepithelial neoplasia. *Ophthalmology.* 2002;109:542-547.

27. Hawkins AS, Yu J, Hamming NA, Rubenstein JB. Treatment of recurrent conjunctival papillomatosis with mitomycin C. *Am J Ophthalmol.* 1999;128:638-40.

28. Yuen HK, Yeung EF, Chan NR, Chi SC, Lam DS. The use of postoperative topical mitomycin C in the treatment of recurrent conjunctival papilloma. *Cornea.* 2002;21:838-839.

29. Chen HC, Chang SW, Huang SF. Adjunctive treatment with interferon alpha-2b may decrease the risk of papilloma-associated conjunctival intraepithelial neoplasm recurrence. *Cornea.* 2004;23:726-729.

30. Omohundro JM, Elliott JH. Cryotherapy of conjunctival papilloma. *Arch Ophthalmol.* 1970;84:609-610.

31. Bosniak SL, Novick NL, Sachs ME. Treatment of recurrent squamous papillomata of the conjunctiva by carbon dioxide laser vaporization. *Ophthalmology.* 1986;93:1078-1082.

32. Burns RP, Wankum G, Giangiacomo J, Anderson PC. Dinitrochlorobenzene and debulking therapy of conjunctival papilloma. *J Pediatr Ophthalmol Strabismus.* 1983;20:221-226.

33. Tulvatana W, Pisarnkorskul P, Wannakrairot P. Solitary keratoacanthoma of the conjunctiva: report of a case. *J Med Assoc Thai.* 2001;84:1059-1064.

34. Freeman RG, Cloud TM, Knox JM. Keratoacanthoma of the conjunctiva. A case report. *Arch Ophthalmol.* 1961;65:817-819.

35. Roth AM. Solitary keratoacanthoma of the conjunctiva. *Am J Ophthalmol.* 1978;85(pt 1):647-650.

36. Coupland SE, Heimann H, Kellner U, Bornfeld N, Foerster MH, Lee WR. Keratoacanthoma of the bulbar conjunctiva. *Br J Ophthalmol.* 1998;82:586.

37. Perdigao FB, Pierre-Filho Pde T, Natalino RJ, Caldato R, Torigoe M, Cintra ML. Conjunctival keratoacanthoma. *Rev Hosp Clin Fac Med Sao Paulo.* 2004;59:135-137.

38. Munro S, Brownstein S, Liddy B. Conjunctival keratoacanthoma. *Am J Ophthalmol.* 1993;116:654-655.

39. Hughes EH, Intzedy L, Dick AD, Tole DM. Keratoacanthoma of the conjunctiva. *Eye.* 2003;17:781-782.

40. Grossniklaus HE, Martin DF, Solomon AR. Invasive conjunctival tumor with keratoacanthoma features. *Am J Ophthalmol.* 1990;109:736-738.

41. McLean IW, Riddle PJ, Schruggs JH, Jones DB. Hereditary benign intraepithelial dyskeratosis. A report of two cases from Texas. *Ophthalmology.* 1981;88:164-168.

42. Shields CL, Shields JA, Eagle RC Jr. Hereditary benign intraepithelial dyskeratosis. *Arch Ophthalmol.* 1987;105:422-423.

43. Dithmar S, Stulting RD, Grossniklaus HE. Hereditary benign intraepithelial dyskeratosis [in German]. *Ophthalmologe.* 1998;95:684-686.

44. Haisley-Royster CA, Allingham RR, Klintworth GK, Prose NS. Hereditary benign intraepithelial dyskeratosis: report of two cases with prominent oral lesions. *J Am Acad Dermatol.* 2001;45:634-636.

45. Allingham RR, Seo B, Rampersaud E, et al. A duplication in chromosome 4q35 is associated with hereditary benign intraepithelial dyskeratosis. *Am J Hum Genet.* 2001;68:491-494.

46. Grossniklaus HE, Green WR, Luckenbach M, Chan CC. Conjunctival lesions in adults. A clinical and histopathologic review. *Cornea.* 1987;6:78-116.

47. Lee GA, Hirst LW. Ocular surface squamous neoplasia. *Surv Ophthalmol.* 1995;39:429-450.

48. Hirst LW. Randomized controlled trial of topical mitomycin C for ocular surface squamous neoplasia: early resolution. *Ophthalmology.* 2007;114:976-982.

49. Schechter BA, Koreishi AF, Karp CL, Feuer W. Long-term follow-up of conjunctival and corneal intraepithelial neoplasia treated with topical interferon alfa-2b. *Ophthalmology.* 2008;115:1291-1296.

50. Lee GA, Williams G, Hirst LW, Green AC. Risk factors in the development of ocular surface epithelial dysplasia. *Ophthalmology.* 1994;101:360-364.

51. McDonnell JM, Mayr AJ, Martin WJ. DNA of human papillomavirus type 16 in dysplastic and malignant lesions of the conjunctiva and cornea. *N Eng J Med.* 1989;320:1442-1446.

52. Lauer SA, Malter JS, Meier JR. Human papillomavirus type 18 in conjunctival intraepithelial neoplasia. *Am J Ophthalmol.* 1990:110:23-27.

53. Scott IU, Karp CL, Nuovo GJ. Human papillomavirus 16 and 18 expression in conjunctival intraepithelial neoplasia. *Ophthalmology.* 2002;109:542-547.

54. Waddell KM, Lewallen S, Lucas SB, Atenyi-Agaba C, Herrington CS, Liomba G. Carcinoma of the conjunctiva and HIV infection in Uganda and Malawi. *Br J Ophthalmol.* 1996;80:503-508.

55. Napora C, Cohen E, Genvert GI, et al. Factors associated with conjunctival intraepithelial neoplasia: a case control study. *Ophthalmic Surg.* 1990;21:27-30.

56. Goyal JL, Rao VA, Srinivasan R, Agrawal K. Oculocutaneous manifestations in xeroderma pigmentosa. *Br J Ophthalmol.* 1994;78:295-297.

57. Rouberol F, Burillon C, Kodjikian L, Simon P, Bouvier R, Denis P. Conjunctival epithelial carcinoma in a 9-year old child with xeroderma pigmentosum. Case report [in French]. *J Fr Ophthalmol.* 2001;24:639-642.

58. Sanders N, Bedotto C. Recurrent carcinoma in situ of the conjunctiva and cornea (Bowen's disease). *Am J Ophthalmol.* 1972;74:688-693.

59. Waring GO III, Roth AM, Ekins MB. Clinical and pathological descriptions of 17 cases of corneal intraepithelial neoplasia. *Am J Ophthalmol.* 1984;97:547-559.

60. Kaeser PF, Uffer S, Zografos L, Hamedani M. Tumors of the caruncle: a clinicopathologic correlation. *Am J Ophthalmol.* 2006;142:448-455.

61. Brown HH, Glasgow BJ, Holland GN, Foos RY. Keratinizing corneal intraepithelial neoplasia. *Cornea.* 1989;8:220-224.

62. Kaji Y, Hiraoka T, Oshika T. Vital staining of squamous cell carcinoma of the conjunctiva using toluidine blue. *Acta Ophthalmol Scan.* 2006;84:825-826.

63. Jones DB, Wilhelmus KR, Font RL. Beta radiation of recurrent corneal intraepithelial neoplasia. *Trans Am Ophthalmol Soc.* 1991;89:285-301.

64. Dausch D, Landesz M, Schroder E. Phototherapeutic keratectomy in recurrent corneal intraepithelial dysplasia. *Arch Ophthalmol.* 1994;112:22-23.

65. Barbazetto IA, Lee TC, Abramson DH. Treatment of conjunctival squamous cell carcinoma with photodynamic therapy. *Am J Ophthalmol.* 2004;138:183-189.

66. Herbort CP, Zografos L, Zwingli M, Schoeneich M. Topical retinoic acid in dysplastic and metaplastic keratinization of corneoconjunctival epithelium. *Graefes Arch Clin Exp Ophthalmol.* 1988;226:22-26.

67. Frucht-Pery J, Rozenman Y. Mitomycin C therapy for corneal intraepithelial neoplasia. *Am J Ophthalmol.* 1994;117:164-168.

68. Wilson MW, Hungerford JL, George SM, Madreperla SA. Topical mitomycin C for the treatment of conjunctival and corneal epithelial dysplasia and neoplasia. *Am J Ophthalmol.* 1997;124:303-311.

69. Heigle TJ, Stulting R, Palay DA. Treatment of recurrent conjunctival epithelial neoplasia with topical mitomycin C. *Am J Ophthalmol.* 1997;124:397-399.

70. Shields CL, Naseripour M, Shields JA. Topical mitomycin C for extensive, recurrent conjunctival-corneal squamous cell carcinoma. *Am J Ophthalmol.* 2002;133:601-606.

71. Prabhasawat P, Tarinvorakup P, Tesavibul N, et al. Topical 0.002% mitomycin C for the treatment of conjunctival-corneal intraepithelial neoplasia and squamous cell carcinoma. *Cornea.* 2005;24:443-448.

72. Yeatts RP, Engelbrecht NE, Curry CD, Ford JG, Walter KA. 5-Fluorouracil for the treatment of intraepithelial neoplasia of the conjunctiva and cornea. *Ophthalmology.* 2000;107:2190-2195.

73. Sherman MD, Feldman KA, Farahmand SM, Margolis TP. Treatment of conjunctival squamous cell carcinoma with topical cidofovir. *Am J Ophthalmol.* 2002;134:432-433.

74. Karp CL, Moore JK, Rosa RH Jr. Treatment of conjunctival and corneal intraepithelial neoplasia with topical interferon alpha-2b. *Ophthalmology.* 2001;108:1093-1098.

75. Boehm MD, Huang AJ. Treatment of recurrent corneal and conjunctival intraepithelial neoplasia with topical interferon alfa 2b. *Ophthalmology.* 2004;111:1755-1761.

76. Fraunfelder FT, Wingfield D. Management of intraepithelial conjunctival tumors and squamous cell carcinoma. *Am J Ophthalmol.* 1983;95:359-363.

77. Erie JC, Campbell RJ, Liesegang TJ. Conjunctival and corneal intraepithelial and invasive neoplasia. *Ophthalmology.* 1986;93:176-183.

78. Tabin G, Levin S, Snibson G, Loughnan M, Taylor H. Late recurrences and the necessity for long-term follow up in corneal and conjunctival intraepithelial neoplasia. *Ophthalmology.* 1997;104:485-492.

79. Tunc M, Char DH, Crawford B, Miller T. Intraepithelial and invasive squamous cell carcinoma of the conjunctiva: analysis of 60 cases. *Br J Ophthalmol.* 1999;83:98-103.

80. Khong JJ, Muecke J. Complications of mitomycin C therapy in 100 eyes with ocular surface neoplasia. *Br J Ophthalmol.* 2006;90:819-822.

81. Aldave AJ, Nguyen A. Ocular surface toxicity associated with topical interferon alpha-2b. *Br J Ophthalmol.* 2006;91:1087-1088.

82. Shields JA, Shields CL, Gunduz K, Eagle RC Jr. The 1998 Pan American Lecture. Intraocular invasion of conjunctival squamous cell carcinoma in five patients. *Ophthal Plast Reconstr Surg.* 1999;15:153-160.

83. Zhang Z, Li B, Shi J, Xu X, Li L, Gao F. Intraocular extension of conjunctival squamous cell carcinoma. *Ophthalmologica.* 2007;221:200-203.

84. Char DH, Kundert G, Bove R, Crawford JB. 20 MHz high frequency ultrasound assessment of scleral and intraocular conjunctival squamous cell carcinoma. *Br J Ophthalmol.* 2002;86:632-635.

85. Finger Pt, Tran HV, Turbin RE, et al. High-frequency ultrasonographic evaluation of conjunctival intraepithelial neoplasia and squamous cell carcinoma. *Arch Ophthalmol.* 2003;121:168-172.

86. Giaconi JA, Karp CL. Current treatment options for conjunctival and corneal intraepithelial neoplasia. *Ocul Surf.* 2003;1:66-73.

87. Tabbara KF, Kersten R, Daouk N, Blodi FC. Metastatic squamous cell carcinoma of the conjunctiva. *Ophthalmology.* 1988;95:318-321.

88. Tulvatana W, Tirakunwichcha S. Multifocal squamous cell carcinoma of the conjunctiva with intraocular penetration in a patient with AIDS. *Cornea.* 2006;25:745-747.

89. Shelil AE, Shields CL, Shields JA, Eagle RC Jr. Aggressive conjunctival squamous cell carcinoma in a patient following liver transplantation. *Arch Ophthalmol.* 2003;121:280-282.

90. Winward K, Curtin V. Conjunctival squamous cell carcinoma in a patient with human immunodeficiency virus infection. *Am J Ophthalmol.* 1989;107:554-555.

91. Rao NA, Font RL. Mucoepidermoid carcinoma of the conjunctiva: a clinicopathologic study of five cases. *Cornea.* 1976;38:1699-1709.

92. Huntington AC, Langloss JM, Hidayat AA. Spindle cell carcinoma of the conjunctiva. An immunohistochemical and ultrastructural study of six cases. *Ophthalmology.* 1990;97:711-717.

93. Mauriello JA Jr, Abdelsalam A, McLean IW. Adenoid squamous carcinoma of the conjunctiva—a clinicopathological study of 14 cases. *Br J Ophthalmol.* 1997;81:1001-1005.

94. Jay B. Naevi and melanomata of the conjunctiva. *Br J Ophthalmol.* 1965;49:169-204.

95. Shields CL, Fasiuddin A, Mashayekhi A, Shields JA. Conjunctival nevi: clinical features and natural course in 410 consecutive patients. *Arch Ophthalmol.* 2004;122:167-175.

96. Folberg R, Jakobiec FA, Bernardino VB, Iwamoto T. Benign conjunctival melanocytic lesions. Clinicopathologic features. *Ophthalmology.* 1989;96:436-461.

97. Gerner N, Norregaard JC, Jensen OA, Prause JU. Conjunctival naevi in Denmark 1960-1980: A 21-year follow-up study. *Acta Ophthalmol Scan.* 1996;74:334-337.

98. McDonnell JM, Carpenter JD, Jacobs P, Wan WL, Gilmore JE. Conjunctival melanocytic lesions in children. *Ophthalmology.* 1989;96:986-993.

99. Zamir E, Mechoulam H, Micera A, Lev-Schaffer F, Pe'er J. Inflamed juvenile conjunctival nevus: clinicopathologic characterization. *Br J Ophthalmol.* 2002;86:28-30.

100. Kwon JW, Jeoung JW, Kim TI, Lee JH, Wee WR. Argon laser photoablation of conjunctival pigmented nevus. *Am J Ophthalmol.* 2006;141:383-386.

101. Gonder JR, Shields JA, Shakin JL, Albert DM. Bilateral ocular melanocytosis with malignant melanoma of the choroid. *Br J Ophthalmol.* 1981;65:843-845.

102. Swann PG. Iris mammillations in ocular melanocytosis. *Clin Exp Optom.* 2001;84:35-38.

103. Turnbull JR, Assaf CH, Zouboulis C, Tebbe B. Bilateral naevus of Ota: a rare manifestation in a Caucasian. *J Eur Acad Dermatol Venereol.* 2004;18:353-355.

104. Singh AD, De Potter P, Fijal BA, Shields CL, Shields JA, Elston RC. Lifetime prevalence of uveal melanoma in white patients with oculo(dermal) melanocytosis. *Ophthalmology.* 1998;105:195-198.

105. Jakobiec FA, Folberg R, Iwamoto T. Clinicopathologic characteristics of premalignant and malignant melanocytic lesions of the conjunctiva. *Ophthalmology.* 1989;96:147-166.

106. Shields JA, Shields CL, Mashayekhi A, et al. Primary acquired melanosis of the conjunctiva: risks for progression to melanoma in 311 eyes: the 2006 Lorenz E. Zimmerman Lecture. *Ophthalmology.* 2008;115:511-519.

107. Paridaens AD, McCartney AC, Hungerford JL. Multifocal amelanotic conjunctival melanoma and acquired melanosis sine pigmento. *Br J Ophthalmol.* 1992;76:163-165.

108. Jay V, Font RL. Conjunctival amelanotic malignant melanoma arising in primary acquired melanosis sine pigmento. *Ophthalmology.* 1998;105:191-194.

109. Folberg R, Baron J, Reeves RD, Stevens RH, Bogh LD. Animal model of conjunctival primary acquired melanosis. *Ophthalmology.* 1989;96:1006-1013.

110. Folberg R, McLean IW, Zimmerman LE. Malignant melanoma of the conjunctiva. *Hum Pathol.* 1985;16:136-143.

111. Jakobiec FA, Rini FJ, Fraunfelder FT, Brownstein S. Cryotherapy for conjunctival primary acquired melanosis and malignant melanoma. Experience with 62 cases. *Ophthalmology.* 1988;95:1058-1070.

112. Frucht-Pery J, Pe'er J. Use of mitomycin C in the treatment of conjunctival primary acquired melanosis with atypia. *Arch Ophthalmol.* 1996;114:1261-1264.

113. Finger PT, Czechonska G, Liarikos S. Topical mitomycin C chemotherapy for conjunctival melanoma and PAM with atypia. *Br J Ophthalmol.* 1998;82:476-479.

114. Pe'er J, Frucht-Pery J. The treatment of primary acquired melanosis (PAM) with atypia by topical Mitomycin C. *Am J Ophthalmol.* 2005;139:229-234.

115. Kurli M, Finger PT. Topical mitomycin chemotherapy for conjunctival malignant melanoma and primary acquired melanosis with atypia: 12 years' experience. *Graefes Arch Clin Exp Ophthalmol.* 2005;243:1108-1114.

116. Char DH. The management of lid and conjunctival malignancies. *Surv Ophthalmol.* 1980;24:679-689.

117. Graham BJ, Duane TD. Ocular melanoma task force report. *Am J Ophthalmol.* 1980;90:728-733.

118. Grossniklaus HE, Green WR, Luckenbach M, Chan CC. Conjunctival lesions in adults. A clinical and histopathologic review. *Cornea.* 1987;6:78-116.

119. Chau KY, Hui SP, Cheng GP. Conjunctival melanocytic lesions in Chinese: comparison with Caucasian series. *Pathology.* 1999;31:199-201.

120. Seregard S. Conjunctival melanoma. *Surv Ophthalmol.* 1998;42:321-350.

121. Shields CL. Conjunctival melanoma: risk factors for recurrence, exenteration, metastasis, and death in 150 consecutive patients. *Trans Am Ophthalmol Soc.* 2000;98:471-492.

122. Crawford JB. Conjunctival melanomas: prognostic factors a review and an analysis of a series. *Trans Am Ophthalmol Soc.* 1980;78:467-502.

123. Seregard S, Kock E. Conjunctival malignant melanoma in Sweden 1969-91. *Acta Ophthalmol Scand Suppl.* 1992;70:289-296.

124. Norregaard JC, Gerner N, Jensen OA, Prause JU. Malignant melanoma of the conjunctiva: occurrence and survival following surgery and radiotherapy in a Danish population. *Graefes Arch Clin Exp Ophthalmol.* 1996;234:569-572.

125. Paridaens AD, Minassian DC, McCartney AC, Hungerford JL. Prognostic factors in primary malignant melanoma of the conjunctiva: a clinicopathological study of 256 cases. *Br J Ophthalmol.* 1994;78:252-259.

126. Griffith WR, Green WR, Weinstein GW. Conjunctival malignant melanoma originating in acquired melanosis sine pigmento. *Am J Ophthalmol.* 1971;72:595-599.

127. De Potter P, Shields CL, Shields JA, Menduke H. Clinical predictive factors for development of recurrence and metastasis in conjunctival melanoma: a review of 68 cases. *Br J Ophthalmol.* 1993;77:624-630.

128. Anastassiou G, Heiligenhaus A, Bechrakis N, Bader E, Bornfeld N, Steuhl KP. Prognostic value of clinical and histopathological parameters in conjunctival melanomas: a retrospective study. *Br J Ophthalmol.* 2002;86:163-167.

129. Tuomaala S, Eskelin S, Tarkkanen A, Kivela T. Population-based assessment of clinical characteristics predicting outcome of conjunctival melanoma in Whites. *Invest Ophthalmol Vis Sci.* 2002;43:3399-3408.

130. Esmaeli B, Wang X, Youssef A, Gershenwald JE. Patterns of regional and distant metastasis in patients with conjunctival melanoma: experience at a cancer center of four decades. *Ophthalmology.* 2001;108:2101-2105.

131. Tuomaala S, Kivela T. Metastatic pattern and survival in disseminated conjunctival melanoma: implications for sentinel lymph node biopsy. *Ophthalmology.* 2004;111:816-821.

132. Missotten GS, Keijser S, De Keizer RJ, De Wolff-Rouendaal D. Conjunctiva melanoma in the Netherlands: a nationwide study. *Invest Ophthalmol Vis Sci.* 2005;46:75-82.

133. Tuomaala S, Toivonen P, Al-Jamal R, Kivela T. Prognostic significance of histopathology of primary conjunctival melanoma in Caucasians. *Curr Eye Res.* 2007;32:939-952.

134. Lommatzsch PK, Lommatzsch RE, Kirsch I, Fuhrmann P. Therapeutic outcome of patients suffering from malignant melanomas of the conjunctiva. *Br J Ophthalmol.* 1990;74:615-690.

135. Shields JA, Shields CL, De Potter P. Surgical approach to conjunctival tumors. The 1994 Lynn B. McMahan Lecture. *Arch Ophthalmol.* 1997;115:808-815.

136. Choi J, Kim M, Park HS, Lee SY. Clinical follow-up of conjunctival malignant melanoma. *Korean J Ophthalmol.* 2005;19:91-95.

137. Zografos L, Uffer S, Bercher L, Gailloud C. Combined surgery, cryocoagulation and radiotherapy for treatment of melanoma of the conjunctiva [in German]. *Klin Monatsbl Augenheilkd.* 1994;204:385-390.

138. Wuestemeyer H, Sauerwein W, Meller D, et al. Proton radiotherapy as an alternative to exenteration in the management of extended conjunctival melanoma. *Graefes Arch Clin Exp Ophthalmol.* 2006;244:438-446.

139. Demirci H, McCormick SA, Finger PT. Topical mitomycin chemotherapy for conjunctival malignant melanoma and primary acquired melanosis with atypia: clinical experience with histopathologic observations. *Arch Ophthalmol.* 2000;118:885-891.

140. Colby KA, Nagel DS. Conjunctival melanoma arising from diffuse primary acquired melanosis in a young black woman. *Cornea.* 2005;24:352-355.

141. Finger PT, Sedeek RW, Chin KJ. Topical interferon alfa in the treatment of conjunctival melanoma and primary acquired melanosis complex. *Am J Ophthalmol.* 2008;145:124-129.

142. Paridaens AD, McCartney AC, Minassian DC, Hungerford JL. Orbital exenteration in 95 cases of primary conjunctival malignant melanoma. *Br J Ophthalmol.* 1994;78:520-528.

143. Baroody M, Holds JB, Kokoska MS, Boyd J. Conjunctiva melanoma metastasis diagnosed by sentinel lymph node biopsy. *Am J Ophthalmol.* 2004;137:1147-1149.

144. Yu GP, Hu DN, McCormick S, Finger PT. Conjunctival melanoma: is it increasing in the United States? *Am J Ophthalmol.* 2003;135:800-806.

145. Swerdlow AJ. Incidence of malignant melanoma of the skin in England and Wales and its relationship to sunshine. *Br Med J.* 1979;2:1324-1327.

146. Swerdlow AJ, Cooke KR, Skegg DC, Wilkinson J. Cancer incidence in England and Wales and New Zealand an in migrants between the two countries. *Br J Cancer.* 1995;72:326-343.

147. Shuler JD, Holland GN, Miles SA, Miller BJ, Grossman I. Kaposi sarcoma of the conjunctiva and eyelids associated with the acquired immunodeficiency syndrome. *Arch Ophthalmol.* 1989;107:858-862.

148. Brun SC, Jakobiec FA. Kaposi's sarcoma of the ocular adnexa. *Int Ophthalmol Clin.* 1997;37:25-38.

149. Antman K, Chang Y. Kaposi's sarcoma. *N Engl J Med.* 2000;342:1027-1038.

150. Schmid K, Wild T, Bolz M, Horvat R, Jurecka W, Zehetmayer M. Kaposi's sarcoma of the conjunctiva leads to a diagnosis of acquired immunodeficiency syndrome. *Acta Ophthalmol Scan.* 2003;81:411-413.

151. Curtis TH, Durairaj VD. Conjunctival Kaposi sarcoma as the initial presentation of human immunodeficiency virus infection. *Ophthal Plast Reconstr Surg.* 2005;21:314-315.

152. Weiter JJ, Jakobiec FA, Iwamoto T. The clinical and morphologic characteristics of Kaposi's sarcomas of the conjunctiva. *Am J Ophthalmol.* 1980;89:546-552.

153. Moore PS, Chang Y. Detection of herpesvirus-like DNA sequences in Kaposi's sarcoma in patients with and without HIV infection. *N Eng J Med.* 1995;332:1181-1185.

154. Foreman KE, Friborg J Jr, Kong WP, et al. Propagation of a human herpesvirus from AIDS-associated Kaposi's sarcoma. *N Eng J Med.* 1997;336:163-171.

155. Hasche H, Eck M, Lieb W. Immunochemical demonstration of human herpes virus 8 in conjunctival Kaposi's sarcoma. *Ophthalmologe.* 2003;100142-144.

156. Visser OH, Bos PJ. Kaposi's sarcoma of the conjunctiva and CMV-retinitis in AIDS. *Doc Ophthalmol.* 1986;64:77-85.

157. Dugel PU, Gill PS, Frangieh GT, Rao NA. Treatment of ocular adnexal Kaposi's sarcoma in acquired immune deficiency syndrome. *Ophthalmology.* 1992;99:1127-1132.

158. Howard GM, Jakobiec FA, DeVoe AG. Kaposi's sarcoma of the conjunctiva. *Am J Ophthalmol.* 1975;79:420-423.

159. Ghabrial R, Quivey JM, Dunn JP Jr, Char DH. Radiation therapy of acquired immunodeficiency syndrome-related Kaposi's sarcoma of the eyelids and conjunctiva. *Arch Ophthalmol.* 1992;110:1423-1426.

160. Hummer J, Gass JD, Huang AJ. Conjunctival Kaposi's sarcoma treated with interferon alpha-2a. *Am J Ophthalmol.* 1993;116:502-503.

161. Gill PS, Lunardi-Ishkandar Y, Louie S, et al. The effects of preparations of human chorionic gonadotropin on AIDS-related Kaposi's sarcoma. *N Engl J Med.* 1996;335:1261-1269.

162. Pellet C, Chevret S, Blum L, et al. Virologic and immunologic parameters that predict clinical response of AIDS-associated Kaposi's sarcoma to highly active antiretroviral therapy. *J Invest Dermatol.* 2001;117:858-863.

163. Cattelan AM, Calabro ML, Gasperini P, et al. Acquired immunodeficiency syndrome-related Kaposi's sarcoma regression after highly active antiretroviral therapy: biologic correlates of clinical outcome. *J Natl Cancer Inst Monogr.* 2001;28:44-49.

164. Martinez V, Caumes E, Gambotti L, et al. Remission from Kaposi's sarcoma on HAART is associated with suppression of HIV replication and is independent of protease inhibitor therapy. *Br J Cancer.* 2006;94:1000-1006.

165. Knowles DM, Jakobiec FA, McNally L, Burke JS. Lymphoid hyperplasia and malignant lymphoma occurring in the ocular adnexa (orbit, conjunctiva, and eyelids): a prospective multiparametric analysis of 108 cases during 1977 to 1987. *Hum Pathol.* 1990;21:959-973.

166. Farmer JP, Lamba M, Merkur AB, et al. Characterization of lymphoproliferative lesions of the conjunctiva: immunohistochemical and molecular genetic studies. *Can J Ophthalmol.* 2006;41:753-760.

167. Shields CL, Shields JA, Carvalho C, Rundle P, Smith AF. Conjunctival lymphoid tumors: clinical analysis of 117 cases and relationship to systemic lymphoma. *Ophthalmology.* 2001;108:979-984.

168. Coupland SE, Krause L, Delecluse HJ, et al. Lymphoproliferative lesions of the ocular adnexa. Analysis of 112 cases. *Ophthalmology.* 1998;105:1430-1441.

169. Jenkins C, Rose GE, Bunce C, et al. Histological features of ocular adnexal lymphoma (REAL classification) and their association with patient morbidity and survival. *Br J Ophthalmol.* 2000;84:907-913.

170. Shields CL, Shields JA, Eagle RC. Rapidly progressive T-cell lymphoma of the conjunctiva. *Arch Ophthalmol.* 2002;120:508-509.

171. Hatef E, Roberts D, McLaughlin P, Pro B, Esmaeli B. Prevalence and nature of systemic involvement and stage at initial examination in patients with orbital and ocular adnexal lymphoma. *Arch Ophthalmol.* 2007;125:1663-1667.

172. Kim NJ, Khwarg SI. Primary diffuse large B-cell lymphoma of the palpebral conjunctiva. *Can J Ophthalmol.* 2007;42:630-631.

173. Shields CL, Shields JA. Conjunctival tumors in children. *Curr Opin Ophthalmol.* 2007;18:351-360.

174. Johnson TE, Tse DT, Byrne GE Jr, et al. Ocular-adnexal lymphoid tumors: a clinicopathologic and molecular genetic study of 77 patients. *Ophthal Plast Reconstr Surg.* 1999;15:171-179.

175. Bessell EM, Henk JM, Whitelocke RA, Wright JE. Ocular morbidity after radiotherapy of orbital and conjunctival lymphoma. *Eye.* 1987;1(pt 1):90-96.

176. Lachapelle KR, Rathee R, Kratky V, Dexter DF. Treatment of conjunctival mucosa-associated lymphoid tissue lymphoma with intralesional injection of interferon alfa-2b. *Arch Ophthalmol.* 2000;118:284-285.

177. Hoang-Xuan T, Bodaghi B, Toublanc M, Delmer A, Schwartz L, D'Hermies F. Scleritis and mucosal-associated lymphoid tissue lymphoma: a new masquerade syndrome. *Ophthalmology.* 1996;103:631-635.

178. Sarraf D, Jain A, Dubovy S, Kreiger A, Fong D, Paschal J. Mucosa-associated lymphoid tissue lymphoma with intraocular involvement. *Retina.* 2005;25:94-98.

179. Ramulu P, Iliff NT, Green WR, Kuo IC. Asymptomatic conjunctival mucosa-associated lymphoid tissue-type lymphoma with presumed intraocular involvement. *Cornea.* 2007;26:484-486.

180. Jenkins C, Rose GE, Bunce C, et al. Clinical features associated with survival of patients with lymphoma of the ocular adnexa. *Eye.* 2003;17:809-820.

181. Freeman C, Berg JW, Cutler SJ. Occurrence and prognosis of extranodal lymphomas. *Cancer.* 1972;29:252-260.

182. Lahous S, Brownstein S, Laflamme MY. Fibrous histiocytoma of the corneoscleral limbus and conjunctiva. *Am J Ophthalmol.* 1988;106:579-583.

183. Conway RM, Holbach LM, Naumann GO. Benign fibrous histiocytoma of the corneoscleral limbus: unique clinicopathologic features. 2003;121:1776-1779.

184. Kim HJ, Shields CL, Eagle RC Jr, Shields JA. Fibrous histiocytoma of the conjunctiva. *Am J Ophthalmol.* 2006;142:1036-1043.

185. Arora R, Monga S, Mehta DK, Raina UK, Gogi A, Gupta SD. Malignant fibrous histiocytoma of the conjunctiva. *Clin Exp Ophthalmol.* 2006;34:275-278.

186. Allaire GS, Corriveau C, Teboul N. Malignant fibrous histiocytoma of the conjunctiva. *Arch Ophthalmol.* 1999;117:685-687.

187. Kass LG, Hornblass A. Sebaceous carcinoma of the ocular adnexa. *Surv Ophthalmol.* 1989;33:477-490.

188. Chao AN, Shields CL, Krema H, Shields JA. Outcome of patients with periocular sebaceous gland carcinoma with and without conjunctival intraepithelial invasion. *Ophthalmology.* 2001;108:1877-1883.

189. Shields JA, Shields CL, Marr BP, Eagle RC Jr. Sebaceous carcinoma of the caruncle. *Cornea.* 2006;25:858-859.

190. Margo CE, Lessner A, Stern GA. Intraepithelial sebaceous carcinoma of the conjunctiva and skin of the eyelid. *Ophthalmology.* 1992;99:227-231.

191. Rao NA, Hidayat AA, McLean IW, Zimmerman LE. Sebaceous carcinomas of the ocular adnexa: A clinicopathologic study of 104 cases, with five-year follow-up data. *Hum Pathol.* 1982;13:113-122.

192. Putterman AM. Conjunctival map biopsy to determine pagetoid spread. *Am J Ophthalmol.* 1986;102:87-90.

193. Shields JA, Demirci H, Marr BP, Eagle RC Jr, Stefanyszyn M, Shields CL. Conjunctival epithelial involvement by eyelid sebaceous carcinoma. The 2003 J. Howard Stokes lecture. *Ophthal Plast Reconstr Surg.* 2005;21:92-96.

194. Lisman RD, Jakobiec FA, Small P. Sebaceous carcinoma of the eyelids. The role of adjunctive cryotherapy in the management of conjunctival pagetoid spread. *Ophthalmology.* 1989;96:1021-1026.

195. Shields CL, Naseripour M, Shields JA, Eagle RC Jr. Topical mitomycin-C for pagetoid invasion of the conjunctiva by eyelid sebaceous gland carcinoma. *Ophthalmology.* 2002;109:2129-2133.

196. Tumuluri K, Kourt G, Martin P. Mitomycin C in sebaceous gland carcinoma with pagetoid spread. *Br J Ophthalmol.* 2004;88:718-719.

197. Nunery WR, Welsh MG, McCord CD. Recurrence of sebaceous carcinoma of the eyelid after radiation therapy. *Am J Ophthalmol.* 1983;96:10-15.

198. De Potter P, Shields CL, Shields JA. Sebaceous gland carcinoma of the eyelids. *Int Ophthalmol Clin.* 1993;33:5-9.

199. Conway RM, Chew T, Golchet P, Desai K, Lin S, O'Brien J. Ultrasound biomicroscopy: role in diagnosis and management in 130 consecutive patients evaluated for anterior segment tumours. *Br J Ophthalmol.* 2005;89:950-955.

200. Gunduz K, Hosal BM, Zilelioglu G, Gunalp I. The use of ultrasound biomicroscopy in the evaluation of anterior segment tumors and simulating conditions. *Ophthalmologica.* 2007;221:305-312.

201. Shields CL, Manquez ME, Ehya H, Mashayekhi A, Danzig CJ, Shields JA. Fine-needle aspiration biopsy of iris tumors in 100 consecutive cases: technique and complications. *Ophthalmology.* 2006;113:2080-2086.

202. Bechrakis NE, Foerster MH, Bornfeld N. Biopsy in indeterminate intraocular tumors. *Ophthalmology.* 2002;109:235-242.

203. Finger PT, Latkany P, Kurli M, Iacob C. The Finger iridectomy technique: small incision biopsy of anterior segment tumours. *Br J Ophthalmol.* 2005;89:946-949.

204. Hogan MJ, Alvarado JA, Weddell JE. *Histology of the Human Eye: An Atlas and Textbook.* Philadelphia, Pa: W.B. Saunders Company; 1971.

205. Eagle RC Jr. Iris pigmentation and pigmented lesions: an ultrastructural study. *Trans Am Ophthalmol Soc.* 1988;86:581-687.

206. Nik NA, Hidayat A, Zimmerman LE, Fine BS. Diffuse iris nevus manifested by unilateral open angle glaucoma. *Arch Ophthalmol.* 1981;99:125-127.

207. Territo C, Shields CL, Shields JA, Augsburger JJ, Schroeder RP. Natural course of melanocytic tumors of the iris. *Ophthalmology.* 1988;95:1251-1255.

208. Harbour JW, Augsburger JJ, Eagle RC Jr. Initial management and follow-up of melanocytic iris tumors. *Ophthalmology.* 1995;102:1987-1993.

209. Michelson JB, Shields JA. Relationship of iris nevi to malignant melanoma of the uvea. *Am J Ophthalmol.* 1977;83:694-696.

210. Horn EP, Hartge P, Shields JA, Tucker MA. Sunlight and risk of uveal melanoma. *J Natl Cancer Inst.* 1994;86:1476-1478.

211. Harbour JW, Brantley MA Jr, Hollingsworth H, Gordon M. Association between posterior uveal melanoma and iris freckles, iris naevi, and choroidal naevi. *Br J Ophthalmol.* 2004;88:36-38.

212. Demirci H, Mashayekhi A, Shields CL, Eagle RC Jr, Shields JA. Iris melanocytoma: clinical features and natural course in 47 cases. *Am J Ophthalmol.* 2005;139:468-475.

213. Shields JA, Shields CL, Eagle RC Jr. Melanocytoma (hyperpigmented magnocellular nevus) of the uveal tract: the 34th G. Victor Simpson lecture. *Retina.* 2007;27:730-739.

214. Fineman MS, Eagle RC Jr, Shields JA, Shields CL, De Potter P. Melanocytomalytic glaucoma in eyes with necrotic iris melanocytoma. *Ophthalmology.* 1998;105:492-496.

215. Shields JA, Annesley WH Jr, Spaeth GL. Necrotic melanocytoma of iris with secondary glaucoma. *Am J Ophthalmol.* 1977;84:826-829.

216. Nakazawa M, Tamai M. Iris melanocytoma with secondary glaucoma. *Am J Ophthalmol.* 1984;97:797-799.

217. Kiratli H, Bilgic S, Gedik S. Late normalization of melanocytomalytic intraocular pressure elevation following excision of iris melanocytoma. *Graefes Arch Clin Exp Ophthalmol.* 2001;239:712-715.

218. Cialdini AP, Sahel JA, Jalkh AE, Weiter JJ, Zakka K, Albert DM. Malignant transformation of an iris melanocytoma. A case report. *Graefes Arch Clin Exp Ophthalmol.* 1989;227:348-354.

219. Shields JA, Kline MW, Augsburger JJ. Primary iris cyst: a review of the literature and report of 62 cases. *Br J Ophthalmol.* 1984;68:152-166.

220. Lois N, Shields CL, Shields JA, Mercado G, De Potter P. Primary iris stromal cysts. A report of 17 cases. *Ophthalmology.* 1998;105:1317-1322.

221. Shields JA, Shields CL, Lois N, Mercado G. Iris cysts in children: classification, incidence, and management. The 1998 Torrence A Makley Jr Lecture. *Br J Ophthalmol.* 1999;83:334-338.

222. Grutzmacher RD, Lindquist D, Chittum ME, Bunt-Milam AH, Kalina RE. Congenital iris cysts. *Br J Ophthalmol.* 1987;71:227-234.

223. Paridaens AD, Deuble K, McCartney AC. Spontaneous congenital non-pigmented epithelial cysts of the iris stroma. *Br J Ophthalmol.* 1992;76:39-42.

224. Cowan A. Congenital and familial cysts and flocculi of the iris. *Am J Ophthalmol.* 1936; 19:287-291.

225. Sallo FB, Hatvani I, Milibak T, Gyetvai T. Surgical treatment of symptomatic primary pupillary pigment epithelial iris cysts. *Acta Ophthalmol Scan.* 2003;81:191-192.

226. Oner HF, Kaynak S, Kocak N, Cingil G. Management of free floating iris cysts in the anterior chamber: a case report. *Eur J Ophthalmol.* 2003;13:212-214.

227. Shen CC, Netland PA, Wilson MW, Morris WR. Management of congenital nonpigmented iris cyst. *Ophthalmology.* 2006;113:1639-1644.

228. Scheie HG. Gonioscopy in the diagnosis of tumors of the iris and ciliary body, with emphasis on intraepithelial cysts. *Trans Am Ophthalmol Soc.* 1953;51:313-331.

229. Pavlin CJ, McWhae JA, McGowan HD, Foster FS. Ultrasound biomicroscopy of anterior segment tumors. *Ophthalmology.* 1992;99:1220-1228.

230. Gogos K, Tyradellis C, Spaulding AG, Kranias G. Iris cyst simulating melanoma. *J AAPOS.* 2004;8:502-503.

231. Shin SY, Stark WJ, Haller J, Green WR. Surgical management of recurrent iris stromal cyst. *Am J Ophthalmol.* 2000;130:122-123.

232. Xiao Y, Wang Y, Niu G, Li K. Transpupillary argon laser photocoagulation and Nd:YAG laser cystotomy for peripheral iris pigment epithelium cyst. *Am J Ophthalmol.* 2006;142:691-693.

233. Duan X, Zhang Y, Wang N. Laser treatment to large iris cyst secondary to trabeculectomy. *Can J Ophthalmol.* 2007;42:316-317.

234. Crowston JG, Medeiros FA, Mosaed S, Weinreb RN. Argon laser iridoplasty in the treatment of plateau-like iris configuration as result of numerous ciliary body cysts. *Am J Ophthalmol.* 2005;139:381-383.

235. Jensen OA. Malignant melanomas of the human uvea. Recent follow-up of cases in Denmark, 1943-1952. *Acta Ophthalmol Scand Suppl.* 1970;48:1113-1128.

236. Shields CL, Shields JA, Materin M, Gershenbaum E, Singh AD, Smith A. Iris melanoma: risk factors for metastasis in 169 consecutive patients. *Ophthalmology.* 2001;108:172-178.

237. Rootman J, Gallagher RP. Color as a risk factor in iris melanoma. *Am J Ophthalmol.* 1984; 98:558-561.

238. Demirci H, Shields CL, Shields JA, Eagle RC, Honavar SG. Diffuse iris melanoma: a report of 25 cases. *Ophthalmology.* 2002;109:1553-1560.

239. Ashton N. Primary tumours of the iris. *Br J Ophthalmol.* 1964;48:650-668.

240. Jakobiec FA, Silbert G. Are most iris "melanomas" really nevi? A clinicopathologic study of 189 lesions. *Arch Ophthalmol.* 1981;99:2117-2132.

241. Rones B, Zimmerman LE. The prognosis of primary tumors of the iris treated by iridectomy. *Arch Ophthalmol.* 1958;60:193-205.

11

CORNEAL TRAUMA AND BURNS

Pedram Hamrah, MD and Richard A. Eiferman, MD, FACS

Trauma to the eye can result in minor to severe damage. Proper response to injury and an understanding of the healing response is necessary for a positive outcome. Here we review the most common trauma cases encountered: corneal abrasions, foreign bodies, blunt trauma, lacerations, and chemical injuries.

CORNEAL ABRASION

Corneal abrasions are one of the most common ophthalmic injuries (Figure 11-1). Damage to the corneal epithelium exposes the superficial nerve endings causing severe pain, photophobia, foreign body sensation and tearing. The epithelial defect can often be visualized with a pen light because of the distortion of the light reflex, or found with the slit lamp because of the brilliant fluorescein uptake when viewed with a cobalt blue filter. The classic treatment of corneal abrasions is cycloplegia, antibiotics, and a tight patch to splint the lid.[1] This approach has been challenged by a study from England that shows no difference in healing rates with or without a patch.[2] Furthermore, the need for patching may be obviated by topical NSAIDS, which reduce the need for oral narcotics and do not significantly impair wound healing. While their mechanism of action is to mediate prostaglandins, they are actually mild anesthetics. Bandage soft contact lenses are an alternative treatment for corneal abrasions since they protect the damaged epithelium and allow passage of drugs while preserving vision.[3]

Antibiotics are mandatory in the treatment of corneal abrasions. Disruption of the epithelium can potentially provide a portal of entry for bacteria. Studies have shown that bacteria (especially *Pseudomonas*[4]) will preferentially attach to areas of disrupted epithelium. Topical antibiotic ointment can be applied at the time of patching or frequent topical antibiotics can be prescribed. If Bowman's layer is unaffected, most corneal abrasions heal uneventfully. However, recurrent corneal erosions can occur if there is poor adherence of the epithelial cells to the basement membrane.[5]

Trattler WB, Majmudar PA, Luchs JI, Swartz TS, eds.
Cornea Handbook (pp. 191-200)
© 2010 SLACK Incorporated

Figure 11-1. Corneal abrasion. (Courtesy of Tracy S. Swartz, OD, MS.)

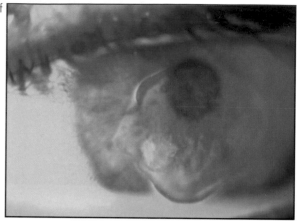

Figure 11-2. Debris resulting from a blast injury. (Courtesy of Eric D. Donnenfeld, MD.)

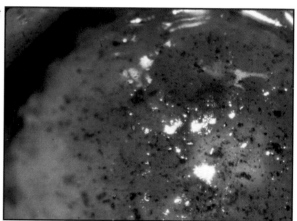

FOREIGN BODIES

Good clinical acumen is required in the management of corneal foreign bodies since a wide variety of organic and inorganic materials can become implanted at all depths in the cornea (Figure 11-2). A breach in Bowman's layer can heal as a minor epithelial facet or dense fibrous tissue. Very superficial materials can be removed with a sterile cotton bud or fine jeweler's forceps. Foreign bodies lodged in the anterior stroma can be removed with a bent needle or spud. Ferrous foreign bodies can be complicated by the development of rust rings due to the interaction with the tears. The rust is usually removed with a handheld drill and a fine burr. The risk of removing deep foreign bodies must be balanced against the development of scar tissue. For example, inert material such as glass slivers can be safely observed.

Corneal foreign bodies from plants can be contaminated with bacteria or fungi, which may lead to infectious keratitis. These wounds should be vigorously debrided and the excised material sent for culture. Some plants are highly antigenic (eg, yucca species) and cause a severe inflammatory response that requires intensive steroid treatment.

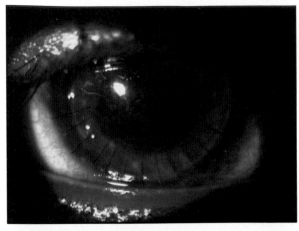

Figure 11-3. Blunt trauma resulted in a graft dehiscence that was successfully sutured. (Courtesy of Tracy S. Swartz, OD, MS.)

Foreign bodies from insects such as caterpillars and tarantulas can evoke an acute and chronic keratitis.[6,7] If possible, barbed hairs should be removed and the inflammation treated with topical steroids. Corneal stings from bees and wasps are complicated by an immediate reaction to the venom.[8] There is associated lid swelling, conjunctival injection and a massive infiltrate around the stinger. Rarely, there may be iritis with keratitic precipitates; there is one report of a hyphema. The prognosis is usually good, although there may be residual iris damage or atrophy.

BLUNT TRAUMA

The cornea can suffer serious injury without direct impact. Concussive injuries such as explosions or blasts cause the cornea to be rapidly flattened and displaced posteriorly causing stromal edema and striate keratopathy. The swelling is usually transient and resolves as the endothelium recovers.[9] However, if sufficient endothelial cells are lost, there may be irreversible damage necessitating a corneal transplant.[10,11]

Contusive injuries caused by blunt objects (eg, fists, clubs) can cause a similar picture (Figure 11-3). Blunt trauma should be treated with intensive topical steroids and cycloplegia.

LACERATIONS

Sharp trauma can lacerate the cornea and adnexa, and usually requires surgical repair. Good clinical judgment and a variety of techniques are required to achieve an optimal result.

Stromal injuries may be full- or partial-thickness. A nonpenetrating corneal flap should be copiously irrigated, debrided, and then repositioned. The flap can be covered with a bandage soft contact lens or anchored in place with fibrin or cyanoacrylate glue (Figure 11-4). More severe injuries or avulsions may require sutures to re-approximate the tissue.

Full-thickness corneal lacerations are especially serious. The hallmark is a positive Seidel test in which aqueous can be seen streaming from the anterior chamber when fluorescein strips are applied to the wound. It is essential to apply mild external pressure to the globe since some wound leaks are only visible with

Figure 11-4. Corneal laceration sealed with fibrin glue in an 8-year-old boy. Full vision recovery to 20/20 unaided vision was achieved after 3 months. (Courtesy of Tracy S. Swartz, OD, MS.)

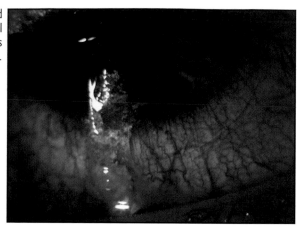

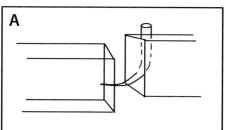

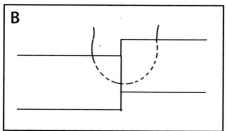

Figure 11-5. (A) If the needle is not passed through the same depth on both ends of the suture, an override of the tissue may result. (B) A superficially placed suture will cause the posterior surface to gape with the possibility of incarceration of intraocular structures.

Figure 11-6. More oblique incisions cause override as the suture is tightened.

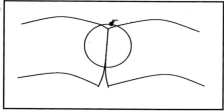

this maneuver. Oblique full-thickness lacerations can be self-sealing and managed with a bandage soft contact lens or cyanoacrylate glue. The authors' favored technique is to use fine dental applicators to deliver a minute amount of adhesive over the external portion of the wound. After polymerization, a bandage contact lens is applied to cover the glue.

More severe injuries require suturing. The preferred material for cornea repair is 10-0 monofilament nylon because it causes minimal tissue reaction; absorbable sutures such as vicryl or dexon can be used to close the sclera. Repair of lacerated corneas requires careful re-approximation of tissue planes. Conventional teaching recommends placement of a 10-0 nylon suture at the level of Descemet's membrane. However, if the needle is not passed through the same depth on both ends, this will lead to an override of the tissue (Figure 11-5). Furthermore, a superficially placed suture will cause the posterior surface to gape with the possibility of incarceration of intraocular structures. More oblique incisions cause override as the suture is tightened (Figure 11-6).

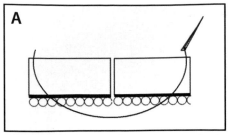 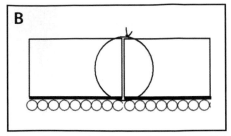

Figure 11-7. (A) Entering and exiting the anterior chamber with the needle gives optimal alignment of tissue. (B) The 10-0 nylon with cheese wire through the endothelium should come to rest on the distal portion of Descemet's membrane

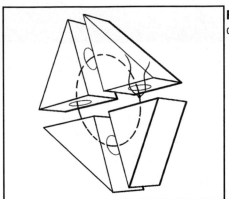

Figure 11-8. Stellate wounds are more complicated, as conventional techniques cause further gaping.

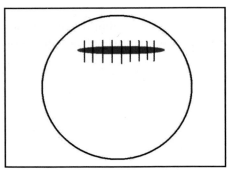 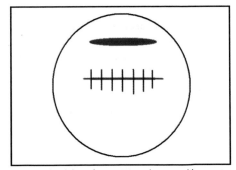

Figure 11-9. Complex wounds that are difficult to oppose or are associated with loss of tissue (A) can be repaired by creating a parallel relaxing incision that releases the tension on the wound (B).

One approach is to utilize full-thickness suturing. Entering and exiting the anterior chamber with the needle gives optimal alignment of tissue (Figure 11-7). It should be noted that the 10-0 nylon with cheese wire through the endothelium should come to rest on the distal portion of Descemet's membrane. The endothelium will heal by sliding over the suture.

Stellate wounds represent a more complicated situation since conventional techniques cause further gaping. The authors believe these are best re-approximated using an intralamellar suture (Figure 11-8). Complex wounds that are difficult to oppose or are associated with loss of tissue can be repaired by creating a parallel relaxing incision which releases the tension on the wound (Figure 11-9).

Figure 11-10. Conjunctivalization of the cornea following a chemical injury. (Courtesy of Tracy S. Swartz, OD, MS.)

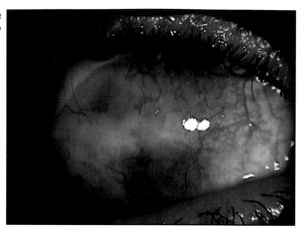

Extremely severe injuries with loss of tissue can sometimes be managed with amniotic membrane grafts. The defect can be filled with pieces of amniotic membrane (stacked like poker chips) or the tissue can be folded like a blanket and placed in the gap. If the injury causes large defects, lamellar or patch grafts from donor tissue may be used to restore the globe until a definitive repair is performed at a later date.

CHEMICAL INJURIES

Chemical injuries are divided into alkali or acid burns, and are considered true emergencies. The severity of ocular injuries in chemical burns is pH-dependent, and can be caused by liquids, powders, solids, or vapors. Additionally, injuries from sparklers and flares containing magnesium hydroxide, as well as tear gas or mace, should be managed as chemical burns.

Alkali Burns

Alkali burns have a rapid penetration through the corneal and anterior chamber, and are in general more severe than acid burns. Basic substances such as lye, ammonia (present in household cleaner), caustic potash, fresh lime, plaster, cement, mortar, whitewash, fertilizers, and refrigerant may cause more serious chemical burns. The rise in tissue pH by these compounds causes saponification of fatty acids in cell membranes, with subsequent disruption of cells and stromal mucopolysaccharides and tissue softening. Once alkali reaches the corneal stroma, it destroys collagen fibers and the stromal matrix. Permanent injury is determined by the concentration of the chemical, as well as the delay in time before initial irrigation. Visual prognosis is dictated by the extent of limbal epithelial and stem cell damage, as well as by the degree of intraocular penetration. Cases with limbal ischemia have the worst prognosis, as re-epithelialization of the cornea is dependent on the limbal stem cells (Figure 11-10). Extensive limbal ischemia results in corneal scarring, neovascularization, conjunctivalization, corneal melting, as well as uveitis and secondary glaucoma.

Table 11-1

HUGHES-ROPER-HALL CLASSIFICATION OF CHEMICAL BURNS

A. Clear cornea, no limbal ischemia, epithelial damage; good prognosis.

B. Less than one-third limbal ischemia, hazy cornea with iris detail visible; good prognosis.

C. One-third to one-half limbal ischemia, total epithelial loss, stromal haze blurring iris details; guarded prognosis.

D. More than one-half limbal ischemia, opaque cornea; poor prognosis.

Acid Burns

Acid burns cause their main damage within the first few minutes to hours of exposure. They are less progressive than alkaline agents, due to lower penetration. Offending agents include battery acid, industrial cleaner, laboratory glacial acetic acid, preservatives, bleach, refrigerant, industrial solvents, mineral refining agents, silicone production agents, and glass-etching agents. Acids cause precipitation and denaturation of tissue proteins, which leads to a rapid set up of barriers against further penetration of the agent. In contrast to alkali, acids burns do not lead to a loss of corneal matrix. Therefore, the tissue damage is localized to the area of contact. Burns from hydrofluoric acid or from acids containing heavy metals are the exception, because they are able to penetrate the cornea and anterior chamber, leading to scarring and membrane formation.

Mace

Tear gas compounds and mace have a variable toxic content, leading to variable clinical results. Generally, they cause only minor chemical conjunctivitis. Mace burns should be managed similar to alkali burns, as a direct spray toward the eyes can result in severe alkali burn-like ocular injuries.

Classification

Classification and prognosis of chemical burns is useful for alkali burns, but may also apply to other chemical injuries of the eye. A common classification system is the Hughes-Roper-Hall classification of Chemical Burns,[12-15] which is described in Table 11-1.

Rather than remember the levels of a particular classification, others categorize the severity of tissue damage. Mild alkali burn with scattered superficial punctate keratitis (SPK) or focal epithelial cell loss may result in slow re-epithelialization and mild corneal haze, leading to a minimum decrease in vision. Moderately severe burns with large epithelial defects and presence of limbal ischemia have a more variable course, depending on the extent of the ocular injury. Stromal opacification, increase in corneal thickness, and anterior chamber inflammation may follow. Persistent epithelial defects may then lead to corneal neovascularization, stromal thinning, and possible corneal perforation, all of which may result in permanent vision loss. Iritis, however, may be severe and sometimes goes undetected. During re-epithelialization, collagenases, elastases, and other enzymes are released from the epithelium, keratocytes, and polymorphonuclear cells (PMN). This leads to decreased collagen synthesis secondary to severe ascorbate deficiency in alkali-burned eyes, and subsequent ulceration and perforation of the cornea.

Therapy

Chemical burns should be copiously irrigated, using water or normal saline solution, as any delay in irrigation will lead to a worse prognosis. The initial lavage should continue for several minutes and done for both eyes.

Once a patient is taken to an emergency room, treatment should be started immediately. Proparacaine should be instilled to relieve pain, and lavage should be started with at least 2 L of normal saline 0.9% or Ringer lactate solution, over a minimum period of 30 minutes. Irrigation can be performed by using a handheld intravenous tubing, a Morgan lens, or an irrigated lid speculum, with the help of lid retractors if necessary. A sterile cotton-tipped applicator, moistened with 0.05 mol/L of 10% EDTA to make sticky CaOH easier to remove, should be used to sweep the conjunctival fornices and palpebral conjunctiva. Double eversion of the upper lid should then be performed to exclude foreign material in the upper fornix. In case embedded chemicals are found in the fornices, 0.05 mol/L EDTA solution should be used for irrigation. After lavage, careful slit-lamp examination should be performed to rule out any perforating ocular injury. If laceration of the globe is suspected, direct pressure on the globe should be avoided. Irrigation should be continued until a normal pH of 7.0 is achieved. However, pH should be checked again in 5 to 10 minutes to ascertain that the pH is not changing.

After stabilization of the pH, eyes should be dilated with a cycloplegic agent, such as atropine 1% or scopolamine 0.25%, to prevent posterior synechiae, as well as to decrease ciliary spasm and associated pain. Phenylephrine should be avoided in chemical burns due to its vasoconstrictive effects. Broad-spectrum topical antibiotics such as moxifloxacin, gatifloxacin, levofloxacin, ciprofloxacin, ofloxacin, tobramycin, or polymyxin–bacitracin ointment should be started to protect against super-infection. For alkali or more severe acid burns, an immediate increase in IOP may occur secondary to shrinkage of scleral collagen fibers. Carbonic anhydrase inhibitors such as intravenous or oral acetazolamide should therefore be given immediately. The fundus should then be examined to rule out necrotic retinopathy from intraocular penetration of the agent. Pain management can be achieved by systemic administration of analgesics. Acetaminophen and oxycodone, 1 to 2 tablets every 4 hours, or meperidine, 50 to 100 mg intramuscularly or by mouth every 4 hours, are generally effective.

If indicated, an emergency physical examination should also be performed by an otolaryngologist and an internist due to possible aspiration or ingestion of chemicals at the time of injury, potentially leading to concomitant chemical burns of the respiratory or upper gastrointestinal tract. The affected eye(s) may be pressure-patched and the patient should be followed daily until the cornea is re-epithelialized. For severe burns, the patient may be hospitalized for close monitoring. Topical antibiotic ointments or drops should be continued every 4 to 6 hours along with the mydriatic-cycloplegics. If the patient's eye is not patched, preservative-free artificial tears or gel should be started hourly.

Topical antibiotic drops should initially be used frequently, then tapered to 4 times daily, while cycloplegia should be maintained as long as anterior segment inflammation persists. Several days to weeks postburn, an increase in IOP may be noted, which is likely secondary to prostaglandin release, although long-term elevation of pressure may result from scarring of outflow channels. Carbonic anhydrase inhibitors, such as oral acetazolamide (250 mg qid) or methazolamide (50 mg tid), are generally effective in reducing the IOP. Topical beta-blockers such as timolol 0.5% twice daily, and an alpha-adrenergic agonist such as brimonidine twice daily, or a combination thereof, may be added if needed. Intravenous mannitol 20% solution, at a dose of 2.5 mL per kg, may be given for short-term pressure control in those patients who cannot take oral medication in the emergency room. However, before using any hyperosmotic agent, the cardiac and renal status should be assessed. Further, long-term carbonic anhydrase inhibitors should be avoided in patients with a history of renal stones.

Topical steroids such as 1% prednisolone every 1 to 4 hours should be used for the first 2 weeks after injury in order to control anterior segment inflammation and limit matrix degradation. After this period, if a persistent epithelial defect is present, steroids should be reduced or stopped in order to prevent infection or corneal melting and perforation, which may result from collagenolytic enzyme release. In these cases, systemic steroids such as prednisone (by mouth) may be substituted if anterior segment inflammation is still present.

In moderately severe and severe alkali burns, Ca^{2+} chelators such as ascorbate or citrate are important adjuncts. Ten percent citrate and 10% ascorbate solution applied every 2 hours for 1 week, followed by every 4 hours thereafter, inhibits PMN activity and inflammatory chemotaxis, which may slow or prevent melting. These eyes may become rapidly scorbutic, potentially interfering with collagen synthesis, and resulting ulceration. Two grams of ascorbate (Vitamin C, orally) should also be given daily until complete re-epithelialization, to promote collagen synthesis.[16] However, ascorbate should not be used in nonalkali burn situations, because the ciliary body concentration of the drug will enhance, rather than inhibit, corneal melting.[16] Additionally, ascorbate should be used with caution in patients with compromised renal function. Oral tetracyclines (eg, doxycycline 100 mg twice daily) should also be used for several weeks, because they chelate Ca^{2+} and thus collagenase. Moreover, 1% medroxyprogesterone has been shown to be effective in suppression of collagen breakdown.[17] If corneal melting is suspected, other collagenase inhibitors, eg, 10% or 20% acetylcysteine, may be used 6 times daily.

Therapeutic soft contact bandage lenses with high water content may be of great benefit in assisting epithelial healing. Re-epithelialization, in turn, will inhibit enzyme release and stromal melting. With delayed epithelial healing, lenses may be placed, and are generally left in place for 6 to 8 weeks. However, immediately after injury, lenses should be used with caution, as they may trap the offending agent and prevent epithelial healing, further increasing the infection rate. Alternatively, in severe burns a temporary tarsorrhaphy or PROKERA amniotic membrane lens (Bio-Tissue, Inc., Miami, FL) may be used. PROKERA is an amniotic membrane placed into a dual concave polycarbonate ring, which when placed on the eye, acts as a symblepharon ring. Further, a scleral ring could be used to maintain the fornices, if symblepharon begin to develop (Figure 11-11).

Depending on the severity of the chemical burn, long-term management may vary from antibiotic and artificial tears coverage to surgical reconstruction of the eye with conjunctival flaps or transplants, amniotic membrane grafts, autologous conjunctival or limbal stem cell transplants, patch grafts, PK, or keratoprosthesis. These procedures may be performed as soon as 2 weeks following the injury.

Figure 11-11. Symblepharon in a patient who suffered a chemical burn secondary to a fireworks injury. (Courtesy of Tracy S. Swartz, OD, MS.)

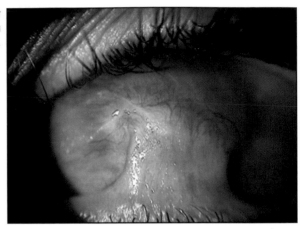

REFERENCES

1. Parrish CM, Chandler JW. Corneal trauma. In: Kaufman HE, Barron BA, McDonald MB, Waltman SR, eds. *The Cornea.* New York: Churchill Livingstone; 1988.

2. Michal JG, Hug D, Dowd MD. Management of corneal abrasion in children: a randomized clinical trial. *Ann Emerg Med.* 2002;40:67-72.

3. Sabri K, Pandit JC, Thaller VT, Evans NM, Crocker GR. National survey of corneal abrasion treatment. *Eye.* 1998;12:278-281.

4. Klotz SA, Yue-Kong A, Raghunath PM. A partial-thickness epithelial defect increases the adherence of *Pseudomonas aeruginosa* to the cornea. *Invest Opthalmol Vis Sci.* 1989;30(6): 1069-1074.

5. Weene LE. Recurrent corneal erosion after trauma: a statistical study. *Ann Opthalmol.* 1985;17:521-524.

6. Chang PC, Soong HK, Barnett JM. Corneal penetration by tarantula hairs. *Br J Ophthalmol.* 1991;75(4):253-254.

7. Conrath J, Hadjadj E, Balansard B, Ridings B. Caterpillar setae-induced acute anterior uveitis: a case report. *Am J Ophthalmol.* 2000;130(6):841-843.

8. Chen CJ, Richardson CD. Bee sting-induced ocular changes. *Am Ophthalmol.* 1986;18:285-286.

9. Slingsby JG, Forstot SL. Effect of blunt trauma on the corneal endothelium. *Arch Ophthalmol.* 1981;99:1041-1043.

10. Roper-Hall MJ, Wilson RS, Thompson SM. Changes in endothelial cell density following accidental trauma. *Br J Opthalmol.* 1982;66:518-519.

11. Liston RL, Olson RJ, Mamalis, N. A comparison of rust-ring removal methods in a rabbit model: small-gauge hypodermic needle versus electric drill. *Ann Ophthalmol.* 1991;23:24-27.

12. Hughes WF Jr. Alkali burns of the eye. I. Review of the literature and summary of present knowledge. *Arch Ophthalmol.* 1946;35:423-428.

13. Hughes WF Jr. Alkali burns of the eye. II. Clinical and pathological course. *Arch Ophthalmol.* 1946;36:189.

14. Ballen PH. Treatment of chemical burns of the eye. *Eye Ear Nose Throat Mon.* 1964;43:57.

15. Roper-Hall MJ. Thermal and chemical burns. *Trans Ophthalmol Soc UK.* 1965;85:631-633.

16. Pfister RR, Paterson CA. Ascorbic acid in the treatment of alkali burns of the eye. *Ophthalmology.* 1980;87(10):1050-1057.

17. Hicks CR, Crawford GJ. Melting after keratoprosthesis implantation: the effects of medroxyprogesterone. *Cornea.* 2003;22(6):497-500.

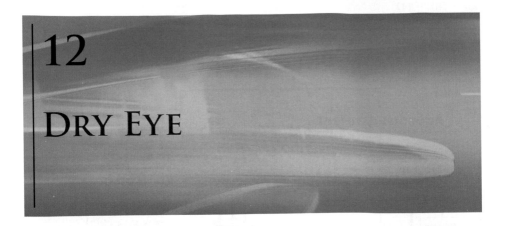

12

DRY EYE

Sanjay N. Rao, MD

Dry eye disease is one of the most common problems facing eye care professionals. Despite the common nature of this problem, our understanding of the pathophysiology has been limited. Fortunately, our understanding of the disease process has advanced significantly in the last decade. Both basic science research on dry eye as well as important expert workshops have elucidated our understanding that dry eye is a progressive inflammatory disease. This increased understanding has heightened the need for improved classification schemes, diagnostic approaches, and targeted therapies for the treatment of dry eye disease and meibomian gland dysfunction. This chapter will discuss a consensus definition, classification scheme, epidemiology, pathophysiology, diagnosis, and treatment approaches for dry eye disease. This chapter will also summarize the current thinking in dry eye disease, reinforce a stepwise approach in diagnosis, and establish treatment strategies based on disease severity.

The definition of dry eye disease has been the source of considerable debate. To address this confusion, as well as consolidate clinical opinion on the definition, the National Eye Institute (NEI) gathered a group of dry eye experts in 1993 and 1994 and formed a workshop to discuss the current understanding of dry eye. This NEI group defined dry eye as "a disorder of the tear film due to tear deficiency or excessive tear evaporation, which causes damage to the interpalpebral ocular surface and is associated with symptoms of ocular discomfort."[1] This broad definition incorporated multiple pathophysiologic mechanisms while emphasizing their common final expression as ocular surface disease. Since this initial definition was proposed, additional research has elucidated more of the pathophysiology of the disease. The current definition adds that dry eye "… results from a localized immune-mediated inflammatory response affecting both the lacrimal gland and the ocular surface." This addition reflects a new understanding of the causes of disease and emphasizes that the condition is mediated by the immune system and involves inflammation of the lacrimal glands and ocular surface.

In 2007, results of the work of the International Dry Eye Workshop (DEWS) were presented. The mission of this group was to "consider current knowledge on all aspects of dry eye disease and to update, in critical and evidence-based fashion,

Trattler WB, Majmudar PA, Luchs JI, Swartz TS, eds.
Cornea Handbook (pp. 201-224)
© 2010 SLACK Incorporated

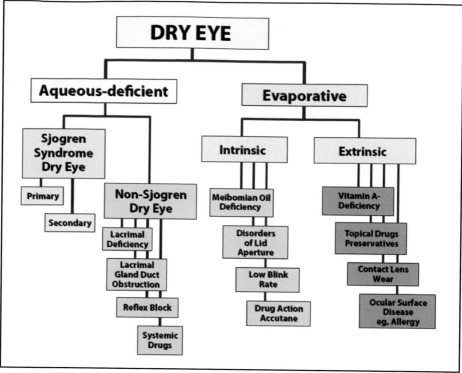

Figure 12-1. The DEWS Definition and Classification Subcommittee updated the work of the NEI Workshop to create this classification system of dry eye disease.

the concepts and information presented in the 1995 NEI Industry Workshop."[2] This group produced a final consensus regarding its definition:

> *Dry eye is a multifactorial disease of the tears and ocular surface that results in symptoms of discomfort,[2-4] visual disturbance,[5-7] and tear film instability[8-10] with potential damage to the ocular surface. It is accompanied by increased osmolarity of the tear film[11-14] and inflammation of the ocular surface.[15,16]*

This comprehensive definition is important in that it emphasizes the central mechanisms present in all forms of dry eye disease: hyperosmolarity of tears and inflammation of the ocular surface. These concepts will be discussed in more detail in the pathophysiology section. The definition also emphasizes key features that define the nature and severity of the disease: tear film instability and ocular surface damage.

CLASSIFICATION OF DRY EYE DISEASE

The DEWS Definition and Classification Subcommittee updated the work of the NEI Workshop to create a classification system of dry eye disease. This classification scheme is presented in Figure 12-1. They reinforced the concept that there are 2 categories of dry eye disease: aqueous tear-deficient and evaporative dry eye. Aqueous tear-deficient dry eye suggests that the disease is due to a failure of lacrimal tear secretion.[17,18] Aqueous tear-deficient dry eye has 2 major subgroupings: Sjögren syndrome dry eye and non-Sjögren syndrome dry eye. Evaporative dry eye is due to excessive tear loss from the ocular surface in the presence of normal lacrimal tear secretion. Evaporative dry eye may be caused by intrinsic factors such as compromised eyelid health, or extrinsic causes such as topical medications. It is important to recognize that these groups are not mutually exclusive and that disease initiated in one major group may coexist with or lead to events that cause dry eye by another mechanism.

Aqueous Tear-Deficient Dry Eye

Lacrimal tear secretion failure is the basis for aqueous tear-deficient dry eye. This failure causes tear hyperosmolarity, because, although the water evaporates from the ocular surface at normal rates, it is from a reduced aqueous pool. Tear film hyperosmolarity causes hyperosmolarity of the ocular surface epithelial cells and stimulates a cascade of inflammatory events involving mitogen-activated protein (MAP) kinases and NFkB signaling pathways resulting in the generation of inflammatory cytokines (interleukin-1α; 1β; tumor necrosis factor-α, and matrix metalloproteinases [MMP-9]).[19-21]

Sjögren Syndrome Dry Eye

Sjögren syndrome (SS) is an autoimmune disease in which the lacrimal and salivary glands are targeted by inflammatory cells. The lacrimal and salivary glands are infiltrated by activated T-cells, which cause glandular cell death and hyposecretion of tears or saliva. Inflammatory activation within the glands leads to autoexpression of antigens at the surface of epithelial cells (eg, fodrin, Ro and La) and the retention of tissue-specific CD4 and CD8 T-cells.[22,23] There are 2 forms of SS, and the classification criteria have recently been harmonized in a European-American collaboration.[24] Primary SS consists of the occurrence of aqueous tear-deficient dry eye in combination with symptoms of dry mouth, in the presence of autoantibodies, evidence of reduced salivary secretion, and with a positive focus score on minor salivary gland biopsy.[25,26] Details of the criteria are presented in Table 12-1. Secondary SS consists of the features of primary SS together with the features of an overt autoimmune connective disease, such as rheumatoid arthritis.[27] The ocular dryness in SS is due to lacrimal hyposecretion and the accompanying characteristic inflammatory changes in the lacrimal gland, together with the presence of inflammatory mediators in the tears and within the conjunctiva.

Non-Sjögren Syndrome Dry Eye

Non-Sjögren syndrome dry eye is a form of aqueous tear-deficient dry eye due to lacrimal dysfunction, where the systemic autoimmune features characteristic of SS have been excluded. The most common form is age-related dry eye. The different forms of non-Sjögren syndrome dry eye are shown in Table 12-2.

Evaporative Dry Eye

Evaporative dry eye is due to excessive water loss from the exposed ocular surface in the presence of normal secretory function. Its causes can be intrinsic, where they are due to disease affecting lid structures or dynamics, or extrinsic, where ocular surface disease occurs due to some external exposure. The major

Table 12-1

REVISED INTERNATIONAL CLASSIFICATION FOR OCULAR MANIFESTATIONS OF SJÖGREN SYNDROME

Ocular symptoms: a positive response to at least 1 of the following questions:

- Have you had daily, persistent, troublesome dry eyes for more than 3 months?
- Do you have a recurrent sensation of sand or gravel in the eyes?
- Do you use tear substitutes more than 3 times a day?

Oral symptoms: a positive response to at least 1 of the following questions:

- Have you had a daily feeling of dry mouth for more than 3 months?
- Have you had recurrently or persistently swollen salivary gland as an adult?
- Do you frequently drink liquids to aid in swallowing dry food?

Ocular signs: that is, objective evidence of ocular involvement defined as a positive result for at least 1 of the following 2 tests:

- Schirmer I test, performed without anesthesia (less than or equal to 5 mm in 5 minutes)
- Rose bengal score or other ocular dye score (less than or equal to 4 according to van Bijsterveld's scoring system)

Histopathology: In minor salivary glands (obtained through normal-appearing mucosa) focal lymphocytic sialadenitis, evaluated by an expert histopathologist, with a focus score of greater than or equal to 1, defined as a number of lymphocytic foci (which are adjacent to normal-appearing mucous acini and contain more than 50 lymphocytes) per 4 mm^2 of glandular tissue

Salivary gland involvement: objective evidence of salivary gland involvement defined by a positive result for at least 1 of the following diagnostic tests:

- Unstimulated whole salivary flow less than or equal to 1.5 mL in 5 minutes
- Parotid sialography showing the presence of diffuse sialectasias (punctate, cavitary, or destructive pattern), without evidence of obstruction in the major ducts
- Salivary scintigraphy showing delayed uptake, reduced concentration, or delayed excretion of tracer

Autoantibodies: presence in the serum of the following autoantibodies:

- Antibodies to Ro(SSA) or La(SSB) antigens or both

Reprinted with permission from Vitali C, Bombardieri S, Jonsson R, et al. Classification criteria for Sjögren's syndrome: a revised version of the European criteria proposed by the American-European Consensus Group. *Ann Rheum Dis.* 2002;61:554-558.

intrinsic causes of evaporative dry eye are meibomian gland dysfunction, poor lid congruity and lid dynamics, low blink rate, and the effects of drug action, such as that of systemic retinoids.

Meibomian gland dysfunction (MGD), or posterior blepharitis, is a condition of meibomian gland obstruction and is the most common cause of evaporative dry eye.[28-30] Its multiple causes and associations include acne rosacea, seborrhoeic dermatitis, atopic dermatitis, and treatment of acne vulgaris with isotretinoin. The diagnosis of MGD is based on morphologic features of the gland acini and duct orifices, presence of orifice plugging, and thickening or absence of expressed excreta. MGD is associated with a deficient tear film lipid layer, an increase in tear evaporation, and the occurrence of evaporative dry eye.

Evaporative dry eye also occurs in disorders where eyelid aperture, position, or eyelid dynamics are affected. Disorders such as craniostenosis, proptosis, and

Table 12-2

CONDITIONS ASSOCIATED WITH NON-SJÖGREN'S SYNDROME DRY EYE

Primary lacrimal gland deficiencies

- Age-related dry eye
- Congenital alacrima
- Familial dysautonomia

Secondary lacrimal gland deficiencies

- Lacrimal gland infiltration
- Sarcoidosis
- Lymphoma
- AIDS
- Graft-versus-host disease
- Lacrimal gland ablation
- Lacrimal gland denervation

Obstruction of the lacrimal gland ducts

- Trachoma
- Cicatricial pemphigoid and mucous membrane pemphigoid
- Erythema multiforme
- Chemical and thermal burns

Reflex hyposecretion

- Reflex sensory block
  - Contact lens wear
  - Diabetes
  - Neurotrophic keratitis

Reflex motor block

- VII cranial nerve damage
- Multiple neuromatosis
- Exposure to systemic drugs

high myopia increase the exposed evaporative surface and can cause dry eye. Endocrine exophthalmos is also associated with ocular drying and tear hyperosmolarity.[31] Poor lid apposition or lid deformity also can lead to exposure-related dry eye.[32] Increasing palpebral fissure width correlates with increased tear film evaporation. Evaporative dry eye can also be caused by problems of lid congruity after blepharoplasty.[33] Drying of the ocular surface may also be caused by a reduced blink rate, which lengthens the period during which the ocular surface is exposed to water loss before the next blink. This may occur during performance of certain tasks of concentration (eg, computer work) or may be a feature of an extrapyramidal disorder such as Parkinson's disease.[34]

The major extrinsic causes of dry eye are vitamin A deficiency, the action of toxic topical agents such as preservatives, contact lens wear, and certain ocular surface diseases, including allergic eye disease. Vitamin A deficiency may cause dry eye by 2 different mechanisms. First, vitamin A is essential for the development of goblet cells and the expression of glyocalyx mucins.[35,36] Second, vitamin A deficiency can cause lacrimal acinar damage and aqueous deficient dry eye.[37] Topical eye drops with epithelial toxic agents can also induce evaporative dry eye. The most common offenders are preservatives, such as benzalkonium chloride, which cause surface epithelial cell damage and punctate epithelial keratitis. Topical anesthetics can also cause dry eye by reducing lacrimal secretion by reducing sensory drive to the lacrimal gland and also reduce the blink rate. In allergic conjunctivitis, the release of inflammatory cytokines via an Ig-E mediated pathway can promote the development of evaporative dry eye.[38]

The purpose of utilizing a simplified classification scheme is two-fold. First, it helps to clarify the pathophysiologic mechanisms at work. Second, it helps to direct therapy to more specifically target the etiologic causes.

PATHOPHYSIOLOGY OF DRY EYE DISEASE

Tear production is regulated by neural communication between the ocular surface and lacrimal glands, also known as the *integrated lacrimal functional unit*. The integrated lacrimal functional unit consists of ocular surface afferent sensory nerves, efferent autonomic and motor nerves that stimulate tear secretion and blinking, and the tear-secreting glands (main and accessory lacrimal glands, conjunctival goblet cells, and meibomian glands). In dry eye disease, this communication becomes disrupted, leading to tear hyperosmolarity and a self-perpetuating cycle of inflammation. The core sequence of events leading to dry eye symptomatology involves tear hyperosmolarity causing damage to ocular surface epithelium leading to tear film instability.

The initiating factor in this pathologic process is secretory dysfunction of the tear-secreting glands caused by multiple factors, including age, hormonal deficiencies (particularly androgen deficiency), use of anticholinergic medications, surgeries that sever the corneal nerves (eg, LASIK), and systemic autoimmune disease.[39-43] This dysfunction of the tear-secreting glands alters the balance of tear film components that stabilize the tear film and support and protect the ocular surface. This secretory dysfunction leads to the production of abnormal, hyperosmolar tears. Hyperosmolar tears simulate the production of inflammatory mediators and leads to the cascade of inflammation.

The changes in tear composition promote inflammation on the ocular surface by several mechanisms (Figure 12-2). First, there is decreased secretion of natural anti-inflammatory factors such as lactoferrin by the dysfunctional lacrimal glands.[44] Second, there is increased production of certain proinflammatory cytokines (interleukin-1 [IL-1] and tumor necrosis factor-α [TNF-α]), increased production of proteolytic enzymes by stressed ocular surface and glandular epithelial cells, and T-cell infiltration of glandular tissues.[45-47] Third, there is activation of latent inactive cytokines and proteases that are normally present in the tear fluid that serves as an early defense mechanism for the ocular surface.[46,47]

Hyperosmolarity of the tears that accompanies dysfunction of the tear-secreting glands is a critical stimulus in the inflammatory process.[48,49] Several studies have shown that exposure of cultured human corneal epithelial cells to media of increasing sodium chloride concentration results in a concentration-dependent increase in the production of the same proinflammatory factors that have been detected in the conjunctival epithelium and tear fluid of dry eye patients.[49-52]

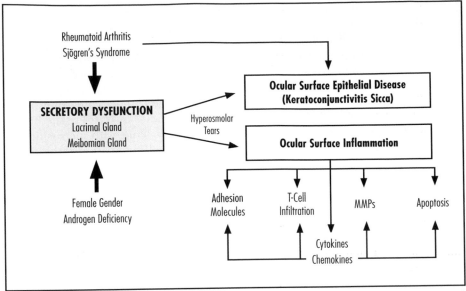

Figure 12-2. Changes in tear composition promote inflammation on the ocular surface by several mechanisms, illustrated here.

Evidence from additional studies indicates that hyperosmolarity stimulates the production of these inflammatory mediators by activating a group of intercellular signaling molecules called *mitogen-activated protein kinases*.[50,52]

The increase in inflammatory mediators in the tear fluid, conjunctiva, and lacrimal glands initiates an inflammatory cascade on the ocular surface.[53] This inflammation is evidenced by increased expression of immune activation and adhesion molecules (HLA-DR and ICAM-1) by the conjunctival epithelium.[54] These molecules function to attract and retain inflammatory cells in the conjunctiva. Another pathologic change is an increased concentration and activity of MMPs in the tear fluid.[46,47] These enzymes, particularly MMP-9, play a role in maintaining corneal epithelial barrier function, regulating corneal epithelial desquamation, and promoting corneal surface regularity.[55-57] Another inflammatory mechanism in dry eye disease is increased apoptosis of the conjunctival and glandular epithelium.[58,59] Though the exact mechanism of apoptosis has not been elucidated, it may occur as a result of exposure to inflammatory cytokines, such as TNF-α, or to decreased expression of antiapoptotic proteins, such as BCL-2.[59]

In summary, the central mechanisms of dry eye are tear hyperosmolarity and tear film instability. Tear hyperosmolarity causes damage to the surface epithelium by activating a cascade of inflammatory events at the ocular surface and a release of inflammatory mediators into the tears. Epithelial damage involves cell death by apoptosis, a loss of goblet cells, and disturbance of mucin expression, leading to tear film instability. This instability exacerbates ocular surface hyperosmolarity and completes the vicious circle.

EPIDEMIOLOGY OF DRY EYE DISEASE

The American Academy of Ophthalmology places chronic dry eye among the most common reasons for visiting ophthalmologists in the United States.

Epidemiologic studies have reported that more than 6% of the population over the age of 40 suffers from dry eye, with the prevalence increasing to 15% of the population over the age of 65.[60-62]

Based on data from the largest studies of dry eye to date, the Women's Health Study,[63] the Physician's Health Study,[64] and other studies, it has been estimated that about 3.23 million women and 1.68 million men, for a total of 4.91 million Americans 50 years and older, have dry eye.[63,64] In the United States, prevalence estimates range from 7.8% in the Women's Health Study[63] to 14.4% in the Beaver Dam Study.[65] Most studies have shown a greater prevalence with increasing age and among women.[66] Approximately 80% of the overall population with dry eye is female. Asians and Hispanics also experience high rates of dry eye.[66] Incidence data extracted from the Medicare/Medicaid databases suggest also that dry eye incidence is increasing. Ellwein and colleagues found that the dry eye case incidence per 100 fee-for-service Medicare beneficiaries increased by 57.4% from 1.22 in 1991 to 1.92 in 1998.[67]

Based on large population-based studies including the Beaver Dam Eye Study,[65] the Salisbury Eye Evaluation study,[62] and the Melbourne study,[60] several risk factors for dry eye have been established[66] (Table 12-3). Substantiated risk factors for dry eye include female sex, older age, postmenopausal estrogen therapy, a diet low in omega-3 essential fatty acids or a diet with a high ratio of omega-6 to omega-3 fatty acids, LASIK and refractive excimer laser surgery, vitamin A deficiency, medications such as antihistamines, connective tissue disease, radiation therapy, and hematopoietic stem cell transplantation.[66] Other less established risk factors include diabetes mellitus, arthritis, thyroid disease, human immunodeficiency virus, systemic cancer chemotherapy, and other medications such as isotretinoin.[65] The strongest risk factors are that of older age and female sex. Total cholesterol to high-density lipoprotein (HDL) cholesterol ratio has been reported to be protective against dry eye. Cigarette smoking is associated with a two-fold increase in the odds of dry eye.[65] Antidepressants and aspirin are also significantly associated with dry eye.[65] The relationship between sex hormones and dry eye is complex. The data suggest that women who use hormone replacement therapy, particularly estrogen alone, are at increased risk of dry eye syndrome.[65]

DIAGNOSIS OF DRY EYE DISEASE

The symptoms of dry eye and MGD can overlap with other ophthalmic diseases. Diagnostic testing should be performed based upon its utility to classify the type of dry eye and characterize the severity of disease. More specifically, diagnostic testing should be performed to establish a level of disease severity to guide treatment decisions and monitor progress. Several tests and tools have been established to aid in the diagnosis of dry eye and meibomian gland disease. Though many of these tests have some utility, performing all of them is not clinically practical. The 2007 DEWS report outlined a practical sequence of tests: clinical history, symptom questionnaire, fluorescein breakup time, ocular surface staining grading, Schirmer testing, and lid and meibomian expression[68] (Table 12-4). The goals of this testing should focus on the characterization of several critical indicators of disease severity including level of discomfort, visual symptoms, ocular surface inflammation, lid and meibomian gland dysfunction, tear production, and tear stability. The following discussion will outline the sequence of tests, explain how they are performed, and highlight the key questions to be answered by each test.

Table 12-3

RISK FACTORS FOR DRY EYE DISEASE

- Older age
- Female sex
- History of arthritis
- Smoking status
- Caffeine use
- History of thyroid disease
- History of gout
- Total to high-density lipoprotein cholesterol ratio
- Diabetes
- Multivitamin use

Table 12-4

PRACTICAL SEQUENCE OF TESTS

- Clinical history
- Symptom questionnaire
- Fluorescein BUT
- Ocular surface staining grading with fluorescein/yellow filter
- Schirmer I test without anesthetic, or a basic secretion test with anesthetic, and/or Schirmer II with nasal stimulation
- Lid and meibomian morphology
- Meibomian expression
- Other tests may be added according to availability

Adapted from Foulks G, Bron AJ. A clinical description of meibomian gland dysfunction. *Ocul Surf.* 2003:107-126.

Clinical History

Because the symptoms of dry eye and meibomian gland dysfunction can overlap with many other ophthalmic diseases, diagnosis requires a thorough and systematic approach. Clinical history is critical in establishing the answers to several important questions that inform characterization of the disease. History-taking should attempt to establish severity and frequency of discomfort as well as the effect of symptoms on vision. The proper workup includes identification of a subjective symptom set that enters the patient into the dry eye diagnostic algorithm.[69] These symptoms may include blurriness, stickiness, burning, stinging, foreign-body sensation, grittiness, dryness, photophobia, and itching. Secondly, an attempt should be made to grade the severity of the disease. Third, it is helpful to establish exacerbating factors. Key exacerbating factors in dry eye syndrome include exposure to smoke, wind, heat, low humidity, and prolonged visual tasking.[69] Fourth, a complete list of patient medications should be obtained because many medications affect tear secretion. Finally, a review of systems should be performed to identify patients with symptoms associated with SS or other systemic diseases associated with dry eye. The primary goals of the clinical history for dry eye are to establish the level of discomfort and to determine whether the symptoms are episodic or constant.

Symptom Questionnaires

Symptom questionnaires can be very helpful in establishing a level of disease severity as well as a benchmark for monitoring therapy. Seven validated questionnaires have been created for use with dry eye patients, including the Women's Health Study, International Sjögren's Classification, Schein, McMonnies, OSDI, Candees, Dry Eye Questionnaire (DEQ), and IDEEL.[68] These questionnaires vary in length from 3 questions to 57 questions. These questionnaires can help to establish the diagnosis of dry eye, identify precipitating factors, and determine the impact on quality of life.[68] The choice of questionnaire should reflect the needs as well as the time constraints of the individual practitioner.

Fluorescein Breakup Time

Tear film breakup time (TFBUT) is indicative of tear film stability and is perhaps the simplest clinical test for dry eye diagnosis. Considered by many as a hallmark of dry eye, a reduced tear film breakup time is shared by all the different conditions that can cause dry eye. A few authors have suggested that noninvasive TFBUT can perhaps differentiate aqueous tear deficiency from evaporative dry eye associated with meibomian gland disease.[69] TFBUT measures tear film quality. Essentially, TFBUT can be performed either utilizing fluorescein dye or without fluorescein dye (noninvasive). TFBUT is measured using a technique originally described by Norn[70] and later by Lemp and Holly.[71] These authors measured TFBUT by utilizing fluorescein dye and measuring the time between a complete blink and the appearance of the first dry spot in the tear film. Several authors have since established that using a controlled amount of fluorescein as well as using a yellow filter to enhance observation of the tear film over the corneal surface improves the reliability of the test.[68] Sensitivity of the fluorescein-aided TFBUT has been shown to be 72.2% with a specificity of 61.6%.[72] Noninvasive TFBUT is performed by imaging a regular pattern on the corneal surface and measuring the time it takes before it distorts or breaks up after a blink. The main advantage of the noninvasive technique is that it minimizes the effect of any confounding factors that affect the tear film such as fluorescein itself or the reflex tearing caused by the instilled fluorescein. If this test is performed consistently, noninvasive TFBUT measurements give moderately high sensitivity (83%) with good overall accuracy (85%).[68] The established TFBUT cutoff for dry eye diagnosis has been less than 10 seconds since the report of Lemp and Hamill in 1973.[73] More recently, values of less than 5 and less than 10 seconds have been adopted based upon the Abelson report, which suggested that the diagnostic cutoff falls to less than 5 seconds when small volumes of fluorescein are instilled (eg, 5 μL of 2.0% fluorescein).[74] For purposes of establishing the severity level of disease, a simplified goal of the TFBUT should be to quantify the level of tear film instability as variable, less than or equal to 10, less than or equal to 5, or immediate.

Ocular Surface Staining Grading

Diagnostic dye instillation is a common and helpful method to detect ocular surface disease associated with dry eye. The most commonly utilized dyes are fluorescein, rose bengal, and lissamine green B. Fluorescein is the most commonly used diagnostic dye due to its easy availability, lack of intrinsic epithelial toxicity, rapid speed of diffusion, and short duration of effect. This dye penetrates corneal epithelial intercellular spaces and staining indicates increased epithelial permeability due to disruption of cell-to-cell junctions. Rose bengal is a water-soluble dye specific for altered conjunctival and corneal epithelium and mucous filaments. Feenstra and Tseng showed that rose bengal, unlike fluorescein, stains healthy epithelial cells when they are not protected by a healthy layer of mucin. Rose bengal dye has the unique property of showing the protective effect of the preocular tear film.[75] Rose bengal also stains dead or degenerating cells, lipid-contaminated mucous strands, and corneal epithelial filaments. Rose bengal, however, can cause significant ocular irritation, and this property has limited its clinical use. Lissamine green B has also been investigated as a diagnostic tool for ocular surface disease and has been used in several clinical trials for dry eye. Less irritating than rose bengal, lissamine green B detects dead or degenerated cells and produces less irritation after topical administration than rose bengal.[76]

Diagnostic dyes can be useful for dry eye diagnosis as well as monitoring disease severity. Several studies have shown that dye staining correlates well with the level of aqueous tear deficiency, tear breakup time, and mucus production by goblet cells.[77-79]

Location of the staining pattern can be very helpful in differentiating various etiologic causes of dry eye. The classic pattern of staining with rose bengal for dry eye is the interpalpebral conjunctiva, which appears in the shape of 2 triangles whose bases are at the limbus.

For monitoring disease severity as well as evaluating response to therapy, the use of an ocular stain grading system can prove helpful. Three systems have been established for quantifying staining of the ocular surface: the van Bijsterveld system, the Oxford system, and a standardized version of the NEI Workshop system. The van Bijsterveld system uses a grading scale that evaluates the intensity of staining based on a scale of 0 to 3 in 3 areas: nasal conjunctiva, temporal conjunctiva, and cornea. The maximum possible score with this grading system is 9.83. The Oxford and the NEI Workshop system use a wider range of scores, allowing for the detection of smaller steps of change.

Schirmer Testing

The most commonly utilized test of aqueous tear production is the Schirmer test. The Schirmer test is performed by introducing a piece of standard filter paper into the lower lid of the eye and the amount of wetting is measured with or without the use of topical anesthesia. The Schirmer test without anesthesia, also known as Schirmer I, is the best standardized of any of versions performed. Van Bijsterveld established a diagnostic cutoff for dry eye at less than 5.5 mm of wetting without anesthesia.[80] More recently, many authors and clinical trialists have adopted a diagnostic cutoff of less than or equal to 5 mm.[68] Jones established the use of topical anesthesia with Schirmer testing (Schirmer II) and defined a measurement of less than 10 mm of wetting in 5 minutes as abnormal.[81] Though the Schirmer test is easy to perform, clinicians must recognize that its variability and poor reproducibility limit the actual value of the number measured. Several authors have shown that the Schirmer test, with and without anesthesia, is highly variable when the test is repeated. Lucca evaluated the sensitivity and specificity of the Schirmer test without anesthesia for the diagnosis of dry eye and found a 25% sensitivity and 90% specificity for this test.[82] When used in the context of a diagnostic algorithm, however, the Schirmer test can prove valuable. This is particularly true in the diagnosis of SS aqueous tear deficiency where 95% of patients have a Schirmer test less than 5 mm.[69]

If aqueous tear deficiency is demonstrated, then additional tests are needed to differentiate Sjögren's and non-Sjögren's etiologies. The following 3 objective findings are useful to document the ocular component of Sjögren's syndrome, as well as to confirm this systemic diagnosis: (1) the absence of the nasal-lacrimal reflex tearing, (2) the degree of ocular surface alteration demonstrated by rose bengal or fluorescein staining, and (3) the presence of serum autoantibodies.[69] The nasal-lacrimal reflex can be elicited by stimulating the nasal mucosa under the middle turbinate with a cotton-tipped applicator.

Lid and Meibomian Gland Evaluation

Evaluating the eyelids is a critical step in the diagnosis of dry eye disease in terms of establishing etiology, determining level of severity, and choosing therapeutic options. The presence of significant meibomian gland dysfunction aids in the determination that the etiologic cause of dry eye is evaporative and intrinsic (Figure 12-3). Also, establishing the severity of meibomian gland dysfunction is important in therapeutic decision making. Several therapies such as tetracyclines, topical azithromycin, and secretagogues such as diquafosol tetrasodium may have specific therapeutic benefit in cases where meibomian gland dysfunction is a major etiologic factor.

Slit-lamp evaluation allows detailed observation of the ocular surface and eyelids, which can reveal several signs of dry eye disease such as the height of tear film meniscus on lower lid; loss, misdirection, or scaling of the lashes; dilation of blood vessels in the lid margins; status of the meibomian gland orifice; debris in the tear film; and appearance of the puncta. Lid margin morphology and turbidity of secretions can be graded to assess disease severity. Transillumination of the meibomian glands can reveal acinar dropout, meibomian cysts, or scarring.

Additional Testing

There are a number of laboratory tests used for diagnosing dry eye diseases that are not readily available in the clinical setting. These tests include tear osmolarity, tear lysozyme, lactoferrin content, fluorescein dilution tests, tear mucin measurement, and impression cytology. Of these tests, tear osmolarity may be the most important because a pathophysiologic hallmark of dry eye disease is hyperosmolarity. A number of studies suggest that the diagnostic cutoff for dry eye disease is greater than 316 MOsm/L.[68] Though the place of tear osmolarity measurement in dry eye diagnosis is well supported by the literature, its general utility as a test has been hindered by the need for a special laboratory to process tear film samples. The development of instruments to measure tear osmolarity and other dry eye parameters may make such measurements in the office feasible in the near future.

A systematic approach to testing should establish several different aspects of the disease. First, testing should help establish the etiology of the disease. In

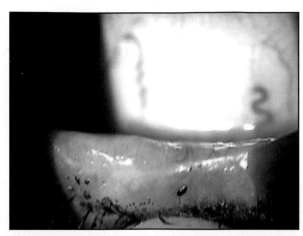

Figure 12-3. Meibomian gland dysfunction is associated with posterior hordeolum. (Courtesy of Tracy S. Swartz, OD, MS.)

particular, utilizing a test of both tear stability and tear production can suggest an etiology of aqueous tear deficiency or evaporative dry eye. Normal tear production is usually seen in dry eye secondary to meibomian gland dysfunction. Second, testing should determine a level of severity. In the next section, a detailed discussion of utilizing both symptoms and signs to establish level of severity will be discussed. Both symptom questionnaires and ocular surface staining are most helpful for this determination. Third, testing can establish a benchmark from which response to therapy can be monitored.

Determining Level of Severity

In 2006, the International Task Force (ITF) Delphi panel on dry eye presented a dry eye severity grading scheme.[83] For the purposes of determining treatment recommendations, the Delphi panel established dry eye severity levels. As important as the treatment recommendations, their findings established an organized plan of evaluating the dry eye patient. Their findings codified and summarized important dry eye parameters, including level of discomfort, visual symptoms, conjunctival injection and staining, corneal staining, lid pathology, TFBUT, and Schirmer score. Determining severity level is a critical exercise in the evaluation of the dry eye patient because it not only provides a reference point to determine treatment but also a benchmark to monitor progress.

TREATMENT

There are a number of treatment options for dry eye disease. All of these options should be tailored to the individual patient based on the etiology and the severity of the disease. Both the International Dry Eye Workshop and the International Task Force Delphi Panel on dry eye have recommended an approach to treatment based on disease severity. This section will discuss the menu of treatment options, recommendations of therapeutic options based on severity of disease, and the current pipeline of dry eye treatments.

Table 12-5 lists a number of potential options for the treatment of dry eye disease. Until recently, treatment options for dry eye have centered on increasing lubrication of the ocular surface, improving conservation of existing natural tears, and treating eyelid and meibomian gland inflammation. Lubrication

Table 12-5

DRY EYE MENU OF TREATMENTS

- Artificial tears
- Gels/ointments
- Moisture chamber spectacles
- Anti-inflammatory agents (topical CsA and corticosteroids, omega-3 fatty acids)
- Tetracyclines
- Plugs
- Secretagogues
- Serum
- Contact lenses
- Systemic immunosuppressives
- Surgery (amniotic membrane transplant, lid surgery, tarsorrhaphy, mucous membrane, and salivary gland transplant)
- CsA

options include artificial tears, ointments, and gels. Tear retention strategies include plugging of the puncta, moisture chamber goggles, contact lenses, surgery such as tarsorrhaphy, and changes in lifestyle to minimize drying. Treating eyelid disease consists of eyelid cleansing regimens, antibiotic/steroid ointments, and oral antibiotics. More recently, the use of anti-inflammatory therapy and biological tear substitutes for the treatment of dry eye has increased as our understanding of the pathophysiology of dry eye disease has improved.

Tear Supplementation

Artificial tears, whether in drop or gel formulations, contain water-soluble polymers to lubricate the ocular surface and increase tear retention time. They may be preserved or nonpreserved and generally are the first step in treatment for dry eye. Most formulations of artificial tears are limited in that they replace only the aqueous portion of tears, do not provide growth factors or other proteins needed for a healthy ocular surface, and require frequent instillation. The main variables in the formulation of ocular lubricants regard the concentration and choice of electrolytes, the osmolarity and type of viscosity/polymeric system, and the presence or type of preservative. The most critical advance in the treatment of dry eye came with the elimination of preservatives, such as benzalkonium chloride, from topical lubricants.[84] The epithelial toxic effects of benzalkonium have been well established and in patients with moderate to severe dry eye, the potential for benzalkonium chloride toxicity is high due to decreased tear secretion and decreased turnover.[85] Preservative-free formulations are necessary for patients with severe dry eye with ocular surface disease and impairment of lacrimal gland secretion, or for patients on multiple, preserved topical medications for chronic eye disease. Although many topical lubricants may improve ocular signs and symptoms, there is no evidence that any agent is superior to another. The elimination of preservatives and the development of newer, less toxic preservatives have made ocular lubricants better tolerated. Ocular lubricants, however, have not been demonstrated in controlled clinical trials to be sufficient to resolve the ocular surface dysfunction and inflammation seen in most dry eye sufferers.[84]

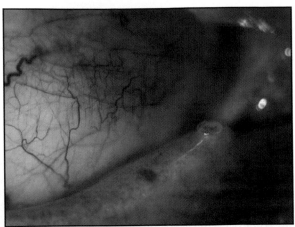

Punctal Occlusion

The rationale behind punctal occlusion is to inhibit tear drainage in order to retain tears on the ocular surface for longer. Punctal occlusion can be accomplished by solid gelatin rods, cyanoacrylate adhesives, silicone or collagen plugs, cautery, or laser. The most common type of punctal occlusion is by punctal plugs (Figure 12-4). The Freeman type of punctal plug, which rests on the opening of the punctum and extends into the cannaliculus, is the most common style of plug in use today. Punctal plugs are divided into 2 main types: absorbable plugs made of collagen or polymers, and nonabsorbable plugs made of silicone. There is significant literature documenting the beneficial effect of punctal plugs in the management of dry eye disease of various etiologies including Sjögren and non-Sjögren aqueous tear deficient dry eye, filamentary keratitis, contact lens intolerance, Stevens-Johnson disease, trachoma, neurotrophic keratopathy, postpenetrating keratoplasty, diabetic keratopathy, and postphotorefractive keratoplasty or laser in situ keratomileusis.[86-90] Beneficial outcomes in dry eye symptoms have been reported in 74% to 86% of patients treated with punctal plugs. Several reports have suggested, however, that punctal plug placement may affect the regulation of tear production and may cause a short-term decrease in tear production.[91,92] Caution should be taken if the patient has significant ocular surface inflammation because punctal occlusion may help retain dysfunctional tears on the surface.

Biological Tear Substitutes

The use of serum or saliva has been reported in humans as a biological tear substitute, particularly in cases of severe ocular surface disease. This option has the advantage of providing factors that promote corneal and conjunctival epithelial health and homeostasis. There is evidence that these tear substitutes maintain the morphology and support the proliferation of primary human corneal epithelial cells better than pharmaceutical tear substitutes.[93] Autologous serum in particular contains a number of anti-inflammatory factors that have the potential to inhibit soluble mediators of the ocular surface inflammatory cascade of dry eye. These include inhibitors of inflammatory cytokines and matrix metalloproteinases inhibitors.[94-96] Autologous serum drops have been reported to improve ocular irritation and conjunctival and corneal dye staining in SS associated dry eye in several small clinical trials.[97-99] Until recently, however, there was no consensus on the concentration or the production protocol for autologous serum. Liu and colleagues recently published an optimized protocol for the production of autologous serum.[100] Studies have demonstrated efficacy at concentrations of 20% to 100% and the effect on ocular surface disease appears to be concentration-dependent.[84]

Anti-inflammatory Therapy

With increasing awareness and understanding that dry eye is an inflammatory disease, more physicians have begun utilizing anti-inflammatory therapy in the treatment of dry eye. The main examples of anti-inflammatory therapy in dry eye are topical cyclosporine, topical corticosteroids, and tetracyclines.

CsA is a fungal-derived peptide that prevents activation and nuclear translocation of cytoplasmic transcription factors that are required for T-cell activation and inflammatory cytokine production. The potential for CsA for treating dry eye disease was initially recognized in dogs that developed spontaneous keratoconjunctivitis sicca. The therapeutic efficacy of CsA for treatment of human dry eye disease has been evaluated in several large multicenter, randomized double-masked clinical trials. Two independent FDA phase 3 clinical trials compared twice-daily treatment with CsA (0.05% or 0.1%) or vehicle for 5 months in 877 patients with moderate to severe dry eye disease.[101] Patients treated with CsA 0.05% or 0.1% showed significantly greater improvement in 2 objective signs of dry eye disease (corneal fluorescein staining and Schirmer values) than those treated with vehicle. Fifteen percent of CsA-treated patients experienced an increase in tear production compared with 5% of vehicle-treated patients. The clinical improvements noted in these clinical trials were accompanied by decreased expression of immune activation markers, apoptosis markers, and inflammatory cytokines. The numbers of T-lymphocytes in the conjunctiva decreased in CsA-treated eyes, whereas vehicle-treated eyes showed an increase in the number of cells. On the strength of these 2 phase 3 clinical trials, cyclosporine .05% ophthalmic emulsion (Restasis, Allergan Inc) was approved in 2004. The exact role of CsA in the treatment of dry eye has yet to be established. Most physicians utilize CsA for patients with moderate to severe dry eye disease, although there is emerging evidence that CsA may have benefit at earlier stages of disease or may limit the progression of disease.

Corticosteroid therapy has been reported to improve both the signs and symptoms of dry eye in several short-term clinical studies.[102-104] Corticosteroids have multiple biologic activities that may have some effect on the inflammatory process prevalent in dry eye. Corticosteroids inhibit inflammatory cytokine and chemokine production, decrease the synthesis of matrix metalloproteinases and lipid mediators of inflammation (for example, prostaglandins), decrease expression of cell adhesion molecules (eg, ICAM-1), and stimulate lymphocyte apoptosis. Though few corticosteroid-related complications were observed in these short-term clinical trials, there is the potential for toxicity with long-term use. This may limit the use of more potent corticosteroids as chronic therapy for dry eye. The risk-benefit ratio may be better with "soft corticosteroids" such as fluorometholone and loteprednol etabonate that have less intraocular activity and a lower likelihood of raising IOP. A randomized, double-masked, placebo-controlled study of loteprednol etabonate and its vehicle was conducted on 64 patients with dry eye.[105] After 2 and 4 weeks of treatment, patients with the most severe inflammatory signs at entry showed a significantly greater decrease in central corneal fluorescein staining scores when treated with loteprednol (31%) compared with its vehicle (0%). There was no change in IOP in the corticosteroid-treated group. Studies such as this one have given physicians more confidence in utilizing corticosteroids to rapidly decrease the symptoms related to inflammatory dry eye. Care should still be taken in using corticosteroids for longer term use, particularly in patients with a history of herpetic eye disease or a history of steroid pressure response.

Oral tetracycline analogs (minocycline, doxycycline) have significant potential efficacy in dry eye disease, in particular because they can improve meibomian gland dysfunction. They have antibacterial, anti-inflammatory, and antiangiogenic properties, all of which may contribute to their efficacy. Tetracyclines decrease bacterial flora producing lipolytic exoenzymes and inhibition of lipase production. These agents also decrease the activity of collagenase, phospholipase A2, and several matrix metalloproteinases. They also decrease the production of IL-1 and TNF-α in conjunctival and corneal tissues. From a clinical perspective, tetracyclines have shown particular efficacy for ocular rosacea and chronic posterior blepharitis. Use of tetracycline in patients with meibomianitis has been shown to decrease lipase production with an associated clinical improvement. Though the optimal dose of tetracyclines has not been established, the most commonly utilized dosing regimen is 100 mg of doxycycline twice a day.

Treatment Based on Severity

The International Task Force Delphi panel on dry eye disease established treatment recommendations for dry eye based on severity level. Table 12-6 shows the dry eye severity-grading scheme that was formulated by the International Task Force Delphi Panel and recommended by the DEWS report. The panel consensus was that there are 4 levels of dry eye severity based upon both signs and symptoms of dry eye disease. Each set of treatment recommendations builds upon the previous level such that if improvement in signs and symptoms is not achieved, additional treatments are employed. Level 1 dry eye patients have mild or episodic symptoms that are exacerbated under environmental stress and have mild ocular signs. For level 1 patients, education, elimination of environmental factors, including offending medications, and utilizing artificial tear substitutes are the mainstay of therapy. For level 2 patients, symptoms and signs are moderate. These patients are treated with anti-inflammatories, tetracyclines, or punctal plugs. Tetracyclines in this setting are particularly useful for patients with significant posterior blepharitis and dry eye. For level 3 patients, symptoms are signs are chronic. Treatments for this level include autologous serum, permanent punctal occlusion, or contact lenses. Level 4 patients have severe symptoms and potentially destructive ocular surface signs. For these patients, systemic anti-inflammatory agents or surgery should be considered.

Future Treatments

Several approaches for targeted therapy for dry eye disease are currently in clinical trials. These approaches can be categorized into 3 groups: secretagogues,

Table 12-6

TREATMENT RECOMMENDATIONS BY SEVERITY LEVEL

Level 1

- Education and environmental/dietary modifications
- Elimination of offending systemic medications
- Artificial tears substitutes, gel/ointments
- Eyelid therapy

Level 2

If level 1 treatments are inadequate, add:

- Anti-inflammatories
- Tetracyclines (for meibomianitis, rosacea)
- Punctal plugs
- Secretogogues
- Moisture chamber spectacles

Level 3

If level 2 treatments are inadequate, add:

- Serum
- Contact lenses
- Permanent punctual occlusion

Level 4

If level 3 treatments are inadequate, add:

- Systemic anti-inflammatory agents
- Surgery (lid surgery, tarsorrhaphy, mucus membrane, salivary gland, amniotic membrane transplantation)

Adapted from International Task Force Guidelines for Dry Eye. Behrens A, Doyle JJ, Stern L, et al. Dysfunctional tear syndrome study group. Dysfunctional tear syndrome: a Delphi approach to treatment recommendations. *Cornea.* 2006;25:900-907.

immunomodulators, and hormonal treatments. Among these future therapies, the most common variety is known as *secretagogues*. Secretagogues combat deficiencies in 1 or more layers of the tear film by stimulating the production of tear components. Secretagogues in development include mucin secretagogues such as 15(S)-HETE and ecabet sodium and compounds such as diquafosol tetrasodium, a P2Y2 agonist that stimulates mucin secretion from goblet cells in the conjunctiva.

Immunomodulators act on different components of the inflammatory cascade in dry eye such as adhesion molecule activity, T-cell infiltration, matrix metalloproteinase activity, apoptosis, and expression of cytokines and chemokines. Examples of currently FDA-approved ophthalmic immunomodulators for dry eye include cyclosporine (Restasis), topical corticosteroids, and oral tetracycline. There are several immunomodulators in clinical trials and in development.

The third major category of targeted therapy for dry eye is hormonal treatments. These treatments seek to address one of the initiating causes for secretory dysfunction of the lacrimal gland apparatus. This category of therapy appears to be the most challenging because the interaction with hormones and the ocular surface is complex. Several hormonal treatments are in clinical trials and in development.

It is unlikely that a single targeted therapy can address all the mechanisms at play in dry eye syndrome. The ideal interventions in dry eye disease would treat the underlying immune-based inflammation of the ocular surface and lacrimal gland, decreasing ocular surface inflammation, and cause the lacrimal glands to secrete tears in a more normal volume and composition.

SUMMARY OF DRY EYE DISEASE

Significant advances in our understanding of dry eye disease have established several important concepts. The classification of dry eye disease as either aqueous-deficient or evaporative helps guide both diagnostic testing as well as therapy. The pathophysiology of dry eye disease has a final common pathway of tear hyperosmolarity leading to ocular surface inflammation and tear film instability. The stepwise diagnostic approach involving history, symptom questionnaires, testing, and clinical evaluation can establish both etiology and severity. Finally, therapy should be based on the severity level of the disease. Our evolving understanding that dry eye is a progressive inflammatory disease should continue to encourage clinicians and researchers to treat the problem aggressively as well as develop targeted therapies for treatment.

REFERENCES

1. Lemp MA. Report of the National Eye Institute/Industry Workshop on Clinical Trials in Dry Eye. *CLAO J.* 1995;21:221-232.

2. Adatia FA, Michaeli-Cohen A, Naor J, et al. Correlation between corneal sensitivity, subjective dry eye symptoms and corneal staining in Sjögren's syndrome. *Can J Ophthalmol.* 2004; 39:767-771.

3. Begley CG, Chalmers RL, Abetz L, et al. The relationship between habitual patient-reported symptoms and clinical signs among patients with dry eye of varying severity. *Invest Ophthalmol Vis Sci.* 2003;44:4753-4761.

4. Vitale S, Goodman LA, Reed GF, Smith JA. Comparison of the NEI-VFQ and OSDI questionnaires in patients with Sjögren's syndrome-related dry eye. *Health Qual Life Outcome.* 2004;2:44.

5. Rieger G. The importance of the precorneal tear film for the quality of optical imaging. *Br J Ophthalmol.* 1992;76:157-158.

6. Liu Z, Pflugfelder SC. Corneal surface irregularity and the effect of artificial tears in aqueous tear deficiency. *Ophthalmology.* 1999;106:936-943.

7. Goto E, Yagi Y, Matsumoto Y, Tsubota K. Impaired functional visual acuity of dry eye patients. *Am J Ophthalmol.* 2002;133:181-16.

8. Holly F, Lemp MA. Formation and rupture of the tear film. *Exp Eye Res.* 1973;15:515-525.

9. Bron AJ. Diagnosis of dry eye. *Surv Ophthalmol.* 2001;45(suppl 2):221-226.

10. Goto T, Zheng X, Klyce SD, et al. A new method for tear film stability using videokeratography. *Am J Ophthalmol.* 2003;135:607-612.

11. Farris RL, Stuchell RN, Mandel ID. Tear osmolarity variation in the dry eye. *Trans Am Ophthalmol Soc.* 1986;84:250-268.

12. Gilbard JP. Human tear film electrolyte concentrations in health and dry eye disease. *Int Ophthalmol Clin.* 1994;34:27-36.

13. Murube J. Tear osmolarity. *Ocul Surf.* 2006;1:62-73.

14. Tomlinson A, Khanal S, Ramaesh K, et al. Tear film osmolarity: determination of a referent for dry eye diagnosis. *Invest Ophthalmol Vis Sci.* 2006;47:4309-4315.

15. Pflugfelder SC, Jones D, Ji Z, et al. Altered cytokine balance in the tear fluid and conjunctiva of patients with Sjögren's syndrome keratoconjunctivitis sicca. *Curr Eye Res.* 1999; 19:201-211.

16. Tsubota K, Fujihara T, Saito K, Takeuchi T. Conjunctival epithelium expression of HLA-DR in dry eye patients. *Ophthalmologica.* 1999;213:16-19.

17. Mishima S, Gasset A, Klyce S, Baum J. Determination of tear volume and tear flow. *Investig Ophthalmol.* 1966;5:264-276.

18. Scherz W, Dohlman CH. Is the lacrimal gland dispensable? Keratoconjunctivitis sicca after lacrimal gland removal. *Arch Ophthalmol.* 1975;93:81-83.

19. Li DQ, Chen Z, Song XJ, et al. Stimulation of matrix metalloproteinases by hyperosmolarity via a JNK pathway in human corneal epithelial cells. *Invest Ophthalmol Vis Sci.* 2004; 45:4302-4311.

20. Luo L, Li DQ, Corrales RM, Pflugfelder SC. Hyperosmolar saline is a proinflammatory stress on the mouse ocular surface. *Eye Contact Lens.* 2005;31:186-193.

21. De Paiva CS, Corrales RM, Villarreal AL, et al. Corticosteroid and doxycycline suppress MMP-9 and inflammatory cytokine expression, MAPK activation in the corneal epithelium in experimental dry eye. *Exp Eye Res.* 2006;83:526-535.

22. Nakamura H, Kawakamu A, Eguchi K. Mechanisms of autoantibody production and the relationship between autoantibodies and the clinical manifestations in Sjögren's syndrome. *Trans Res.* 2006;148(6):281-288.

23. Hayashi Y, Arakaki R, Ishimaru N. The role of caspase cascade on the development of primary Sjögren's syndrome. *J Med Invest.* 2003;50:32-38.

24. Vitali C, Bombardieri S, Jonsson R, et al. Classification criteria for Sjögren syndrome: a revised version of the European criteria proposed by the American-European Consensus Group. *Ann Rheum Dis.* 2002;61:554-558.

25. Vitali C, Bombardieri S, Moutsopoulos HM, et al. Preliminary criteria for the classification of Sjögren's syndrome. Results of a prospective concerted action supported by the European Community. *Arthritis Rheum.* 1993;36:340-347.

26. Fox RI, Robinson CA, Curd JG, et al. Sjögren's syndrome. Proposed criteria for classification. *Arthritis Rheum.* 1986;29:477-585.

27. Wiik A, Cervera R, Haass M, et al. European attempts to set guidelines for improving diagnostics of autoimmune rheumatic disorders. *Lupus.* 2006;15:391-396.

28. Foulks G, Bron AJ. Meibomian gland dysfunction: a clinical scheme for description, diagnosis, classification, and grading. *Ocul Surf.* 2003;1:107-126.

29. Bron AJ, Tiffany JM. The contribution of Meibomian disease to dry eye. *Cornea.* 2004;2:149-164.

30. Bron AJ, Tiffany JM, Gouveia SM, Yokoi N, Voon LW. Functional aspects of the tear film lipid layer. *Exp Eye Res.* 2004;78:347-360.

31. Gilbard JP, Farris RL. Ocular surface drying and tear film osmolarity in thyroid eye disease. *Acta Ophthalmol.* 1983;61:108-116.

32. Lemp MA. Surfacing abnormalities in the preocular tear film and dry eye syndromes. *Int Ophthalmol Clin.* 1973;13:191-199.

33. Rees TD, Jelks GW. Blepharoplasty and the dry eye syndrome: guidelines for surgery? *Plast Reconstr Surg.* 1981;68:249-252.

34. Tsubota K, Nakamori K. Effects of ocular surface area and blink rate on tear dynamics. *Arch Ophthalmol.* 1995;113:155-158.

35. Tei M, Spurr-Michaud SJ, Tisdale AS, Gipson IK. Vitamin A deficiency alters the expression of mucin genes by the rat ocular surface epithelium. *Invest Ophthalmol Vis Sci.* 2000;41:82-88.

36. Hori Y, Spurr-Michaud S, Russo CL, et al. Differential regulation of membrane-associated mucins in the human ocular surface epithelium. *Invest Ophthalmol Vis Sci.* 2004;45:114-122.

37. Sommer A, Emran N. Tear production in a vitamin A responsive xerophthalmia. *Am J Ophthalmol.* 1982;93:84-87.

38. Kunert KS, Keane-Myers AM, Spurr-Michaud S, et al. Alteration in goblet cell numbers and mucin gene expression in a mouse model of allergic conjunctivitis. *Invest Ophthalmol Vis Sci.* 2001;42:2483-2489.

39. Henderson JW, Prough WA. Influence of age and sex of flow of tears. *Arch Ophthalmol.* 1950; 43:224-231.

40. Sullivan BD, Evans JE, Dana MR, Sullivan DA. Impact of androgen deficiency on lipid profiles in human meibomian gland secretions. *Adv Exp Med Biol.* 2002;506:449-458.

41. Bacman S, Berra A, Sterin-Borda L, Borda E. Muscarinic acetylcholine receptor antibodies as a new marker of dry eye Sjögren syndrome. *Invest Ophthalmol Vis Sci.* 2001;42:321-327.

42. Battat L, Macri A, Dursun D, Pflugfelder SC. Effects of laser in situ keratomileusis on tear production, clearance, and the ocular surface. *Ophthalmology.* 2001;108:1230-1235.

43. Fox RI. Systemic diseases associated with dry eye. *Int Ophthalmol Clin.* 1994;34:71-87.

44. McCollum CJ, Foulks GN, Bodner B, et al. Rapid assay of lactoferrin in keratoconjunctivitis sicca. *Cornea.* 1994;13:505-508.

45. Pflugfelder SC, Jones D, Ji Z, Afonso A, Monroy D. Altered cytokine balance in the tear fluid and conjunctiva of patients with Sjögren's syndrome keratoconjunctivitis sicca. *Curr Eye Res.* 1999;19:201-211.

46. Solomon A, Dursus D, Liu Z, Xie Y, Macri A, Pflugfelder SC. Pro- and anti-inflammatory forms of interleukin-1 in the tear fluid and conjunctiva of patients with dry-eye disease. *Invest Ophthalmol Vis Sci.* 2001;42:2283-2292.

47. Afonso A, Sobrin L, Monroy DC, Selzer M, Lokeshwar B, Pflugfelder SC. Tear fluid gelatinase B activity correlates with IL-1α concentration and fluorescein tear clearance. *Invest Ophthalmol Vis Sci.* 1999;40:2506-2512.

48. Farris RL, Tear osmolarity—a new gold standard? *Adv Exp Med Biol.* 1994;350:495-503.

49. Furuichi S, Hashimoto S, Gon Y, Matsumoto K, Horie T. p38 mitogen-activated protein kinase and c-Jun-NH2-terminal kinase regulate interleukin-8 and RANTES production in hyperosmolarity stimulated human bronchial epithelial cells. *Respirology.* 2002;7:193-200.

50. Li D-Q, Chen Z, Song XJ, Farley W, Pflugfelder SC. Hyperosmolarity stimulates production of MMP-9, IL-1β and TNF-α by human corneal epithelial cells via a c-Jun NH$_2$-terminal kinase pathway [abstract]. *Invest Ophthalmol Vis Sci.* 2002;43:E-Abstract 1981.

51. Luo L, Li D-Q, Doshi A, Farley W, Pflugfelder SC. Experimental dry eye induced expression of inflammatory cytokines (IL-1α and TNF-α), MMP-9 and activated MAPK by the corneal epithelium [abstract]. *Invest Ophthalmol Vis Sci.* 2003;44:E-Abstract 1026.

52. Rosette C, Karin M. Ultraviolet light and osmotic stress activation of the JNK cascade through multiple growth factor and cytokine receptors. *Science.* 1996;274:1194-1197.

53. Pflugfelder SC. Anti-inflammatory therapy for dry eye. *Am J Ophthalmol.* 2004;137:337-342.

54. Boudouin HLA, Brignole F, Pisella PJ, et al. Flow cytometric analysis of inflammatory markers in conjunctival epithelial cells of patients with dry eyes. *Invest Ophthalmol Vis Sci.* 2000;41:1356-1363.

55. Sternlicht MD, Werb Z. How matrix metalloproteinases regulate cell behavior. *Ann Rev Cell Dev Biol.* 2001;17:463-516.

56. Behzadian MA, Wang XL, Windsor LJ, Ghaly N, Caldwell RB. TGF-beta increases retinal endothelial cell permeability by increasing MMP-9 possible role of glial cells in endothelial barrier function. *Invest Ophthalmol Vis Sci.* 2001;42:853-859.

57. Asahi M, Wang X, Mori T, et al. Effects of matrix metalloproteinase-9 gene knock-out on the proteolysis of blood-brain barrier and white matter components after cerebral ischemia. *J Neurosci.* 2001;21:7724-7732.

58. Gao J, Schwalb TA, Addeo JV, Ghosn CR, Stern ME. The role of apoptosis in the pathogenesis of canine keratoconjunctivitis sicca the effect of topical cyclosporin A therapy. *Cornea.* 1998;17:654-663.

59. Yeh S, Song XJ, Farley W, Li DQ, Stern ME, Pflugfelder SC. Apoptosis of ocular surface cells in experimentally induced dry eye. *Invest Ophthalmol Vis Sci.* 2003;44:124-129.

60. McCarty CA, Bansal AK, Livingston PM, Stanislavsky YL, Taylor HR. The epidemiology of dry eye in Melbourne, Australia. *Ophthalmology.* 1998;105:1114-1119.

61. Bjerrum KB. Keratoconjunctivitis sicca and primary Sjögren's syndrome in a Danish population aged 30-60 years. *Acta Ophthalmol Scand.* 1997;75:281-286.

62. Schein OD, Munoz B, Tielsch JM, Bandeen-Roche K, West S. Prevalence of dry eye among the elderly. *Am J Ophthalmol.* 1997;124:723-728.

63. Schaumberg DA, Sullivan DA, Buring JE, Dana MR. Prevalence of dry eye syndrome among US women. *Am J Ophthalmol.* 2003:136;318-326.

64. Miljanovic B, Dana MR, Sullivan DA, Schaumberg DA. Prevalence and risk factors for dry eye syndrome among older men in the United States [abstract]. *Invest Ophthalmol Vis Sci.* 2007;48:E-abstract 4293. Presented at Annual Meeting of the Association for Research in Vision and Ophthalmology (ARVO); May 6-10, 2007; Ft Lauderdale, FL.

65. Moss SE, Klein R, Klein B. Prevalence of and risk factors for dry eye syndrome. *Arch Ophthalmol.* 2000;118:1264-1268.

66. The epidemiology of dry eye disease: Report of the Epidemiology Subcommittee of the International Dry Eye WorkShop. *Ocul Surf.* 2007;5(2):93-107.

67. Ellwein LB, Urato CJ. Use of eye care and associated charges among the Medicare population: 1991-1998. *Arch Ophthalmol.* 2002;120:804-811.

68. Bron AJ, Smith JA, Calonge M. Methodologies to diagnose and monitor dry eye disease: report of the Diagnostic Methodology Subcommittee of the International Dry Eye Work Shop (2007). *Ocul Surf.* 2007;5(2):108-152.

69. Murillo-Lopez F, Pflugfelder SC. Disorders of tear production and the lacrimal system. In: Krachmer, Mannis, Holland, eds. *Cornea.* St. Louis, MO: Mosby; 2005.

70. Norn MS. Dessication of the precorneal tear film. I. Corneal wetting time. *Acta Ophthalmol.* 1969;47:865-880.

71. Lemp MA, Holly FJ. Recent advances in ocular surface chemistry. *Am J Optom Arch Am Acad Optom.* 1970;47:669-672.

72. Vitali C, Moutsopoulos HM, Bombardieri S. The European Community Study Group on diagnostic criteria for Sjögren's syndrome. Sensitivity and specificity of tests for ocular and oral involvement in Sjögren's syndrome. *Ann Rheum Dis.* 1994;53(10):637-647.

73. Lemp MA, Hamill JR. Factors affecting tear film breakup in normal eyes. *Arch Ophthalmol.* 1973;89:103-105.

74. Abelson M, Ousler G III, Nally LA, et al. Alternate reference values for tear film break-up time in normal and dry eye populations. *Adv Exp Med Biol.* 2002;506(pt B):1121-1125.

75. Feenstra RPF, Tseng SCG. Comparison of fluorescein and rose bengal staining. *Ophthalmology.* 1992;99:605-617.

76. Norn MS. Lissamine green. Vital staining of cornea and conjunctiva. *Acta Ophthalmol.* 1973; 69:79-86.

77. Lemp MA, Dohlman CH, Kuwabara T, Holly FJ, Carroll JM. Dry eye secondary to mucus deficiency. *Trans Am Acad Ophthalmol Otolaryngol.* 1971;75:1223-1227.

78. Dohlman CH, Friend J, Kalevar V, Yagoda D, Balazs E. The glycoprotein (mucus) content of tears from normals and dry eye patients. *Exp Eye Res.* 1976;22:359-365.

79. Holly FJ, Patten JT, Dohlman CH. Surface activity determination of aqueous tear components in dry eye patients and normals. *Exp Eye Res.* 1977;24:479-491.

80. van Bijsterveld OP. Diagnostic tests in sicca syndrome. *Arch Ophthalmol.* 1969;82:10-14.

81. Jones LT. The lacrimal secretory system and its treatment. *Am J Ophthalmol.* 1966;62:47-60.

82. Lucca JA, Nunez JN, Farris RL. A comparison of diagnostic tests for keratoconjunctivitis sicca: lactoplate, Schirmer and tear osmolarity. *CLAO J.* 1990;16:109-112.

83. Behrens A, Doyle JJ, Stern L, et al. Dysfunctional tear syndrome. A Delphi approach to treatment recommendations. *Cornea.* 2006;25:90-97.

84. Management and therapy of dry eye disease: Report of the Management and Therapy Subcommittee of the International Dry Eye Work Shop (2007). 2007;5(2):163-178.

85. Smith L, George M, Berdy G, Abelson M. Comparative effects of preservative free tear substitutes on the rabbit cornea: a scanning electron microscopic evaluation [abstract]. *Invest Ophthalmol Vis Sci.* 1991;32(suppl):733.

86. Tuberville AW, Frederick WR, Wood TO. Punctal occlusion in tear deficiency syndromes. *Ophthalmology.* 1982;89:1170-1172.

87. Willis RM, Folberg R, Krachmer JH, et al. The treatment of aqueous-deficient dry eye with removable punctal plugs. A clinical and impression cytological study. *Ophthalmology.* 1987; 94:514-518.

88. Gilbard JP, Rossi SR, Azar DT, Gray KL. Effect of punctal occlusion by Freeman silicone plug insertion on tear osmolarity in dry eye disorders. *CLAO J.* 1989;15:216-218.

89. Balaram M, Schaumberg DA, Dana MR. Efficacy and tolerability outcomes after punctal occlusion with silicone plugs in dry eye syndrome. *Am J Ophthalmol.* 2001;131:30-36.

90. Baxter SA, Laibson PR. Punctal plugs in the management of dry eyes. *Ocul Surf.* 2004;2:255-265.

91. Paulsen F. The human nasolacrimal glands. *Adv Anat Embryol Cell Biol.* 2003;170:iii-xi, 1-106.

92. Yen MT, Pflugfelder SC, Feuer WJ. The effect of punctal occlusion on tear production, tear clearance, and ocular surface sensation in normal subjects. *Am J Ophthalmol.* 2001;131:314-323.

93. Geerling G, Daniels JT, Dart JK, et al. Toxicity of natural tear substitutes in a fully defined culture model of human corneal epithelial cells. *Invest Ophthalmol Vis Sci.* 2001;42948-42956.

94. Liou LB. Serum and in vitro production of IL-1 receptor antagonist correlate with C-reactive protein levels in newly diagnosed, untreated lupus patients. *Clin Exp Rheumatol.* 2001;19:515-523.

95. Ji H, Pettit A, Ohmura K, et al. Critical roles for interleukin 1 and tumor necrosis factor alpha in antibody-induced arthritis. *J Exp Med.* 2002;196:77-85.

96. Paramo JA, Orbe J, Fernandez J. Fibrinolysis/proteolysis balance in stable angina pectoris in relation to angiographic findings. *Thromb Haemost.* 2001;86:636-639.

97. Fox RI, Chan R, Michelson JB, Belmont JB, Michelson PE. Beneficial effect of artificial tears made with autologous serum in patients with keratoconjunctivitis sicca. *Arthritis Rheum.* 1984;27:459-461.

98. Kono I, Kono K, Narushima K, et al. Beneficial effect of the local application of plasma fibronectin and autologous serum in patients with keratoconjunctivitis sicca of Sjögren's syndrome. *Ryumachi.* 1986;26:339-343.

99. Tsubota K, Goto E, Fujita H, et al. Treatment of dry eye by autologous seum application in Sjögren's syndrome. *Br J Ophthalmol.* 1999;83:390-395.

100. Liu L, Hartwig D, Harloff S, et al. An optimised protocol for the production of autologous serum eyedrops. *Graefes Arch Clin Exp Ophthalmol.* 2005;243:706-714.

101. Sall K, Stevenson OD, Mundorf TK, Reis BL. Two multicenter, randomized studies of the efficacy and safety of cyclosporine ophthalmic emulsion in moderate to severe dry eye disease. *Ophthalmology.* 2000;107:631-639.

102. Marsh P, Pflugfelder SC. Topical non-preserved methylprednisolone therapy of kerato-conjunctivitis sicca in Sjögren's syndrome. *Ophthalmology.* 1999;106:811-816.

103. Sainz de la Maza Serra SM, Simon Castellvi C, Kabbani O. Nonpreserved topical steroids and punctual occlusion for severe keratoconjunctivitis sicca. *Arch Soc Esp Oftalmol.* 2000;75:751-756.

104. Maskin SL, Anderson B, Chodosh J, et al. Loteprednol etabonate 0.5% (Lotemax) versus vehicle in the management of patients with KCS and at least moderate inflammation [abstract]. *Invest Ophthalmol Vis Sci.* 2003;44:E-Abstract 686.

105. Solomon A, Rosenblatt M, Li DQ, et al. Doxycycline inhibition of interleukin-1 in the corneal epithelium. *Invest Ophthalmol Vis Sci.* 2000;41:2544-2557.

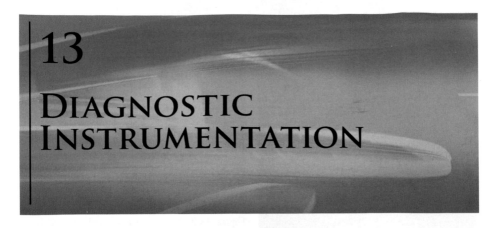

13

DIAGNOSTIC INSTRUMENTATION

Emil William Chynn, MD, MBA and Conswalla Shavers, MD

Advances in technology used to evaluate the cornea have increased our understanding of corneal physiology, biomechanical properties, and pathology. Such technology includes confocal microscopy, ultrasound biomicroscopy, topography, tomography, optical coherence tomography (OCT), pachymetry, and ocular response analysis.

CONFOCAL MICROSCOPY

Conventional microscopes suffer from several limitations. Such instruments collect the light reflected back from an object, along with light from above and below the focal plane. This creates noisy, unsatisfactory images in all but the thinnest of specimens when viewed under high magnification.[1] In order to use it, specimens must be mechanically prepared, embedded, or stained. This makes it impossible to view undisturbed physiologic processes and introduces artifacts into the subject during the handling process.

Confocal microscopy avoids these problems by focusing the incident light in the same plane as the objective lens of the microscope.[2] The pinhole source of light and its conjugate pinhole detector limit the passage of light from outside of the focal plane. Both the condenser lens and the objective lens are focused at the same point, hence the term *confocal*.[2]

The resulting field of view is small, and a full field of view must be created by scanning. This can be achieved by rotating discs with thousands of optically conjugate source-detector pinholes, using a scanning mirror system, or using a laser light source scanned across a specimen in a raster pattern. Regardless of the method, it gives the clinician the ability to optically section living or in vitro tissues noninvasively over time.

Its primary advantage is its high resolution. Confocal microscopes image cells within corneal epithelium, the epithelial nerve plexus, various layers of stroma, and endothelium in the range of 1.5 to 4 µm. Unfortunately, multiple sections are required to evaluate larger areas of cornea, which requires a large amount of time for image acquisition and processing. Time to acquire a single image is typically

Trattler WB, Majmudar PA, Luchs JI, Swartz TS, eds.
Cornea Handbook (pp. 225-248)
© 2010 SLACK Incorporated

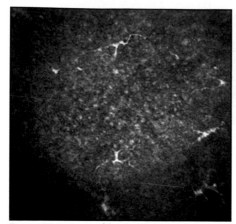

Figure 13-1. Image of basal epithelium and Langerhans cells, obtained using laser confocal microscopy. (Courtesy of Heidelberg Engineering, Heidelberg, Germany.)

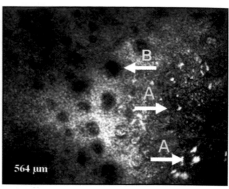

Figure 13-2. Image of pigment granules (A) and irregular guttata (B), obtained using laser confocal microscopy. (Courtesy of Heidelberg Engineering, Heidelberg, Germany.)

less than 1/30 second, and the observation time in clinical settings is around 5 minutes.[1]

In clinical practice, confocal microscopy has been used to identify *Acanthamoeba* cysts and trophozoites, bacteria, fungi, and other pathogens within the cornea. It can also be used to study corneal flap thickness, analyze the LASIK interface, and count endothelial cells. In clinical research, it can be used for the evaluation of corneal healing processes and various corneal diseases.

The Heidelberg Retina Tomograph, known for its posterior-segment applications, is capable of anterior segment imaging using a combination of software and hardware added to the HRT-II (Heidelberg, Germany). It provides black-and-white images with a 400 μm field of view at 600× magnification with a resolution of 2 μm. Tissue layers are evaluated along the *z* axis in real time and saved as digital images (Figures 13-1 through 13-3). It has been used to evaluate corneal physiology in relation to healing,[3] corneal dystrophies, and degenerations.[4,5]

CORNEAL ENDOTHELIAL CELL ANALYSIS: SPECULAR MICROSCOPY

An experienced ophthalmologist may be able to examine the corneal endothelium using only a slit lamp; however, specular microscopes allow for a more magnified, direct view of the endothelial cell structure, morphology, and number. Modern specular microscopes can obtain high-quality images of the corneal endothelial layer within seconds, using noncontact techniques that are comfortable for the patient as well as easy for the ophthalmic technician.

The earliest specular microscopes date back to work by Vogt and Goldmann that allowed ophthalmologists to visualize the endothelium at a very low magnification. The term *Spiegelmikroskopie* or *specular microscopy* was coined by Vogt. The invention of the modern specular microscope is credited to David Maurice, who in 1968 developed a microscope to photograph endothelial cells at a high magnification (500×). Bourne and Liang later adapted the microscope for clinical use. The first specular microscopes were used primarily for in vitro research

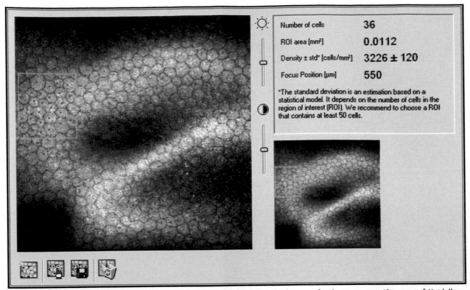

Number of cells	36
ROI area [mm²]	0.0112
Density ± std* [cells/mm²]	3226 ± 120
Focus Position [µm]	550

*The standard deviation is an estimation based on a statistical model. It depends on the number of cells in the region of interest (ROI). We recommend to choose a ROI that contains at least 50 cells.

Figure 13-3. Image of endothelial cell count software available using the laser confocal microscope. (Courtesy of Heidelberg Engineering, Heidelberg, Germany.)

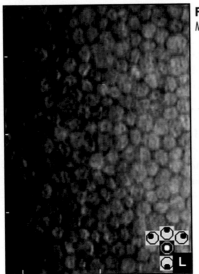

Figure 13-4. Normal corneal endothelial cell pattern. (Courtesy of Parag Majmudar, MD.)

studies but are now increasingly used in clinical practice for a variety of reasons (Figure 13-4).

Specular microscopy may guide the physician's decision-making process in the management of corneal disorders from Fuchs' endothelial dystrophy (Figure 13-5) to bullous keratopathy, as well as other endothelial dystrophies such as posterior polymorphous dystrophy. In addition, endothelial cell counts should be monitored carefully in patients who have undergone phakic intraocular lens implantation.

Modern specular microscopes not only magnify the endothelial monolayer for close inspection, but computer algorithms may also enable an accurate cell

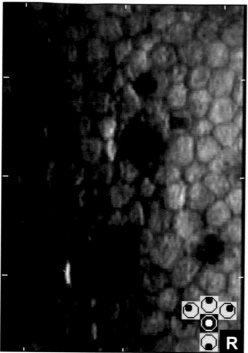

Figure 13-5. Fuchs' dystrophy: note the dark "guttae" that have replaced the normal endothelial cells. (Courtesy of Parag Majmudar, MD.)

density measurement, corneal pachymetry, and morphometric analysis such as the percentage of hexagonal cells and coefficient of variation. These indices are helpful in determining the amount of polymegathism (Figure 13-6) and pleomorphism and may reflect more closely the health of the endothelium.

ULTRASOUND BIOMICROSCOPY

Ophthalmic ultrasonography uses high-frequency sound waves transmitted into the eye using a probe. Sound is emitted in a parallel, longitudinal wave pattern, similar to that of light. The frequency of the sound wave is the number of cycles, or oscillations, per second measured in hertz.[6] For sound to be considered ultrasound, it must have a frequency of greater than 20,000 oscillations per second, or 20 kHz.[7] As the sound waves strike intraocular structures, they are reflected back to the probe and converted into an electric signal. The signal is reconstructed as an image, allowing dynamic evaluation of the eye and photographic documentation of pathology. Higher frequency ultrasound is associated with shorter wavelength. A direct relationship exists between wavelength and depth of tissue penetration. The shorter the wavelength, the shallower the penetration and the better the resolution. Because ophthalmic examinations require little tissue penetration and high tissue resolution, ultrasound probes used for ophthalmic B-scan are manufactured with very high frequencies (10 MHz). Recently, high-resolution ophthalmic B-scan probes (ultrasound biomicroscopy, or UBM) of 20 to 50 MHz have been manufactured that penetrate only about 5 to 10 mm into the eye for incredibly detailed resolution of the anterior segment.[8] The tissue resolution of 5 to 20 μm distinguishes the layers of the cornea and the corneal flap after LASIK

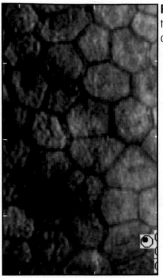

Figure 13-6. Polymegathism: note the large size of endothelial cells compared to those in Figure 13-4. This is an indicator of corneal endothelial dysfunction. (Courtesy of Parag Majmudar, MD.)

and characterizes the 3-dimensional structure of the cornea at this precision level under normal or pathologic conditions. The major advantage of UBM is its ability to image the anterior segment through edematous or scarred corneal tissue.

ARTEMIS

The Artemis system is a very high-frequency (VHF) ultrasound eye scanner that employs a 50-MHz transducer. Scans are made in several arcs over the cornea using a novel reverse immersion technique. A computer digitizes the signal, yielding measurement of the thickness of individual corneal layers over an 8-mm to 10-mm zone in 3 dimensions. This technology has been used to evaluate corneal flap integrity,[9] residual stromal surfaces,[10,11] and anterior and posterior chamber structures (Figure 13-7).

This is the only ultrasound technology available that can produce topographic maps of the individual corneal layers, such as the epithelium, the flaps, and the stroma (Figures 13-8 and 13-9). The topographic information has been used to correct a poorly positioned free cap following LASIK based on epithelial irregularities in the flap.[13] In addition, topographical information may enable diagnosis of keratoconus at an earlier stage than tomography or conventional topography. Epithelium often compensates for stromal surface irregularities such as keratoconus; that is, epithelium overlying the cone becomes progressively thinner as the cone become more elevated. The epithelium becomes invaginated by the underlying bulging stromal surface and the anterior surface remains regular. Epithelial thickness profiles derived from Artemis VHF digital ultrasound scans can help in differentiating true keratoconus from apparent keratoconus as well as in cases of so-called forme fruste keratoconus by observing back surface asymmetry accompanied by coincident thinning of the epithelium. The thinning over the anterior stromal cone is accompanied by thickening of the epithelium circumferentially to the cone.[12]

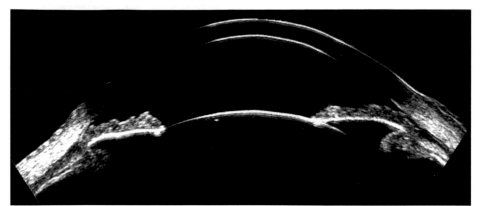

Figure 13-7. Full anterior segment horizontal Artemis VHF digital ultrasound B-scan encompassing a 15-mm wide sector. The anterior retina can be seen within this scan. The angle-to-angle and sulcus-to-sulcus diameters are easily measured directly. Printed with permission from Wang M, ed. *Corneal Topography in the Wavefront Era.* Thorofare, NJ: SLACK Incorporated; 2006.

Figure 13-8. 3D pachymetric map of the epithelium (top left map) digitally superimposed onto Tomey front surface topography (bottom right map). The topography map is shown at different levels of transparency to demonstrate the coincidence of the irregular topography with the epithelial irregularities. Printed with permission from Wang M, ed. *Corneal Topography in the Wavefront Era.* Thorofare, NJ: SLACK Incorporated; 2006.

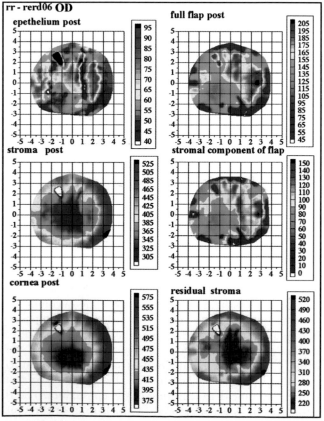

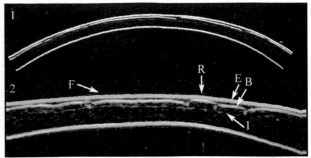

Figure 13-9. Horizontal VHF digital ultrasound corneal B-scan through the visual axis. The upper image (1) shows the geometrically corrected image, while the lower image (2) shows the raw ultrasound data with axial zoom to better appreciate the interfaces. The surface of epithelium (E), Bowman's (B), the keratectomy interface (I) are labeled. It is clearly noted that Bowman's surface is highly irregular, with numerous true microfolds (*) which were only very faintly visible on slit-lamp examination, due to the impressive epithelial compensation producing excellent smoothing of the corneal surface. Printed with permission from Wang M, ed. *Corneal Topography in the Wavefront Era.* Thorofare, NJ: SLACK Incorporated; 2006.

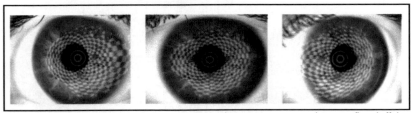

Figure 13-10. Placido targets, simple rings, or more complex ring patterns as seen here are reflected off the cornea and digitally analyzed to determine corneal curvature. (Courtesy of Tracy S. Swartz, OD, MS.)

CORNEAL TOPOGRAPHY

Corneal topography is the measurement of corneal curvature using computerized imaging. Various methods can be used, including placido disc (computerized video keratoscopy), fluorescein profilometry (stereo photogrammetry), and interference techniques. The last is limited to research. Axial and meridional curvature of the cornea are directly measured by most commercial systems, which typically compute elevation data from the curvature data to produce elevation maps.

Placido Imaging

Most corneal topography instruments used in clinical practice are based on placido reflective image analysis (Figure 13-10). This method uses analysis of reflected images of multiple concentric rings projected on the cornea to evaluate the anterior cornea. Corneal ectasias such as keratoconus and pellucid marginal degeneration may be seen on topography well before they manifest clinically, and topography is performed prior to any keratorefractive procedure for this reason. Topography is also important when considering patients for presbyopic lens implantation where proper alignment and a regular corneal surface are crucial for successful outcomes (Figure 13-11). Misalignment of the corneal apex or

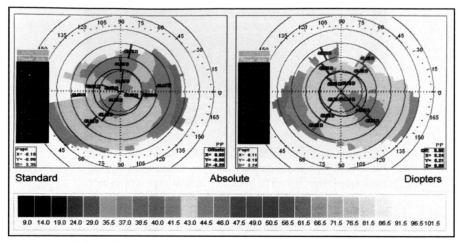

Figure 13-11. Slight irregular astigmatism in this patient who underwent a ReStor lens implant (Alcon Laboratories, Fort Worth, TX) and suffered severe subjective symptoms that improved only with a gas-permeable lens in the affected eye. (Courtesy of Tracy S. Swartz, OD, MS.)

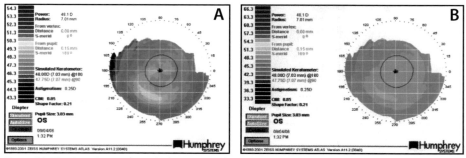

Figure 13-12. (A) Axial map using a scale of 0.5 D. (B) Axial map using a scale of 1.5 D. (Courtesy of Tracy S. Swartz, OD, MS.)

irregular astigmatism can reduce vision both objectively and subjectively, resulting in unhappy patients.

Scaling is important in topography, because each system uses a slightly different scale, making comparisons between machines complicated. It is best to monitor corneal changes using the same system, with verification of the scale used each time. Too large a step size can minimize abnormalities, and too small a step can exaggerate a small, possibly insignificant change (Figure 13-12). A step scale of 1.5 D for curvature and power maps and 5-μm steps for elevation maps are generally recommended.

Map types will also vary, so attention must be paid to the type of map before making a diagnosis. The most common map used is the axial or tangential power map. Values at each point on these maps represent the power associated to a sphere that has the same slant as the cornea being examined. The power is calculated in a similar method used in keratometry, with the assumption regarding the index used (1.3375). It is important to remember that these maps are a descriptor of corneal optics rather than shape.

Tangential maps represent the local curvature of the cornea at each point and are often referred to as "local" or "instantaneous curvature" maps. The axis of

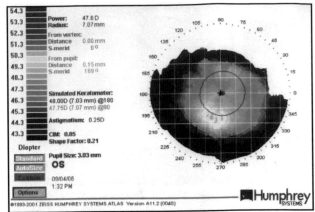

Figure 13-13. Tangential map of the same eye in Figure 13-12. (Courtesy of Tracy S. Swartz, OD, MS.)

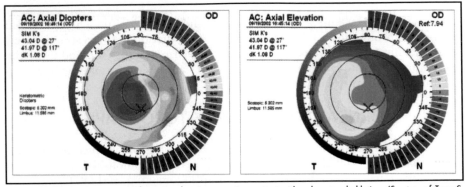

Figure 13-14. Axial curvature and anterior elevation maps in a patient with a decentered ablation. (Courtesy of Tracy S. Swartz, OD, MS.)

reference is different for each point, resulting in a higher degree of variability from point to point. This results in more focal irregularities compared to an axial map of the same eye (Figure 13-13), and tangential maps are preferred by contact lens fitters for this reason.

Elevation maps show the difference in surface height based on a reference sphere and are a better representation of the corneal shape (Figure 13-14). These can be most beneficial for patients following refractive surgery where the elevation has been purposely altered to correct the vision.

Though placido imaging continues to be the most sensitive measure of corneal curvature, evaluation is limited to the anterior corneal surface. Eye position and irregular corneal surfaces may cause errors in data collection, and scaling variability between instruments can complicate clinical use (Figure 13-15).

Fluorescein Prolifometry

In this technique, fluorescein is instilled into the tear film and simultaneous pictures are captured at different angles to create a dimensional view. Surface elevation is created. Though this technique enables measurement onto the sclera and in highly irregular corneas, it is not as sensitive in measuring small distortions and is more invasive. Fluorescein may alter tear volume and chemistry, lead-

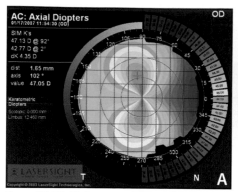 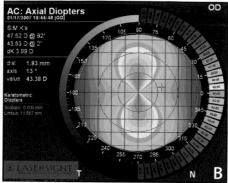

Figure 13-15. (A) Apparent pathology resulting from poor eye alignment. When tilted 7.5 degrees, 0.36 D of astigmatism is induced. (B) When properly aligned, the pattern becomes normal. Printed with permission from Wang M, ed. *Irregular Astigmatism: Diagnosis and Treatment.* Thorofare, NJ: SLACK Incorporated; 2008.

ing to tear film breakup and artifactual irregular astigmatism. Though formal fluorescein prolifometry, taking pictures after installation of fluorescein is rarely used in clinical practice, clinicians commonly utilize a similar method using the slit lamp to calculate tear breakup time (TBUT) and to less formally gain a clinical impression of the ocular surface.

CORNEAL TOMOGRAPHY/TOPOGRAPHY

Corneal tomography/topography is the creation of 3-dimensional models created from 2-dimensional cross-sectional images. It is accomplished using several technologies, including slit-scanning, Scheimpflug imaging, and OCT.

Scanning Slit

The Orbscan IIz (Bausch & Lomb, Rochester, NY) corneal topography system uses a scanning optical slit design to create images of the cornea in combination with a placido disc. The high-resolution video camera captures 40 light slits at the 45 degree angle projected through the cornea (Figure 13-16). The instrument's software analyzes 240 data points per slit to produce elevation maps of the anterior and posterior cornea and calculates the corneal thickness.

This technology was the first to allow evaluation of the cornea's posterior surface. The accuracy and repeatability of the instrument are reported to be below 10 μm and, under optimal conditions, in the range of 4 μm in the central cornea and 7 μm in the peripheral cornea. Limited eye movement, ability of patients to keep the eye wide open, and optically clear cornea are required for data capture. Results are typically presented using the "Quad map," shown in Figure 13-17. This map commonly included 4 maps: axial or tangential curvature, anterior and posterior elevation, and pachymetry.

Scheimpflug Imaging

Scheimpflug imaging is based on the Scheimpflug principle, which occurs when a planar subject is not parallel to the image plane. In typical photography, the film plane, lens plane, and plane of sharp focus are parallel to each other

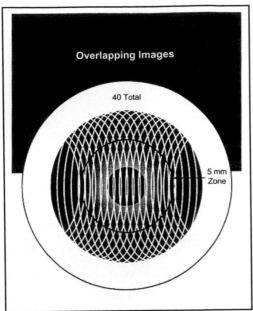

Figure 13-16. Orbscan slit image figure. Printed with permission from Wang M, ed. *Corneal Topography in the Wavefront Era: A Guide for Clinical Application.* Thorofare, NJ: SLACK Incorporated; 2006.

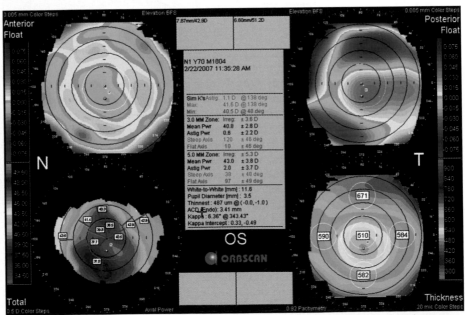

Figure 13-17. A "Quad map" typically includes an anterior elevation, posterior elevation, axial curvature and pachymetry map. (Courtesy of Tracy S. Swartz, OD, MS.)

(Figure 13-18). In Scheimpflug cameras, an oblique tangent can be drawn from the image, object, and lens planes, and the point of intersection is the Scheimpflug intersection, where the image is in best focus (Figure 13-19). With a rotating Scheimpflug camera, the Pentacam can obtain 50 Scheimpflug images in less than 2 seconds. Each image has 500 true elevation points for a total of 25 000 true elevation points for the surface of the cornea.

Figure 13-18. Planes of an ordinary camera. Printed with permission from Wang M, ed. *Corneal Topography in the Wavefront Era: A Guide for Clinical Application.* Thorofare, NJ: SLACK Incorporated; 2006.

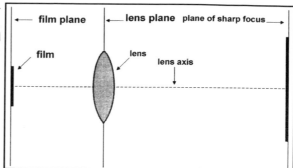

Figure 13-19. Diagram of a Scheimpflug camera. Printed with permission from Wang M, ed. *Corneal Topography in the Wavefront Era: A Guide for Clinical Application.* Thorofare, NJ: SLACK Incorporated; 2006.

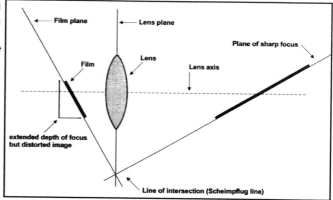

The Pentacam utilizes 2 cameras. One detects and measures the pupil for orientation and fixation. The second camera visualizes the anterior segment and captures the images for analysis. The Pentacam creates anterior and posterior surface topography, including curvature, tangential, and axial maps, anterior chamber maps, pachymetry maps, and cataract densometry as well as corneal wavefront analysis (Figure 13-20). Advantages of the Pentacam include the following: (1) high resolution of the entire cornea, including the center of the cornea, which is interpolated by placido systems; (2) ability to measure corneas with severe irregularities, such as keratoconus, that may not be amenable to placido imaging; and (3) ability to calculate pachymetry from limbus to limbus.

Optical Coherence Tomography

OCT of the cornea and anterior segment is an optical method of cross-sectional scanning based on reflection and scattering of light from the structures within the cornea. In optical interferometry, the light source is split into the reference and measurement beams. The measurement beam is reflected from ocular structures and interrelates with the reference light reflected from the reference mirror. This is called *interference*. The positive interference creates an increased signal which is measured by the interferometer. This enables the position of the structure to be measured. Structures of the anterior segment can be visualized with a high degree of resolution (currently 18 µm axial and 60 µm transverse).[14]

A cross-sectional image of the cornea and other anterior segment structures anterior to the lens is produced (Figure 13-21). OCT is particularly useful in the

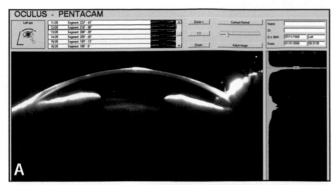

Figure 13-20. (A) Pentacam imaging of a patient with a central scar where slit scanning and placido topography were unable to image the cornea. The Scheimpflug image clearly shows the scar. (B) Topographic and pachymetry analysis in the same patient. (Courtesy of Tracy S. Swartz, OD, MS.)

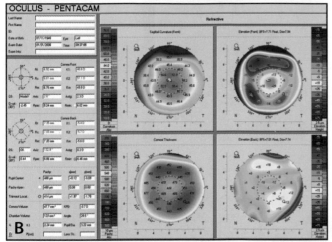

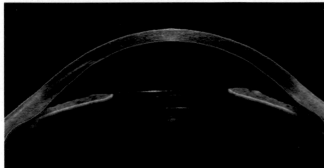

Figure 13-21. Visante imaging of a narrow angle following implantation of a phakic IOL. (Courtesy of Tracy S. Swartz, OD, MS.)

eye because soft tissue cannot be accurately imaged using conventional X-rays or magnetic resonance imaging (MRI). It is also more functional than confocal microscopy because it can provide images of the entire anterior portion of the eye at once. Additional benefits of this technology are that it is noncontact and uses no coupling medium. Therefore, structures such as the angle, iris, and lens can be seen in their natural state.

The use of light as an analysis medium also has its drawbacks. The depth of penetration is limited to the anterior segment, and image quality is greatly reduced when attempting to penetrate corneal opacities such as scarring or pannus. Initial clinical use of anterior segment OCT was mainly focused on measurement

Figure 13-22. Visante image from a patient with a history of LASIK. Flap thickness can be evaluated using the "flap tool." (Courtesy of Tracy S. Swartz, OD, MS.)

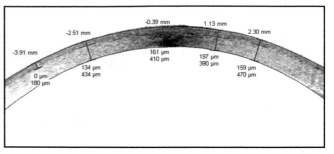

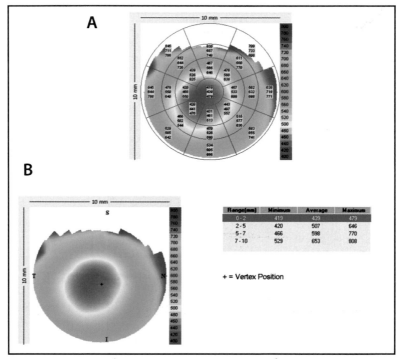

Figure 13-23. Visante pachymetry map in a LASIK patient. (Courtesy of Tracy S. Swartz, OD, MS.)

of phakic IOL placement, angle analysis in glaucoma, and flap detection after LASIK.[15,16] AS-OCT is now used for the detection and management of corneal diseases including keratoconus, pellucid marginal degeneration, and corneal ectasia following refractive surgery (Figure 13-22), angle structures in glaucoma (see Figure 13-22), and optical pachymetry (Figure 13-23).

PACHYMETRY

Pachymetry, a thickness measurement of the cornea, is used to evaluate corneal edema and endothelial dysfunction, for surgical planning to calculate postoperative residual stromal thickness sufficiency, and in diagnosis and management of glaucoma and ocular hypertension. Though ultrasound measurement techniques remain the standard, disadvantages of this technique include lack of precision, variable pressure applied during measurement, spread of infection and epithelial

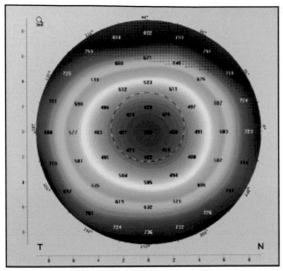

Figure 13-24. Pentacam pachymetry map. (Courtesy of Tracy S. Swartz, OD, MS.)

disruption, and the required anesthetic. Pancorneal thickness maps produced by various optical pachymeters and ultrasound microscopy may be more useful in identifying early corneal ectasia and in directing surgical procedures in the corneal periphery, such as astigmatic keratectomy (AK), LASIK, PRK, and Intacs placement. An example of such a map is shown in Figure 13-24.

Newer technologies are currently being studied for reliability and are not considered interchangeable with ultrasound as a rule at this time. It is generally accepted that Orbscan measurement of corneal thickness is greater than ultrasound; in such cases the acoustic factor used in the Orbscan can be adjusted to better correlate with pachymetry measurement obtained by ultrasound. (Before making this adjustment, it is suggested that you consult your Bausch & Lomb representative.) Specular microscopy appears to yield significantly smaller values than the other methods.[17-19] Other methods have been studied but comparisons are not consistent and results are conflictive. At this time, it is best to monitor corneal disease using the same method and to avoid comparing methods unless pathology requires it such as in cases of corneal haze and scarring.[20-23]

OCULAR RESPONSE ANALYZER

The Ocular Response Analyzer measures biomechanical properties of the cornea using an air jet similar to air-puff tonometry. As the air contacts the cornea, it moves inward, past applanation to slight concavity, and a second applanation occurs as the cornea returns to its normal shape after the air pulse is discontinued. An electrooptical collimation detector system monitors the corneal curvature of the cornea's central 3.0 mm during measurement. The light reflected by the cornea peaks upon applanation. Thus, 2 pressure values are measured. Two measurements are taken within 20 milliseconds such that ocular pulse effects, eye position, or other variables do not affect measurement. The values of the pressure signal at the 2 applanation times are different due to the viscoelastic properties of the cornea.[24] A signal results (Figure 13-25) where the raw signal is red, the filtered applanation is blue, and the pressure signal is green.

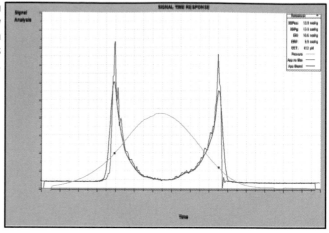

Two biomechanical properties are evaluated: hysteresis and resistance factor. Corneal hysteresis (CH) is related to the viscoelastic structure of the tissue, and it is the difference between the 2 pressure values. Reduced corneal hysteresis has been reported in patients with keratoconus and Fuchs' dystrophy, possibly related to the disorganization of stromal collagen lamellae.[25]

Corneal resistance factor (CRF) is an indicator of the tissue's overall resistance and is a measurement of cumulative effects of both viscous and elastic resistance encountered by the air jet during applanation. It is calculated as a linear function of the pressure values associated with each applanation process. It tends to increase with elevated pressure.

In addition to the values for CH and CRF, IOP values are measured. The corneal-compensated IOP (IOPCC) is obtained from the difference between the 2 applanation pressures using the formula $(P2 - kP1)$, where $P1$ and $P2$ represent the applanation pressures and k is constant at 0.43.[26] It is described as the representation of IOP that is free of corneal influence and may be more accurate than Goldmann applanation tonometry, which may be influenced by corneal curvature and pachymetry.

Ortiz et al investigated ORA measurements in 3 groups: normals, keratoconus, and post-LASIK patients. They found that both corneal hysteresis and resistance factor were lower for keratoconic eyes compared to post-LASIK and normal eyes.[27] Examples of signals in eyes with keratoconus can be seen in Figures 13-26 and 13-27. This may result from the biomechanical changes brought about by excimer procedures: reduced pachymetry and changes in biomechanics induced by the flap. Applications for this technology include refractive surgery screening and complication management (Figure 13-28), corneal disease diagnosis and management, and glaucoma. More studies are needed on this technology.

CASE EXAMPLES

Common anterior segment disorders manifest in characteristic patterns using these technologies. Keratoconus manifests with corresponding areas of elevation on the posterior and anterior float and corneal thinning (Figure 13-29). Pellucid marginal degeneration manifests are steepening lower on the cornea due to the

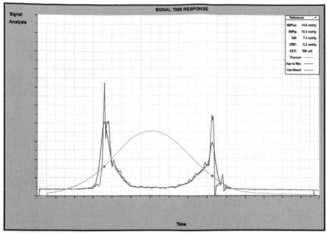

Figure 13-26. ORA signal for a keratoconic patient. Note the reduced CH and CRF values and the "bounce" after the second peak. (Courtesy of Tracy S. Swartz, OD, MS.)

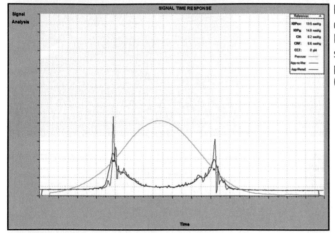

Figure 13-27. An ORA signal in a patient with severe keratoconus. Note the flat peaks, noisy signal, and significant bounce after the second peak. (Courtesy of Tracy S. Swartz, OD, MS.)

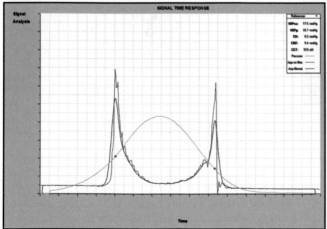

Figure 13-28. An ORA signal of a patient with a mild asymmetry on topography, a manifest refraction of −8.25 D, and a pachymetry of 512 μm. Note that the CH is 9.4, the signal is slightly noisy, and there is a "bounce" after the second peak. This patient may not be a good candidate for keratorefractive surgery. (Courtesy of Tracy S. Swartz, OD, MS.)

Figure 13-29. (A) Keratoconus manifests with inferior steepening, corresponding areas of elevation on the posterior and anterior elevation maps, and corneal thinning. (B) The Scheimpflug image of a keratoconic cornea shows the distortion and central scarring characteristic of the disease. (C) Coma is associated with keratoconus and may be seen in early stages prior to vision loss. (Courtesy of Tracy S. Swartz, OD, MS.)

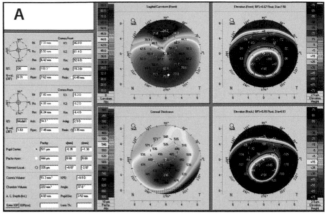

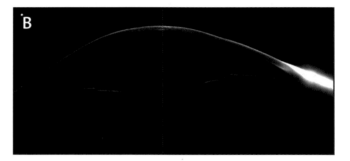

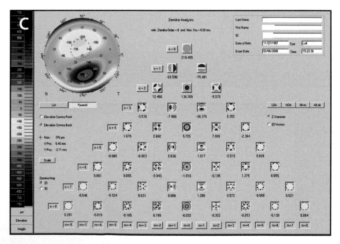

lower area of thinning (Figure 13-30). Trauma may manifest in irregular astigmatism with variable asymmetry (Figure 13-31). Dry eye may result in multifocal irregularities and data loss due to lack of reflection (Figure 13-32).

Refractive surgery directly alters corneal shape, producing predictable patterns. Normal myopic treatments result in central thinning corresponding to the ablation area and a central plateau. This creates positive spherical aberration (Figure 13-33). Hyperopic treatments result in central steepening and negative spherical aberration (Figure 13-34).

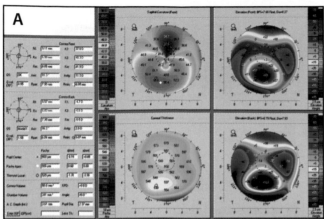

Figure 13-30. (A) Pellucid marginal degeneration manifests are steepening lower on the cornea due to the lower area of thinning. The crab claw pattern is characteristic but may also be seen in keratoconus. (B) The truncated bowtie pattern may be an early sign of ectatic disease and may precede the typical crab claw pattern. (Courtesy of Tracy S. Swartz, OD, MS.)

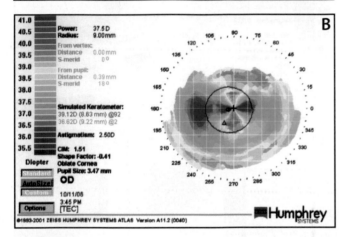

Figure 13-31. Trauma may manifest in irregular astigmatism with variable asymmetry. This patient had a corneal scar inferiorly. (Courtesy of Tracy S. Swartz, OD, MS.)

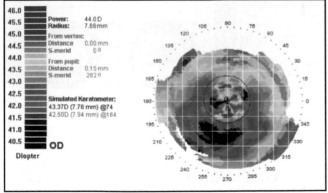

Complications from keratorefractive surgery tend to produce the most irregular corneal surfaces. If the excimer ablation is decentered during PRK, epithelial LASIK (epi-LASIK), or LASIK, the patient may present with decreased visual acuity, complaints on poor quality of vision, and aberrations due to the irregular topography (Figure 13-35). Ectasia following keratorefractive surgery manifests similarly to keratoconus in an eye with a history of surgical correction (Figure

Figure 13-32. (A) Dry eye may result in multifocal irregularities. (B) Data loss due to lack of reflection is also common in dry eye patients. (Courtesy of Tracy S. Swartz, OD, MS.)

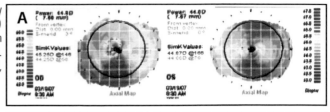

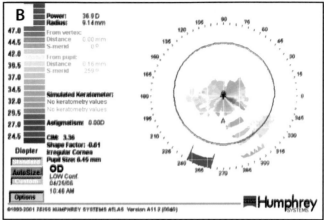

Figure 13-33. (A) Normal myopic treatments result in central thinning and a central plateau corresponding to the ablation area. (Courtesy of Tracy S. Swartz, OD, MS.)

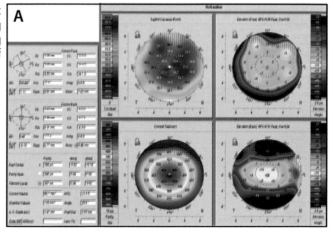

13-36). Radial keratotomy may cause severe irregularity, often in a petal shape, secondary to the incisions (Figure 13-37).

CONCLUSION

Refractive surgery has necessitated advances in the technologies used to evaluate the cornea, and all subspecialties of ophthalmology have benefited. As our understanding of the posterior surface, corneal biomechanics, and pathology expand using these technologies, and as newer technologies become better understood and clinically studied, our practice patterns will continue to progress.

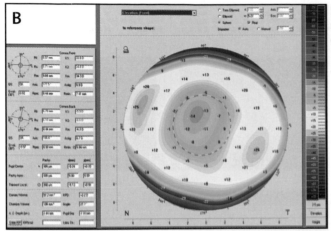

Figure 13-33. (B) The anterior elevation should show a central depression following myopic LASIK. (Courtesy of Tracy S. Swartz, OD, MS.)

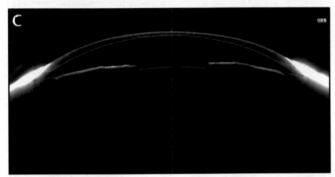

Figure 13-33. (C) The central thinning secondary to the ablation. (D) The myopic treatment results in positive spherical aberration. (Courtesy of Tracy S. Swartz, OD, MS.)

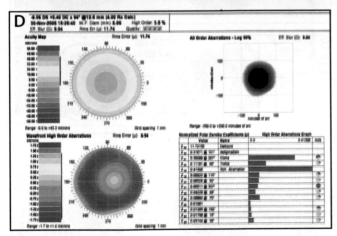

Figure 13-34. Hyperopic treatments result in central steepening (A), and negative spherical aberration (B). (Courtesy of Tracy S. Swartz, OD, MS.)

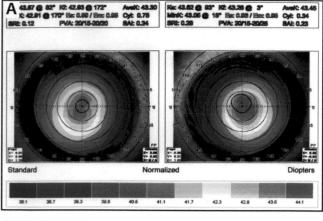

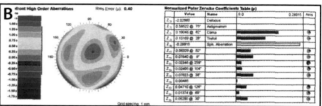

Figure 13-35. (A) If the excimer ablation is decentered during PRK, epithelial LASIK (epi-LASIK), or LASIK, the patient may present with decreased visual acuity, complaints on poor quality of vision, and aberrations due to the irregular topography. Here, the myopic ablation was decentered. (B) Note the improved topography following a topographically based custom treatment in the left eye. (Courtesy of Tracy Swartz, OD, MS).

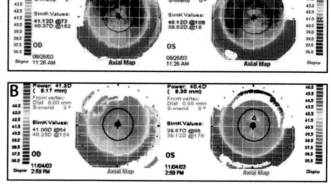

Figure 13-36. Ectasia following keratorefractive surgery resembles keratoconus but is found in an eye with a history of surgical correction. The right eye suffers from ectasia while the left shows the characteristic, albeit decentered ablation zone. (Courtesy of Tracy S. Swartz, OD, MS.)

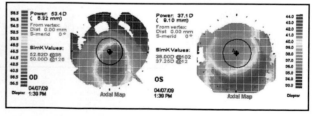

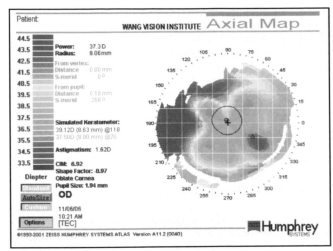

Figure 13-37. Radial keratotomy may cause severe irregularity, often in a petal shape, secondary to the incisions. (Courtesy of Tracy S. Swartz, OD, MS.)

REFERENCES

1. Gills J, Sanders DR, Thornton SP, et al. *Corneal Topography: The State of the Art.* Thorofare, NJ: SLACK Incorporated; 1995.

2. Thomas J, Wang J, Rollins AM, Sturm J. Comparison of corneal thickness measured with optical coherence tomography, ultrasonic pachymetry, and a scanning slit method. *J Refract Surg.* 2006;22:671-678.

3. Doga AV, Mushkova IA, Maychuk NV. Confocal microscopy of corneal wound healing after thermokeratoplasty. *J Refract Surg.* 2007;23(suppl 9):1046-1049.

4. Erdurmus M, Selcoki Y, Yagci R, Hepsen IF. Amiodarone-induced keratopathy: full-thickness corneal involvement. *Eye Contact Lens.* 2008;34:131-132.

5. Iordanidou V, Sultan G, Boileau C, Raphael M, Baudouin C. In vivo corneal confocal microscopy in marfan syndrome. *Cornea.* 2007;26:787-792.

6. Cusumano A, Coleman DJ, Silverman RH, et al. Three-dimensional ultrasound imaging—clinical applications. *Ophthalmology.* 1998;105:300-306.

7. Kaufman HE, Barron BA, McDonald M, Kaufman SC. *Companion Handbook to the Cornea.* Butterworth Heinemann; 2000.

8. Wolffsohn J, Davies L. Advances in ocular imaging. *Expert Rev Ophthalmol.* 2007;2:755-767.

9. Reinstein DZ, Sutton HF, Srivannaboon S, et al. Evaluating microkeratome efficacy by 3D corneal lamellar flap thickness accuracy and reproducibility using Artemis VHF digital unltrasound arc-scanning. *J Refract Surg.* 2006;22:431-440.

10. Reinstein DZ, Srivannaboon S, Archer TJ, Silverman RH, Sutton H, Coleman DJ. Probability model of the inaccuracy of residual stromal thickness prediction to reduce the risk of ectasia after LASIK part I: quantifying individual risk. *J Refract Surg.* 2006;22:851-860.

11. Reinstein DZ, Sutton HF, Srivannaboon S, Silverman RH, Archer TJ, Coleman DJ. Evaluating microkeratome efficacy by 3D corneal lamellar flap thickness accuracy and reproducibility using Artemis VHF digital ultrasound arc-scanning. *J Refract Surg.* 2006; 22:431-440.

12. Reinstein DZ, Archer TJ, Silverman RH. Evaluation of irregular astigmatism with Artemis VHF digital ultrasound scanning. In: Wang MX, ed. *Irregular Astigmatism: Diagnosis and Treatment.* Thorofare, NJ: SLACK Incorporated; 2008.

13. Reinstein DZ, Rothman RC, Couch DG, Archer TJ. Artemis very high frequency digital ultrasound-guided repositioning of a free cap after laser in situ keratomileusis. *J Cataract Refract Surg.* 2006;32:1877-1883.

14. Hirano K, Ito Y, Suzuki T, Kojima T, Kachi S, Miyake Y. Optical coherence tomography for the noninvasive evaluation of the cornea. *Cornea*. 2001;20:281-289.

15. Hirano K, Ito Y, Suzuki T, Kojima T, Kachi S, Miyake Y. Optical coherence tomography for the noninvasive evaluation of the cornea. *Cornea*. 2001;20:281-289.

16. Belin M, Holladay J, Michelson M, Woodhams JT, Ahmed I. The Pentacam: precision, confidence, results and accurate "Ks." *Insert to Cataract & Refractive Surgery Today*. 2007.

17. Ucakhan OO, Ozkan M, Kanpolat A. Corneal thickness measurements in normal and keratoconic eyes: Pentacam comprehensive eye scanner versus noncontact specular microscopy and ultrasound pachymetry. *J Cataract Refract Surg*. 2006;32:970-977.

18. Modis L Jr, Langenbucher A, Seitz B. Corneal thickness measurements with conant and noncontact specular microscopic and ultrasonic pachymetry. *Am J Ophthalmol*. 2001;132: 517-521.

19. Suzuki S, Oshika T, Oki K, et al. Corneal thickness measurements: scanning-slit corneal topography and noncontact specular microscopy versus ultrasonic pachymetry. *J Cataract Refract Surg*. 2003:29:1313-1318.

20. Sanchis-Gimeno JA, Herrera M, Lleo-Perez A, et al. Quantitative anatomical differences in central corneal thickness values determined with scanning-slit corneal topography and noncontact specular microscopy. *Cornea*. 2006;25:203-205.

21. Amano A, Honda N, Amano Y, et al. Comparison of central corneal thickness measurements by rotating Scheimpflug camera, ultrasonic pachymetry, and scanning-slit corneal topography. *Ophthalmology*. 2006;113:937-941.

22. Airiani S, Trokel SL, Lee SM, Braunstein RE. Evaluating central corneal thickness measurements with noncontact optical low-coherence reflectometery and contact ultrasound pachymetry. *Am J Ophthalmology*. 2006;142:164-165.

23. Leung DY, Lam DK, Yeung BY, Lam DS. Comparison between central corneal thickness measurements by ultrasound pachymetry and optical coherence tomography. *Clin Exp Ophthalmol*. 2006;34:751-754.

24. Soergel F, Jean B, Seiler T, et al. Dynamic mechanical spectroscopy of the cornea for measurement of its viscoeleastic properties in vitro. *Ger J Ophthalmol*. 1995;4:151-156.

25. Luce DA. Determining in vivo biomechanical properties of the cornea with an ocular response analyzer. *J Cataract Refract Surg*. 2005;31:156-162.

26. Medeiros, FA, Weinreb RN. Evaluation of the influence of corneal biomechanical properties on intraocular pressure measurements using the ocular response analyzer. *J Glaucoma*. 2006;15:364-370.

27. Ortiz D, Pinero D, Shabayek MH, Arnalich F, Alio JL. Corneal biomechanical properties in normal, post-laser in situ keratomileusis, and keratoconic eyes. *J Cat Refract Surg*. 2007;33:1371-1375.

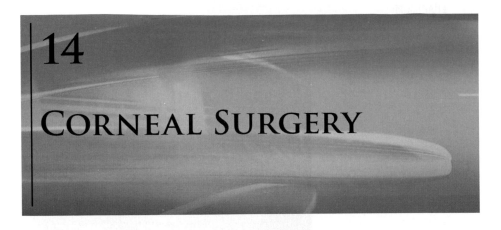

14

CORNEAL SURGERY

Yassine J. Daoud, MD and Terry Kim, MD

Anterior segment surgery encompasses a wide variety of procedures from the straightforward to the complex. The general ophthalmologist should be familiar with the procedures, their indications, and postoperative complications to better serve patients who might not always return to their primary surgeon for follow-up or when acute problems arise.

Corneal transplantation commonly refers to replacement of a portion or the entire diseased host cornea with a healthy donor cornea. Great advancements have occurred in corneal transplantation surgery with improvements in preservation and storage of donor corneas in dedicated eye banks.[1] At the same time, introduction of the operating microscope, improvements in microsurgical instruments and suture materials, and better postoperative care have helped corneal transplantation to become one of the most successful and most common types of transplantation surgery in the United States, with approximately 40 000 corneal transplants performed annually.[1]

PENETRATING KERATOPLASTY

PK refers to full-thickness corneal grafting, whereas lamellar keratoplasty refers to partial-thickness corneal grafting. PK is performed for a variety of corneal conditions. Two recent reviews showed that the most common reasons for PK are failed grafts, pseudophakic or aphakic bullous keratopathy edema (Figure 14-1), Fuchs' dystrophy, keratoconus, and corneal scars (Figure 14-2).[2,3] Other less frequent causes are corneal thinning or perforation secondary to viral or bacterial infection and chemical or physical trauma.

A complete eye exam including visual acuity, color vision or pupillary reaction, and slit-lamp examination should be done prior to the surgery. If fundus exam is not possible secondary to corneal or media opacity, ancillary tests such as ultrasonography may uncover potential vision-threatening retinal abnormalities. Other tests such as visually evoked potentials and laser interferometer may be employed to assess the afferent visual system. Other concomitant eye disease such as glaucoma, active inflammation, or dry eyes should be addressed before proceeding to corneal transplantation.

Trattler WB, Majmudar PA, Luchs JI, Swartz TS, eds.
Cornea Handbook (pp. 249-268)
© 2010 SLACK Incorporated

Figure 14-1. Bullous keratopathy with an epithelial defect. (Courtesy of Tracy S. Swartz, OD, MS.)

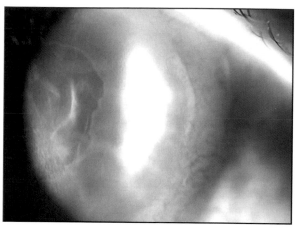

Figure 14-2. Deep corneal scar. (Courtesy of Tracy S. Swartz, OD, MS.)

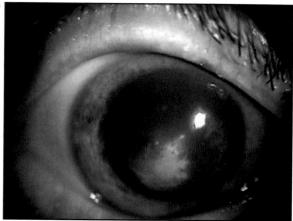

When it is determined that corneal transplantation is required, donor tissue is obtained from an eye bank. Eye banks routinely screen donor tissues for dangerous diseases that may be transmitted to the recipients such as HIV, viral hepatitis, sepsis, rabies, leukemia, Creutzfeldt-Jakob disease, and intraocular tumors.

In general, anesthesia for PK consists of a retrobulbar or peribulbar block and occasionally a facial block in the cooperative and mature patient. In children or uncooperative patients, general anesthesia is advocated. Patients with a corneal perforation are often offered general anesthesia to eliminate the possibility of an expulsive hemorrhage through the perforation as a result of the retrobulbar injection.

First, the IOP is lowered pharmacologically or using digital massage. After the recipient eye is prepped and draped in a sterile fashion, an eyelid speculum that places minimal pressure on the globe is inserted. Scleral support with a Flieringa (or equivalent) ring is needed in pediatric eyes and in aphakic or pseudophakic eyes with previous vitrectomy.

The size of the corneal transplant is checked initially at the slit lamp and verified with calipers at the time of surgery. Based on this measurement, the donor cornea is trephined about 0.25 to 0.50 mm larger in diameter. Although different techniques can be used, the main goal is to excise a uniform donor button with

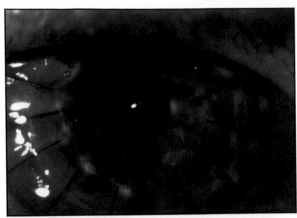

Figure 14-3. PK 1 day postoperative. (Courtesy of Ming Wang, MD, PhD.)

vertical edges. Typical trephination size ranges from 7.5 to 8.5 mm. Smaller grafts may give rise to astigmatism, whereas larger ones might lead to increased IOP, peripheral anterior synechiae, or vascularization postoperatively.

Unless doing a combined procedure, the pupil is usually constricted pharmacologically to prevent injury to the lens. Again, many techniques, including manual, vacuum, or motorized trephines, can be used to trephine the recipient eye. It is extremely important that the trephine be placed exactly where the surgeon intends, usually centered on the pupil unless the pathology or diseased tissue is decentered. Trephination should proceed slowly and carefully until the anterior chamber is entered. Then, corneoscleral scissors are used to remove the recipient corneal button, taking care not to injure the iris or the lens.

The main goals for graft placement and suturing are to secure the wound, reform the anterior chamber, create a relatively smooth corneal contour, and minimize excessive flattening, steepening, and astigmatism. Once the anterior chamber is filled with balanced salt solution or viscoelastic material, the donor button is carefully transferred and secured to the recipient bed with 4 cardinal sutures in the 3-, 6-, 9-, and 12-o'clock positions. Complete wound closure can be achieved with running sutures, interrupted sutures, or a combination of both. Interrupted sutures are preferred if areas of the graft are likely to heal or vascularize before other areas, causing localized areas of suture to loosen. The number of sutures depends on the suture technique used and the size of the graft. Care should be taken to bury the knots to lessen the possibility of vascularization or infection. The wound should be carefully checked to be watertight. Afterwards, the Flieringa ring is removed and suture tension is adjusted to minimize astigmatism in the graft. At the completion of surgery, topical and/or subconjunctival antibiotics and steroids are given and a pressure patch and protective shield are placed over the eye (Figure 14-3).

Postoperatively, topical corticosteroids are extremely important in preventing allograft rejection. Typically, they should be administered 4 times daily for a month and continued 1 time daily for at least 6 months and every other day for another 6 months. The frequency and duration of the topical corticosteroids may vary depending on each situation at the treating physician's discretion. Occasionally, systemic corticosteroids or other immunosuppressive agents may be used.

Adequate postoperative care is crucial to the success of PK. Most postoperative complications, such as endophthalmitis and epithelial downgrowth, are more

Figure 14-4. Graft failure. (Courtesy of Tracy S. Swartz, OD, MS.)

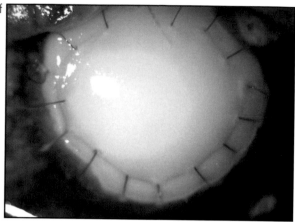

common after PK than cataract surgery. Management of such complications is the same as after cataract surgery.

A wound leak can occur right after PK. It usually presents as a soft globe with shallow anterior chamber. If the anterior chamber is shallow or flat, surgical repair should be performed immediately in order to minimize trauma to the graft. If the anterior chamber is formed, other measures to manage the wound include adding aqueous suppressants, decreasing topical corticosteroids, bandage contact lens, and patching.

Epithelial defects are common in the early postoperative period. These can be managed with bandage contact lens or ophthalmic ointment and usually resolve within 1 to 2 weeks.

Glaucoma can result from pupillary block, choroidal effusion, or aqueous misdirection and malignant glaucoma. Less commonly, it might be caused by epithelial downgrowth or fibrous ingrowth. The cause must be identified and treated medically or surgically as indicated.

Patients who undergo PK are at risk of infectious keratitis or crystalline keratopathy. Crystalline keratopathy is usually caused by *Streptococcus viridans* but may be caused by other gram-positive bacteria or even fungi. It usually arises adjacent to a corneal suture, often, but not always, with an epithelial defect. It typically appears as grey-white infiltrate in the superficial stroma with tiny protruding branches. It is usually treated with frequent topical antibiotics. In case of infectious keratitis, scarring of the infected area and sending the sample for microbiological analysis might be warranted. Fortified, topical broad-spectrum antibiotics should be used frequently. Once the causative agent is identified, organism-specific topical antibiotics should be started. Endophthalmitis is probably the most feared complication after PK. It may arise from donor or host tissue contamination, intraoperative contamination, or postoperative infection. Endophthalmitis should be treated aggressively with intraocular antibiotics, aqueous and vitreous cultures to identify the culprit organism, and possibly vitrectomy. Prognosis is usually guarded in these unfortunate cases.

Graft rejection is the most common cause of graft failure (Figure 14-4). About 50% of graft rejections occur in the first 6 months and the majority occur within 1 year of transplant surgery. Early recognition and aggressive treatment, most commonly with frequent topical corticosteroids, are crucial for a corneal graft to survive a rejection episode. Graft rejection may be epithelial or endothelial. Epithelial rejection accounts for 10% of all rejection episodes and usually presents as a linear epithelial ridge as the host epithelial cells replace those of the donors. It generally occurs within the first postoperative month and is self-limited and treated with topical corticosteroids. Endothelial rejection accounts for most cases of graft rejection.[4] It is also the most serious form of rejection because damaged corneal endothelial cells can only be replaced with another corneal transplant. A migratory line of inflammatory cells may be occasionally seen and is referred to as an *endothelial rejection* or *Khodadoust line*. As endothelial cells are targeted by the immune system, they fail to pump fluid, which leads to corneal edema. Patients may present with conjunctival injection, keratic precipitates, corneal edema, and anterior chamber cell and flare.

Newly diagnosed corneal edema immediately following corneal transplantation is treated with intensive topical corticosteroids. If no improvement is noted, the diagnosis of primary graft failure is made. This is usually due to either preoperative or intraoperative damage to the donor endothelium.

If sutures are loose or exposed, they should be removed immediately to minimize risk of graft rejection or infection. If sutures are tight and causing astigmatism, visual acuity might be suboptimal despite clarity of the graft. Such sutures may be removed after 3 to 12 months postoperatively under the guidance of corneal topography. While taking sutures out, care must be taken not to jeopardize wound stability, especially during the early postoperative period. If astigmatism persists after suture removal, rigid contact lenses may be employed. Other options include limbal-relaxing incisions with or without compression sutures and wedge resection. Recently, LASIK has been successfully used to treat mild to moderate degrees of post-PK astigmatism.[5]

LAMELLAR KERATOPLASTY

Lamellar keratoplasty refers to partial-thickness corneal transplantation. It targets transplantation of diseased corneal tissue while leaving the functioning parts of the cornea in place. In order to understand the indications for lamellar keratoplasty, a brief overview of the corneal anatomy is needed. The average adult cornea is approximately 540 µm thick[6] and consists of (anterior to posterior) epithelium, Bowman's layer, stroma, Descemet's membrane, and endothelium. Some diseases only affect the anterior portions of the cornea (epithelium, Bowman's layer, and anterior stroma), leaving the posterior structures intact. Other diseases only affect the posterior structures (endothelium and/or Descemet's membrane).

Two major forms of lamellar keratoplasty have emerged. Anterior lamellar keratoplasty (ALK) refers to transplantation of the epithelium, Bowman's layer, and anterior stroma. Posterior lamellar keratoplasty (PLK) refers to transplantation of the endothelium and Descemet's membrane with or without posterior stroma.

ANTERIOR LAMELLAR KERATOPLASTY

Several advantages to performing ALK rather than PK exist. ALK is considered a nonpenetrating extraocular procedure and is associated with lower rates of expulsive hemorrhage, cataract formation, glaucoma, endophthalmitis, and

Figure 14-5. Avellino dystrophy. (Courtesy of Eric D. Donnenfeld, MD.)

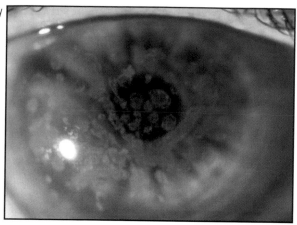

retinal detachment. Because the host endothelium remains intact, the chance for endothelial rejection is greatly reduced, with decreased need for immunosuppression. Finally, ALK heals more rapidly with faster visual recovery than PK.

The main disadvantages of ALK include a longer and technically more challenging procedure, suboptimal visual acuity caused by interface problems, residual scarring, and possible vascularization of the donor–recipient interface. However, the newer techniques of DALK have similar visual acuity outcomes to those of PK[7] with lower long-term IOP and higher number of endothelial cells. DALK may be indicated in patients with superficial disease not involving the corneal endothelium. Such diseases include keratoconus, superficial stromal dystrophies and degenerations (eg, Avellino dystrophy; Figure 14-5), lattice dystrophy, granular dystrophy, Salzmann's nodular degeneration (Figure 14-6), corneal thinning (eg, pellucid marginal degeneration), superficial corneal scars as a result of nonpenetrating trauma or superficial infections, severe ocular surface disease (eg, SJS, OCP, and chemical burns), superficial corneal tumors, and multiple recurrent pterygium (Figure 14-7).

ALK is contraindicated if the corneal edema is secondary to endothelial cell dysfunction, such as in aphakic or pseudophakic bullous keratopathy or Fuchs' dystrophy. Macular dystrophy is a relative contraindication if there is extensive involvement of the corneal stroma and possibly Descemet's membrane.

DALK may be performed under retrobulbar or general anesthesia. The size of the corneal button transplanted should be identified at the slit lamp preoperatively and confirmed with a trephine intraoperatively. It is important to have full-thickness donor corneal tissue available in case of accidental penetration into the anterior chamber, requiring conversion to full-thickness PK.

Initial preparation is similar to that of PK. Multiple techniques have been described to aid in preparing the host corneal bed to minimize postoperative recipient-donor interface and maximize visual potential. These include creating a hinged flap,[8] intrastromal air injection,[9] air injection between Descemet's membrane and the posterior stroma,[10] microkeratome or femtosecond laser-assisted dissection,[11] and injection of air into the anterior chamber to improve visualization,[12] among others. The basic technique, however, is usually the same. Viscoelastic material, air, or saline may be injected into the corneal stroma to aid visualization. The trephine guard is set to the appropriate thickness (usually

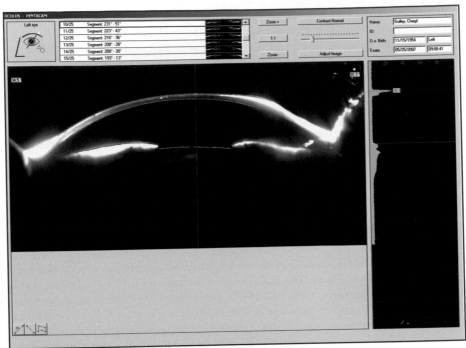

Figure 14-6. Salzmann's nodules. (Courtesy of Tracy S. Swartz, OD, MS.)

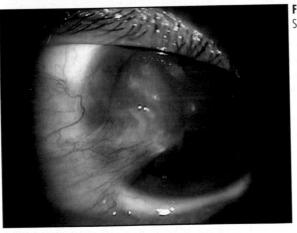

Figure 14-7. Pterygium. (Courtesy of Tracy S. Swartz, OD, MS.)

about 90% corneal depth), often with the aid of ultrasound biomicroscopy and pachymetry. The stroma is then dissected with a rounded-end sharp blade to 0.5 mm peripheral to the trephination to facilitate suture placement.

Donor tissue may be fashioned from a whole donor globe or a corneoscleral button. It is advisable to remove the corneal endothelium by either mechanical debridement or stripping of Descemet's membrane prior to grafting to minimize endothelial rejection and facilitate wound healing. Typically, a limbal cutdown is performed with a rounded-end sharp blade to the desired depth for dissection. This is followed with a lamellar spreader or cyclodialysis spatula in a sweeping motion to create a limbus-to-limbus dissection. A trephine is then used to harvest the donor graft, usually 0.25 mm larger than the recipient button.

The lamellar graft is transferred to the recipient bed and is sutured with interrupted 10-0 nylon sutures. Care must be taken to clear the interface from any debris with irrigation.

If the recipient endothelium remains intact and the anterior chamber is not penetrated, DALK has fewer complications than PK, including glaucoma, endophthalmitis, and endothelial rejection. If the anterior chamber is inadvertently penetrated, the full-thickness wound must be sutured closed. If the wound is large, converting to full-thickness PK is required. Postoperatively, DALK patients may suffer from astigmatism, persistent epithelial defect, infection, and allograft rejection as described for PK. Interface scarring and vascularization might be treated with topical corticosteroids but with modest results.

POSTERIOR LAMELLAR KERATOPLASTY

Posterior lamellar keratoplasty is undergoing major changes as it becomes increasingly popular. One of the most popular techniques for PLK is DSEK. DSEK offers several advantages over PK. DSEK patients enjoy faster visual recovery, improved tectonic support, and less postoperative astigmatism.[13] Because the epithelium and anterior stroma are not violated, minimal suturing is required and the concern for graft dehiscence is markedly reduced. Furthermore, because the host corneal epithelium and stroma remain intact in DSEK, the risk of epithelial or stroma rejection is negated.

DSEK is indicated for patients whose corneal edema is secondary to a diseased endothelium such as aphakic or pseudophakic bullous keratopathy and Fuchs' dystrophy. It has also been used to treat corneal edema associated with endothelial graft failure and in iridocorneal endothelial syndrome.[14,15]

DSEK may be performed under retrobulbar or general anesthesia. Initial preparation is similar to that of PK. Initially, 2 clear corneal limbal incisions are created as access points to the anterior chamber. Acetylcholine chloride intraocular solution (Miochol, Novartis, East Hanover, NJ) is injected to constrict the pupil to protect the lens. After cohesive viscoelastic material inflates the anterior chamber, the desired size and location of the host button is marked on the corneal epithelium. A blunt-tip Sinskey hook (Bausch & Lomb, St. Louis, MO) or a bent 25-gauge needle with a roughened tip is inserted through the paracentesis and lifted anteriorly to score Descemet's membrane 360 degrees in accordance with the epithelial marking. Then, through a clear corneal (or scleral) incision, a Descemet's membrane stripping instrument with a blunt edge is used to strip Descemet's membrane completely off the posterior stroma. Finally viscoelastic material is completely removed from the anterior chamber by irrigation/aspiration.

A whole globe or corneoscleral button with an artificial anterior chamber can be used to harvest the donor button. If using a manual or automated microkeratome, the corneoscleral button is first coated with a thin layer of 1% sodium hyaluronate (Healon, Abbott Medical Optics, Abbott Park, IL) on the endothelial side. It is then transferred and secured endothelial side down to the artificial anterior chamber. An epithelial cap is then removed using the microkeratome. The donor tissue is then transferred and placed endothelial side up and a trephine is used to obtain the endothelial donor button. Finally, a thin strip of 1% sodium hyaluronate is placed on the endothelial surface and the donor graft is folded with the endothelium on the inside.

After the folded donor graft is gently inserted into the anterior chamber with fine nontoothed forceps, balanced salt solution on an irrigating cannula is used to re-form the anterior chamber and manipulate the unfolding of the donor graft to ensure that the correct orientation (ie, endothelial side facing the iris) is maintained. 10-0 Nylon sutures are used to close the corneal incision and the anterior chamber is gently deepened with balanced salt solution, followed by an air bubble to tamponade the donor graft against the posterior stroma. Finally, the pupil is dilated (to lessen risk of papillary block glaucoma) and the patient is instructed to lie flat for approximately 1 hour. After this time period, slit-lamp examination is performed to ensure proper placement of the donor graft and to check IOP.

Graft dislocation is the most frequently reported complication after DSEK.[16] This is usually addressed by repeating the air-injection protocol into the anterior chamber. Graft rejection occurs in about 7.5% of all cases of DSEK.[17] This can be treated with frequent topical corticosteroids. Pupillary block glaucoma is also a concern and may be treated by releasing some air from the anterior chamber after the procedure.

SUPERFICIAL CORNEAL SURGERY

Corneal Biopsy

Corneal biopsy is indicated if there is a need for histophathologic or microbiologic evaluation of corneal tissue in diseases such as unresponsive and culture-negative corneal ulcers or suspicious corneal lesions. It can be performed at the slit lamp or the operating microscope under topical anesthesia. If the lesion is superficial, it may be scraped or peeled. If it is deeper, a handheld trephine can be used to create a partial-thickness trephination that can be removed with a 0.12 forceps and sharp blade. Care must be taken not to penetrate the anterior chamber, especially in cases of corneal thinning. Typically, trephination of the abnormal tissue with a margin of normal tissue is obtained and divided for histological and microbiological analysis. Topical broad-spectrum antibiotics and ointments should be continued until the causative agent is identified.

Anterior Stromal Puncture

The nonsurgical treatment of recurrent corneal erosion (RCE) consists of aggressive lubrication and use of hypertonic agents to promote better adhesion of the epithelium to the basement membrane. When these measures fail, surgical therapy consisting of anterior stromal puncture (ASP) may be helpful.

The primary abnormality in recurrent erosion is an inadequate adhesion between the epithelial cell (via its hemidesmosomes) to the underlying basement membrane. ASP attempts to create "micro-scars" so that in those particular areas, the epithelial attachment will be greater (Figure 14-8). The procedure is performed using topical anesthesia at the slit lamp. It is helpful to know the extent of the erosion so that the application of ASP can be delivered in the correct area. Fluorescein dye may be used to highlight the area of abnormal epithelium. A bent 25-gauge needle may be used to create small punctures through the epithelium

Figure 14-8. ASP is performed at the slit lamp. The appearance is typical for early in the postoperative course. (Courtesy of Roy Rubinfeld, MD.)

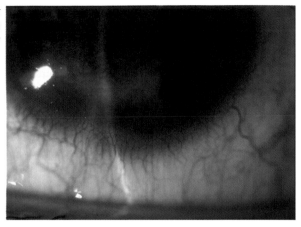

and into the anterior stroma. Alternatively, Roy Rubinfeld, MD, has created a specialized needle for ASP. It is designed with a fixed depth so that the needle cannot penetrate too far into the stroma. There have also been reports of using the Nd: YAG laser to create the stromal scars in ASP.

The application of ASP is carried out in a grid pattern for the entire extent of the involved area. ASP is not recommended for erosions that extend into the central visual axis because the small scars may create a potential for reduced visual acuity.

Care must be taken to distinguish between RCE secondary to traumatic corneal abrasion versus RCE due to corneal dystrophies (such as EBMD [map-dot-fingerprint] or any of the stromal dystrophies [lattice and granular]). In the former, there is usually a localized area of poor epithelial attachment, and this would benefit from ASP. In cases of dystrophy, however, the preferred treatment consists of epithelial debridement, because the area of involvement is more widespread. In addition, EBMD will often require treatment within the central visual axis, and ASP should be avoided in this area.

Superficial Keratectomy

Superficial keratectomy involves surgical or laser-assisted excision of abnormal, especially elevated, corneal tissue to clear and/or smooth the cornea. It is indicated in the treatment of anterior corneal dystrophies, excision of retained foreign body, superficial corneal scar, and removal of hyperplastic tissue. Mechanical superficial keratectomy is done under local anesthesia using a 0.12 forceps, a trephine, or a sharp blade in a lamellar fashion. Care must be taken to ensure an even and smooth dissection plane to aid in epithelial regrowth and prevention of interface scar formation. Superficial keratectomy can also be carried out using the excimer laser with greater precision, especially with concomitant use of viscous liquid as a "masking agent" to smoothen the surface by covering the "valleys" and leaving the "mountain tops" uncovered to be removed by the excimer laser. Use of preoperative oral vitamin C and intraoperative mitomycin C with PRK has been shown to reduce postoperative haze. After the procedure, topical antibiotic and corticosteroid drops along with a bandage contact lens are used until re-epithelialization is completed. Infrequently, corneal haze or scarring, infection, or persistent epithelial defect may ensue. These could be addressed

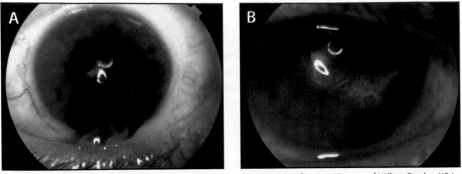

Figure 14-9. (A) Positive Seidel test. (B) Glue utilized to correct the corneal perforation. (Courtesy of William Trattler, MD.)

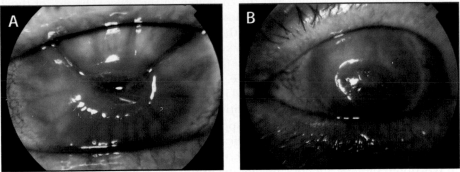

Figure 14-10. (A) Central corneal perforation. (B) Healed perforation corrected with glue. (Courtesy of William Trattler, MD.)

with further photorefractive surgery, aggressive topical antibiotics, or other surgical procedures, respectively.

Corneal Glue

Tissue adhesives, both biologic and synthetic, have been increasing in popularity for use in many anterior segment surgeries including corneal perforations, amniotic membrane graft, pterygium surgery, wound repair, and as sealants in glaucoma and plastics procedures.

Cyanoacrylate-based tissue adhesives are usually used in the management of small (<1.5 mm) corneal ulcerations or perforations due to trauma, infection, or inflammatory thinning alongside systemic or topical antibiotics (Figures 14-9 and 14-10). It is probably contraindicated in cases with iris or vitreous prolapse and is ineffective in large perforations (>2 mm). After topical anesthesia, an eyelid speculum is used to help keep the eye open and any necrotic tissue and overlying or adjacent corneal epithelium should be removed. The epithelium should be denuded up to 2 mm surrounding the involved tissue. The area is then gently dried and cyanoacrylate glue is applied using a 30-gauge needle or on a sterile plastic disc from a sterile plastic drape. The glue polymerizes within 20 to 60 seconds. A bandage contact lens with topical antibiotics is then applied. The patient should be monitored closely and frequently until the epithelium regrows and dislodges the glue.

Cyanoacrylate glue has advantages compared to sutures, including ease of application and reduced time required to perform. In cases of tissue edema or friability, it can provide additional support until healing occurs. Potential suture complications such as infection or neovascularization are virtually eliminated.

Human fibrin-based glue (such as Tisseel, Baxter Corporation, Mississauga, Ontario) has been increasing in popularity as suture substitutes for adhering biologic tissues in certain surgical procedures, especially those involving the conjunctiva or amniotic membrane graft. Fibrin glue consists of 2 main components: fibrinogen/aprotinin and thrombin. When applied together, they lead to a cascade of events during which fibrinogen is converted into fibrin monomers with subsequent cross-linking to form a fibrin adhesive clot. The glue is biocompatible, permeable, easy to apply, and spontaneously dissolves over a 2-week time period.

The fibrin-based glue is usually supplied in an applicator system containing the fibrinogen in one syringe and the thrombin in the other. The tips of the 2 syringes form a common port, which allows delivery of equal volume of each solution upon application. There are 2 methods to apply the fibrin-based glue. The glue can be applied using the applicator system with spontaneous delivery of both components to the area of interest. The fibrin clot starts forming within seconds and holds the biological tissues in place. The main drawback to the dual-chambered syringe technique is the quick and irreversible clotting that occurs once the components are combined, thereby limiting time to position the graft.

In our practice, we have found that applying each component separately leads to a more controlled and elegant application of the glue to a relatively precise location where it is meant to be applied. We have used the technique successfully in pterygium surgery, amniotic membrane graft, as well as lamellar keratoplasty. In pterygium surgery, after removal of the pterygium and successful harvesting of the conjunctival graft, the fibrinogen is applied to the dry scleral bed. The thrombin is applied separately to the underside of the conjunctival graft. Then, the graft is carefully placed into the desired position and held in place for 30 seconds, allowing the mixture of glue components. Diffuse pressure is then applied with WECK-CEL sponges to squeeze out any excess solution. Five to 8 minutes of drying time is allowed for a complete coagulum to form, and excess clot is then excised. A bandage contact lens with topical antibiotics is then applied. If an amniotic membrane graft is used, the technique is slightly modified. First, the fibrinogen is placed on the dried scleral bed and the dehydrated amniotic membrane graft is placed and positioned on the scleral bed and allowed to be rehydrated and activated by the fibrinogen solution. Finally, the thrombin is placed over, and diffuses through, the amniotic membrane graft to combine with the fibrinogen to form the fibrin clot. A bandage contact lens with topical antibiotics is then applied.

Compared to sutures, fibrin-based tissue adhesives are easier and faster to use, leading to improved operating room efficiency. It also leads to better homeostasis because of the clotting components of the adhesive. Fibrin glue also lessens the chances of potential suture complications such as infection and neovascularization. Because it spontaneously dislodges or degrades, there is no need for suture removal. Possible disadvantages include the higher cost of the fibrin glue compared to the sutures. Although it has never been reported, possible transmission of viruses or prions is a theoretical risk of human-derived fibrin-based glue.

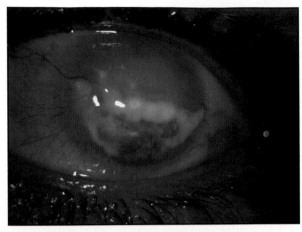

Figure 14-11. Band keratopathy. (Courtesy of Tracy S. Swartz, OD, MS.)

Currently, there are many novel adhesives that are being tested, including modified chondroitin sulfate aldehyde adhesive, acrylic copolymer tissue adhesive, biodendrimers, and dendrtic macromers, among others. The discussion of these is beyond the scope of this chapter.

Band Keratopathy Removal

Band keratopathy is largely composed of calcium secondary to chronic inflammation or hypercalcemia (Figure 14-11). The first step in therapy is identification of the underlying pathology. A neutral chelating agent, 1.5% to 3% disodium EDTA is prepared. After topical anesthesia, the overlying epithelium is scraped to expose the calcium-containing bed. Then a sponge soaked with EDTA is applied to the area repetitively to remove the calcium deposits. Alternatively, a well placed over the cornea is filled with EDTA and left in place for few minutes to chelate the calcium deposits. Finally, a bandage contact lens or ophthalmic ointment is used until complete re-epithelialization occurs.

Limbal Stem Cell Transplant

Limbal stem cells (LSCs) are crucial to the regeneration of corneal epithelial cells and prevention of corneal conjunctivalization. Limbal stem cell transplant (LSCT) procedures may be indicated in cases of chemical or thermal injury, multiple ocular surgeries, SJS, OCP, repeated infections, or prolonged and chronic contact lens wear. In cases of unilateral involvement, the fellow eye can serve as the donor. In cases of bilateral disease, a living relative or a cadaver might serve as the donor. In the latter case, immune-mediated rejection of the LSCT limits the success rate of this procedure. The amount of LSC transplanted is to be determined on individual cases.

LSCT is usually done under retrobulbar anesthesia. A 360 degree peritomy of 2-mm-wide limbal conjunctiva is carried out in the host tissue with removal of the abnormal corneal epithelium, conjunctiva, and pannus tissue, if present. The donor tissue is then harvested including 0.5 mm of superficial clear cornea to 4 mm onto the bulbar conjunctiva. The donor tissue is then transplanted and sutured into the host bed using 10-0 nylon sutures for the corneal wound and 8-0 vicryl sutures for the conjunctival wound. A new procedure where LSCs

Figure 14-12. Amniotic membrane grafting with pterygium removal. (Courtesy of Tracy S. Swartz, OD, MS.)

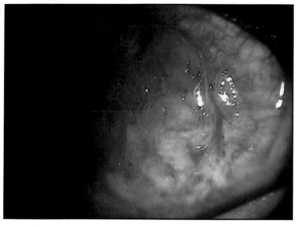

are harvested and expanded on an amniotic membrane graft (AMG) in organ culture medium have also been transplanted with promising results.[18] A bandage contact lens is placed at the end of the procedure. Because LSCs are very immunogenic, aggressive and prolonged systemic immunosuppression therapy is usually needed. Despite adequate immunosuppression, the incidence rate of LSC allograft rejection is 14% to 75%. Early features of rejection include tortuous and engorged limbal blood vessels and a sudden epithelial defect with conjunctival inflammation.[19] If either is observed, aggressive topical and, possibly, systemic immunosuppression should be started. Finally, LSCT may be complicated by poor re-epithelialization of the recipient cornea and infectious or noninfectious keratitis. Bandage contact lens, ophthalmic ointment, and topical antibiotics might help in these situations.

Amniotic Membrane Graft

Amniotic membranes are harvested from placentas after delivery. The amniotic membrane consists of a single layer of epithelium with underlying stroma made of extracellular matrix and collagens. It has been shown to help promote corneal epithelialization and inhibit inflammation, neovascularization and fibrosis. AMG is being used for a widening variety of ocular surface reconstruction procedures. It is now used in conjunction with LSCT (discussed previously), persistent epithelial defects, sterile corneal ulcerations, conjunctival defects, pterygia excision (Figure 14-12), descemetocele formation, and corneal and scleral perforation, among others. It should be noted that the AMG does not have stem cells of its own and thus might not be used as a sole therapy for patients who lack LSCs.

The preparation of the AMG is described elsewhere.[24] Surgically, AMG can be applied in 3 ways.[20] It can be used in the "overlay technique" and sutured with 10-0 nylon sutures as a biological contact lens covering the cornea, limbus, and perilimbal area. For this technique, the orientation of the AMG should be epithelial-basement membrane side facing down. However, for the "inlay technique," the AMG is sized to fit just slightly larger than the size of the defect and must be sutured with the epithelial-basement side facing up. In this technique, the AMG acts like a basement membrane over which new corneal epithelium can grow. Finally, multiple layers of AMG can be used to fill a deep stromal ulceration with the outermost layer oriented basement membrane side up to help re-epithelializa-

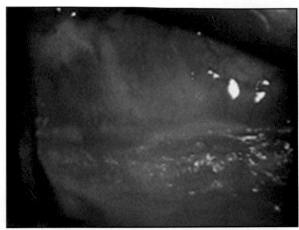

Figure 14-13. Conjunctival flap. (Courtesy of Ming Wang, MD, PhD.)

tion. Aggressive lubrication is employed in the postoperative period. AMG may be complicated by pain, irritation, and AMG dehiscence.

Conjunctival Flap

Once popular, conjunctival flaps are used less frequently today. They still play an important role in the treatment of chronic sterile corneal ulcerations, painful bullous keratopathy in eyes with low vision potential, and indolent corneal infections secondary to fungal or herpetic organisms. Conjunctival flap is contraindicated in active infectious ulcers and corneal perforations. The goal of the surgery is to stabilize the corneal surface and to decrease pain. The procedure is typically performed under local anesthesia (Figure 14-13).

Initially, the entire corneal epithelium is debrided. The superior conjunctiva is preferable to use, but the inferior conjunctiva may be used if there is superior conjunctival scarring or pathology. Local anesthetic is injected into the subconjunctival space to separate the conjunctiva from Tenon's fascia. Then, a small conjunctival incision is made 12 to 14 mm away from the limbus and, subsequently, carried to the limbus and into the temporal and nasal quadrants. Extreme care should be taken not to create buttonholes in the conjunctiva. Once the flap is completely undermined, a 360 degree peritomy is carried out at the limbus to leave a free conjunctival flap with bridges nasally and temporally. In case of the superior conjunctival flap, the inferior edge of the flap is sutured to the inferior corneal limbus and inferior ridge of the conjunctiva. The superior edge of the flap is sutured to the superior episclera. If a buttonhole was created in the process, it should be sutured tight with 11-0 nylon suture. Postoperatively, antibiotic and corticosteroid ointment are applied. Conjunctival flaps might be complicated by retraction of the conjunctival flap, infection (either primary or recurrent in the case of herpes), and a poorly healing buttonhole that can lead to infection, corneal melting, or chronic epithelial defects. It should be noted that conjunctival flaps do not provide an optically clear surface and are usually used in patients with low vision potential or a stabilizing bridge to PK in the future.

Keratoprosthesis

In the rare patient with severe bilateral corneal disease not amenable to PK and ocular surface reconstruction, or in whom such procedures carry a poor

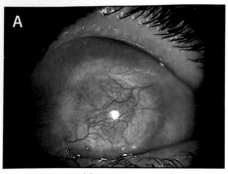
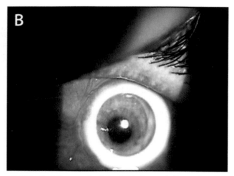

Figure 14-14. (A) Alphacor (Coopervision, Pleasanton, CA) stage I. Note that the prosthesis is visible beneath the conjunctival tissue. (B) Alphacor (Coopervision, Pleasanton, CA) after stage II. (Courtesy of Ming Wang, MD, PhD.)

prognosis, a keratoprosthesis (KPro) surgery may be indicated (Figure 14-14). Such cases include SJS, OCP, LSC deficiency, repeated PK graft failure, and severe keratoconjunctivitis sicca, among others.[26] It is important to note that KPro is a last-effort measure in eyes with complicated corneal blindness but an otherwise functioning posterior segment. This "telescopic lens" provides very good central vision but a severely constricted visual field. Many different KPros and multiple techniques have been described.[21] It is important that any inflammation or active process is brought under control to ensure success of the surgery. KPro surgery is a time-consuming and skill-demanding procedure that is done in few specialized centers around the world.

The procedure involves securing the KPro with autologous tissue, such as periosteum, which must be harvested from the patient prior to the surgery. The entire bulbar and palpebral conjunctiva is excised and the medial and lateral recti are disinserted. Total iridectomy, removal of the crystalline or pseudophakic lens, and core vitrectomy are performed. A small trephine is used to excise a corneal button. The KPro with its supporting plate are inserted and secured either to the cornea or the sclera. Depending on the model and technique, complete tarsorrhaphy might be performed at the end of the procedure. Topical and systemic antibiotics and corticosteroids are given in the postoperative period. The most common postoperative complication is extrusion of the KPro. Other complications include sterile or infectious endophthalmitis, glaucoma, or retroprosthetic membrane formation.

PTERYGIUM EXCISION

Pterygium excision is indicated if there is extension to the visual axis, reduced vision secondary to astigmatism, reduced motility secondary to involvement of the medial rectus, severe irritation not remedied by medical therapy, difficulty with contact lens wear, and cosmesis. The goals for pterygium excision are complete excision of the pterygium, topographically normal and smooth ocular surface, and prevention of recurrence. Patients must be counseled about the recurrent nature of the pterygium and the need for strict compliance with the postoperative medication regimen.

A multitude of techniques have been described, including bare sclera technique, conjunctival autograft with or without mitomycin C, and amniotic membrane

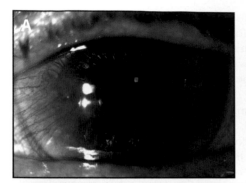

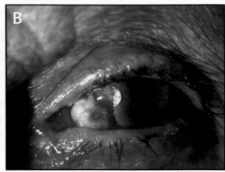

Figure 14-15. (A) Pterygium preoperatively. (B) Pterygium removal using AMT graft and fibrin glue. (C) Three months after removal of pterygium. (Courtesy of Ming Wang, MD, PhD.)

transplantation[22,23] (Figure 14-15). In this section, we will describe pterygium excision with conjunctival autograft and intraoperative mitomycin C.

After local anesthesia, the extent of the pterygium is marked with superficial cautery or a marking pen. A traction 6-0 vicryl suture is placed at the superior limbus. Subconjunctival anesthetic may be used to infiltrate the pterygium and dissect it off the underlying sclera. The conjunctival portion of the pterygium is excised with Westcott scissors down to the bare sclera. Especially in cases of recurrent pterygium, care must be taken not to cut the rectus muscle because it might be adherent to the fibrotic tissue. Then, a sharp rounded-end blade is placed flat against the cornea, just central to the head of the pterygium, and is pushed using a forward-backward motion to peel the pterygium off the cornea to the limbus to join the conjunctival excised portion. It is important to leave the corneal surface as smooth as possible to reduce risk of recurrence. The sharp blade or a diamond burr might be useful for this purpose.

Following the pterygium excision, surgical sponges soaked with mitomycin C (0.02%) are applied directly to the bare sclera for 3 minutes followed by copious irrigation. Then, the conjunctival defect is measured with calipers and the eye is rotated downwards to expose the superotemporal bulbar conjunctiva. Light cautery or a marking pen is used to mark the 4 corners of the conjunctival donor graft. Then, subconjunctival anesthetic material is administered to separate the conjunctiva from Tenon's fascia. The conjunctiva may be removed using Westcott scissors as described previously. Care must be exercised not to create buttonholes and, if they do occur, to tightly close them. The graft is then moved to the host space and sutured to the host conjunctiva, epithelial side up, using absorbable (eg, 8-0 or 9-0 vicryl) or nonabsorbable (eg, 10-0 nylon). It is unclear whether conjunctivolimbal grafts yield better results than conjunctival grafts alone. The superior donor conjunctiva may be left to heal spontaneously. Topical antibiotics and corticosteroids, often in ointment form, are used 3 or 4 times daily in the postoperative period. The antibiotics may be discontinued once the conjunctival defect is healed; however, corticosteroids should be continued to reduce the risk of scarring and recurrence. IOP must be monitored while the patient is on the corticosteroids.

Pterygium recurrence is the most common complication and is usually more aggressive than the previous pterygium. It should be treated with topical corticosteroids or surgical excision. Other complications include infection, delayed healing of the epithelial defect, and delle formation. Less frequently, pyogenic granuloma may develop, especially with large epithelial defects. Rare but serious and potentially sight-threatening complications such as perforation, endophthalmitis, infectious scleritis, and scleral necrosis may develop years after application of mitomycin C during surgery.[24]

CONCLUSION

Anterior segment surgery includes a wide variety of procedures that require detailed preoperative evaluation and exam, meticulous attention to detail perioperatively, excellent surgical skill, and careful postoperative follow-up to ensure the best outcomes and to reduce risk of complications. Although not every ophthalmologist is expected to be facile with these procedures, all ophthalmologists should be aware of the procedures and their potential complications to best serve these patients.

REFERENCES

1. Eye Bank Association of America. How prevalent is corneal transplantation? Available at: http://www.restoresight.org/general/faqs.htm#5. Accessed January 17, 2008.
2. Kang PC, Klintworth GK, Kim T, et al. Trends in the indications for penetrating keratoplasty, 1980-2001. *Cornea*. 2005;24:801-803.
3. Ghosheh FR, Cremona FA, Rapuano CJ, et al. Trends in penetrating keratoplasty in the United States 1980-2005. *Int Ophthalmol*. 2008;28:147-153.
4. Alldredge OC, Krachmer JH. Clinical types of corneal transplant rejection. Their manifestations, frequency, preoperative correlates, and treatment. *Arch Ophthalmol*. 1981;99:599-604.
5. Pereira T, Forseto AS, Alberti GN, Nose W. Flap-induced refraction change in LASIK after penetrating keratoplasty. *J Refract Surg*. 2007;23:279-283.
6. Edelhauser HF. The balance between corneal transparency and edema: the Proctor Lecture. *Invest Ophthalmol Vis Sci*. 2006;47:1755-1767.
7. Shimazaki J, Shimmura S, Ishioka M, Tsubota K. Randomized clinical trial of deep lamellar keratoplasty vs penetrating keratoplasty. *Am J Ophthalmol*. 2002;134(2):159-165.
8. Azar DT, Jain S, Sambursky R. A new surgical technique of microkeratome-assisted deep lamellar keratoplasty with a hinged flap. *Arch Ophthalmol*. 2000;118:1112-1118.
9. Archila EA. Deep lamellar keratoplasty dissection of host tissue with intrastromal air injection. *Cornea*. 1984;3:217-218.
10. Anwar M, Teichmann KD. Big-bubble technique to bare Descemet's membrane in anterior lamellar keratoplasty. *J Cataract Refract Surg*. 2002;28:398-403.
11. Suwan-Apichon O, Reyes JM, Griffin NB, et al. Microkeratome versus femtosecond laser predissection of corneal grafts for anterior and posterior lamellar keratoplasty. *Cornea*. 2006;25:966-968.

12. Melles GR, Lander F, Rietveld FJ, et al. A new surgical technique for deep stromal, anterior lamellar keratoplasty. *Br J Ophthalmol.* 1999;83:327-333.

13. Terry MA, Ousley PJ. Deep lamellar endothelial keratoplasty visual acuity, astigmatism, and endothelial survival in a large prospective series. *Ophthalmology.* 2005;112:1541-1548.

14. Price MO, Price FW Jr. Descemet stripping with endothelial keratoplasty for treatment of iridocorneal endothelial syndrome. *Cornea.* 2007;26:493-497.

15. Price FW Jr, Price MO. Endothelial keratoplasty to restore clarity to a failed penetrating graft. *Cornea.* 2006;25:895-899.

16. Price FW Jr, Price MO. Descemet's stripping with endothelial keratoplasty in 200 eyes: early challenges and techniques to enhance donor adherence. *J Cataract Refract Surg.* 2006; 32:411-418.

17. Allan BD, Terry MA, Price FW Jr, et al. Corneal transplant rejection rate and severity after endothelial keratoplasty. *Cornea.* 2007;26:1039-1042.

18. Tsai RJ, Tseng SC. Human allograft limbal transplantation for corneal surface reconstruction. *Cornea.* 1994;13:389-400.

19. Lee SH, Tseng SC. Amniotic membrane transplantation for persistent epithelial defects with ulceration. *Am J Ophthalmol.* 1997;123:303-312.

20. Sippel KC, Ma JJ, Foster CS. Amniotic membrane surgery. *Curr Opin Ophthalmol.* 2001; 12(4):269-281.

21. Khan B, Dudenhoefer EJ, Dohlman CH. Keratoprosthesis: an update. *Curr Opin Ophthalmol.* 2001;12(4):282-287.

22. Ang LP, Chua JL, Tan DT. Current concepts and techniques in pterygium treatment. *Curr Opin Ophthalmol.* 2007;18(4):308-313.

23. Hirst LW. The treatment of pterygium. *Surv Ophthalmol.* 2003;48(2):145-180.

24. Rubinfeld RS, Pfister RR, Stein RM, et al. Serious complications of topical mitomycin-C after pterygium surgery. *Ophthalmology.* 1992;99:1647-1654.

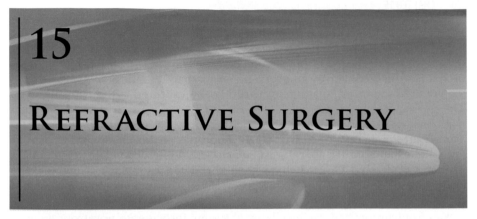

15

REFRACTIVE SURGERY

Jerome Charles Ramos-Esteban, MD; Sonya Bamba, MD;
and Ronald R. Krueger, MD

The surgical correction of refractive errors can be performed by modifying the curvature of the cornea or by altering the internal optics of the eye. Corneal curvature modification can be achieved with corneal incisions or excimer laser tissue ablation. Advances in refractive optics led to the introduction of patient-specific wavefront guided treatments and improved visual outcomes. In presbyopic patients, addressing the correction of refractive errors must also take into account the natural hardening of the crystalline lens and associated loss of accommodation. Developments in IOLs have introduced multifocal and accommodative lenses that correct presbyopia in addition to other refractive errors.

The scope of this chapter is to provide a comprehensive review of excimer laser, IOLs, and other surgical procedures for the correction of refractive errors. Each procedure is described in terms of surgical technique and patient selection, with special emphasis on identification and management of complications associated with each method.

EXCIMER LASER PROCEDURES

The excimer laser operates in the range of UV light at a wavelength of 193 nm. Excimer laser ablation of the cornea for the correction of myopia was first performed in the United States in 1988. The United States FDA granted approval for the use of this medical device for the correction of myopia in 1995 and astigmatism in 1997.[1] Commercially available excimer laser platforms have individual approvals for the correction of different levels of myopia, hyperopia, and astigmatism.

Wavefront Technology

Aberrations inherent to an optical system have been traditionally described using ray tracing methods that assume that the cornea is a spherical structure. These techniques are extremely time-consuming and difficult to apply clinically. Spectacle or contact lens correction of refractive errors is limited to first-order optical aberrations, known as *defocus* and *astigmatism*.

Trattler WB, Majmudar PA, Luchs JI, Swartz TS, eds.
Cornea Handbook (pp. 269-294)
© 2010 SLACK Incorporated

Technological advances in astrophysics, in particular efforts to improve the image resolution and quality from telescopes, led to the advent of wavefront sensing devices. The first applications of wavefront sensing in ophthalmology used a Hartmann-Shack-based aberrometer to analyze optical aberrations from a point light source originating in the retina and captured at the cornea plane.[2] The pattern of light rays coming out of the eye creates a wavefront, which is then mathematically expressed in terms of either Zernicke or Fourier polynomials. The wavefront characterizes the optical properties of the whole eye in terms of lower- and higher-order aberrations, which are highly dependent on pupillary diameter, and some of which have been correlated to clinical symptoms. For example, spherical aberration has been correlated with night vision problems and coma with reading difficulties.[3]

Wavefront-customized excimer laser ablations incorporate wavefront analysis into the ablation profile to correct inherent higher order aberrations of the patient's eye and those induced by refractive surgery procedures.[4] Technological requirements for wavefront guided excimer laser treatments include: (1) scanning spot laser delivery, (2) robust eye tracking, (3) an accurate wavefront sensing device, and (4) wavefront–laser interface.[5]

Laser In Situ Keratomileusis

The creation of a corneal flap followed by excimer laser tissue ablation of the exposed stromal bed is common to LASIK, laser-assisted subepithelial keratomileusis (LASEK), and epithelial LASIK (epi-LASIK) procedures. The techniques differ in the thickness of the flap and the methods used to separate the flap from the stroma. The selection of the procedure is based on the experience of the surgeon and patient-related factors such as corneal thickness, desired depth of ablation, and postoperative comfort. In theory, more superficial ablations may have less impact on corneal biomechanics[6] and wound healing, and therefore, LASEK and epi-LASIK have gained popularity in recent years. Thinner LASIK flaps created by femtosecond lasers, termed *sub-Bowman's keratomileusis* (or SBK) is now becoming more popular.

LASIK is the most common surgical procedure for the correction of refractive errors in the United States.[7] LASIK consists of the creation of a partial-thickness hinged corneal flap and subsequent excimer laser ablation of the exposed stromal bed. LASIK flaps can be created with either mechanical microkeratomes or with the femtosecond laser.[8] The position of the LASIK hinge, which can be either superior or nasal, determines the nomenclature of the flap. Advantages of the femtosecond laser over microkeratomes include more uniform and planar LASIK flaps,[9] better astigmatic neutrality,[10] and a reduction in intraoperative complications such as buttonholes, free flaps, and epithelial defects, among others.[8,10]

The steps for the creation of a femtosecond laser flap include preoperative planning and execution. Preoperative planning should take advantage of the femtosecond laser's ability to create uniplanar flaps of controlled thicknesses.[8] In our center we routinely perform 90-μm flaps with the femtosecond laser in patients with thin corneas who would be otherwise ineligible for LASIK surgery, simulating a sub-Bowman's excimer laser treatment.

Under aseptic conditions, execution of the flap consists of centration of the suction ring over the patient's visual axis and corneal applanation with a plastic cone, which is used to focus the laser energy. The surgeon should be careful to eliminate the tear meniscus that forms along the walls of the suction ring because it can interfere with the suction ring and can also lead to increased opaque bubble layer (OBL) formation. The femtosecond laser utilizes a photodisruptive process, delivering pulses of energy (10^{-15} second duration) that result in a buildup of water, CO_2, and other gas bubbles (the OBL) on the flap interface. Flap creation takes 30 seconds, during which time the patient should experience dimming of vision caused by the suction ring increasing IOP, decreasing perfusion of the retinal vasculature. A 30-minute waiting period is incorporated into the procedure to allow for the OBL to dissipate in order to avoid interference with the tracker system[11] and to provide a smoother stromal surface during the ablation step. This step is not universally followed by all LASIK surgeons. The cleavage plane produced between the flap and the underlying stroma also allows for a smooth stromal optical surface and ensures a uniform flap thickness.[9]

Once the LASIK flap is created, the remaining tissue adhesions at the flap interface are separated with the use of surgical instruments. Preoperative and intraoperative ultrasound pachymetries should be documented in the chart in order to monitor the effects of dehydration and laser ablation of the corneal stroma. This is particularly important in patients with thin corneas to prevent the development of corneal ectasia due to excessive tissue ablation[12] and may also be considered when developing surgical nomograms. Monitoring of tracker functioning, patient fixation, and saccadic eye movements as well as head movements during the tissue ablation is essential. All surgeries should be performed under the same conditions of temperature and humidity and should follow the same sequence of steps in order to increase the reproducibility of results. As mentioned in the previous section, wavefront analysis can be incorporated in the surgical plan in order to reduce and correct higher order aberrations.

Laser-Assisted Subepithelial Keratomileusis

The steps for the LASEK procedure only differ from that of LASIK in the process of flap creation. In this technique, a corneal epithelial flap of 70 μm is created with a mechanical microkeratome following application of 20% ETOH solution for 30 seconds to allow for epithelial separation from the corneal stromal. The flap is then removed, the area is irrigated with balanced salt solution, and the excimer laser ablation is performed following the same steps described for LASIK. The corneal flap is then repositioned over the ablated stromal bed in order to improve patient comfort after surgery.[13]

Epithelial-LASIK

Epi-LASIK consists of a combination between LASIK and LASEK. A corneal flap is created with an epikeratome that detaches the epithelium from Bowman's membrane, followed by blunt dissection of the flap from the corneal stroma with the use of surgical instruments and excimer laser ablation of the stromal bed.[14]

Figure 15-1. Epithelial defect created by PRK. (Courtesy of Tracy S. Swartz, OD, MS.)

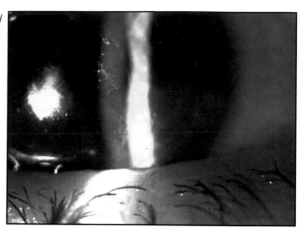

SURFACE ABLATION TECHNIQUES

Photorefractive Keratectomy

PRK was the first excimer laser tissue ablation surgery used for the correction of low levels of myopia. The indications for surgery have since expanded to include the correction of hyperopia and astigmatism. PRK is considered a surface ablation procedure and may lead to increased biomechanical stability after surgery.[15]

After topical anesthetic application, the corneal epithelium is mechanically removed with a beaver blade with or without previous application of 20% ETOH solution for 30 seconds (Figure 15-1). Once the epithelium is scraped, the exposed stromal collagen is ablated with the excimer laser. Ablations greater than –6.00 D may lead to the development of corneal haze, which is usually seen to occur between 1 and 3 months after surgery and may take more than 1 year to clear.[15] Corneal haze development after PRK not only is visually significant for patients but has been associated with refractive regression.[16] The mechanisms for haze development after PRK will be discussed in a later section under complications.

MMC 0.02% has been advocated as a prophylactic treatment for the prevention of corneal haze after high myopic corrections.[17,18] MMC 0.02% is applied over the ablated stroma for 30 seconds to 2 minutes followed by copious irrigation of the surgical field with balanced salt solution. Due to the surface treatment properties of PRK, it can be used in patients with thin corneas who may not be candidates for LASIK. Unlike LASIK, LASEK, and epi-LASIK, PRK does not make use of a flap and therefore may lead to more postoperative patient discomfort due to the presence of an exposed and irritated corneal stroma. Surface irregularities induced by the wound healing process during the early postoperative period may also lead to a slower visual recovery compared to LASIK surgery.

Bandage contact lenses are used for patient comfort after surgery and in some cases may lead to faster re-epithelialization times. Use of topical nonsteriodal medications may lead to delayed healing and increased haze formation after PRK. Customized laser ablations can also be used for the correction of refractive errors with this technique.

Phototherapeutic Keratectomy

PTK is an excimer laser procedure used to correct surface micro-irregularities induced by disorders of the anterior cornea, such as anterior basement membrane dystrophy, opacities occurring from previous trauma, surgery or infection, and surface irregularities induced by previous excimer laser treatments.[19]

PTK is not available in all the excimer laser platforms and can only be performed with lasers with a flat beam profile. The flat beam profile of the excimer laser allows the surgeon to ablate the peaks of the corneal irregularities while sparing the valleys. This procedure is most effective in pathology of the anterior 20% of the cornea.[19]

When performing PTK, the surgeon first estimates the depth of the diseased tissue. The epithelium is then removed, and the tissue is ablated, according to the estimated depth. Following the initial ablation, the amount of remaining diseased tissue is determined by slit-lamp examination, and another treatment is performed, if needed, until the corneal surface is free of lesions.

Transepithelial PTK can be performed prior to a PRK treatment in order to only expose the elevated areas of the irregularity while creating a smoother optical surface.[20] This technique can be further augmented by applying a methylcellulose[21] or a viscoelastic agent (Healon, Alcon Laboratories, Fort Worth, TX) to the surface of the cornea to decrease surface irregularities.[22] Ablative zones can be either central or peripheral and are centered on the area of diseased tissue. In the case of central PTK ablations, the central cornea becomes flatter and the peripheral nonablated corneal stroma becomes thicker, resulting in a hyperopic shift.[23] In such cases, an antihyperopia treatment can be performed, which involves ablating a peripheral area of the cornea that straddles the main ablation zone in order to maintain the preoperative corneal curvature.[24] Despite treatment with PTK, the irregularities of the cornea often recur, such that additional PTK, DALK or PK may be required.

PHAKIC INTRAOCULAR LENS

In patients with very high refractive error, ablative procedures such as LASIK and PRK carry a significant risk of postoperative ectasia due to the extensive amount of corneal tissue that must be removed.[25] In addition, higher corrections have also been correlated with the development of dry eye,[26] higher rates of enhancement,[27] and corneal haze in the case of PRK.[18,21] Placement of a phakic IOL may represent a safe and efficient alternative for patients who cannot undergo keratorefractive procedures for the correction of refractive errors spanning from −8 D of myopia to +5 D of hyperopia.[28]

Patients seeking visual rehabilitation with phakic IOLs should be carefully selected; prepresbyopic patients may enjoy additional benefits due to their ability to accommodate. The major acceptable patient criteria for the implantation of phakic IOLs include (1) age between 21 and 51 years; (2) stable manifest refractive error <0.50 D over 6 months; (3) anterior chamber depth (distance from lens to corneal endothelium) >2.8 mm; (4) open iridocorneal angle >30 degrees as determined by gonioscopy; (5) corneal endothelial cell density more than 2000 mm at 40 years; (6) no previous ocular surgery; (7) ametropia not correctable by other means (spectacles, contact lens intolerance, refractive procedures[28]). Exclusion criteria include (1) age less than 21 years; (2) history or signs of active uveitis; (3)

pigment dispersion syndrome; (4) pregnancy and lactation; (5) unstable corneal ecstatic disorders; (6) other ocular pathologies precluding surgery such as uncontrolled diabetic retinopathy, glaucoma, or ocular hypertension.

Phakic IOLs can be divided into 2 major categories based upon the location of implantation in the eye. Anterior chamber phakic lenses can be either iris-fixated or angle-fixated, whereas posterior chamber lenses are placed in front of the crystalline lens in the sulcus space.[28]

Iris-Claw Lenses (Artisan/Verisyse)

A drop of miotic agent (pilocarpine 1%) is administered to the preanesthetized eye. Two 1.5-mm paracenteses are created at the 2- and 10-o'clock positions with a super sharp blade. Viscoelastic is injected into the anterior chamber prior to the creation of a 5.5 to 6.5 mm superior clear cornea or sclerocorneal tunnel incision. The lens is grabbed with a smooth forceps and inserted into the anterior chamber through the main corneal incision and rotated 180 degrees to ensure centration over the center of the pupil. An "enclavation" needle is used to affix the anterior and posterior iris stroma onto the lens claws. A peripheral surgical iridotomy should be performed with Vannas scissors in order to prevent the occurrence of pupillary block. Irrigation aspiration is then used to remove the remaining viscoelastic material from the anterior segment of the eye. The main clear corneal wound is then sutured with a 10-0 nylon suture.

Angle-Supported Lenses

A drop of miotic agent (pilocarpine 1%) is administered to the preanesthetized eye. A paracentesis is created with a sharp blade followed by injection of viscoelastic into the anterior chamber. A clear corneal temporal incision is then created with a keratome (incision size depends on IOL design and foldable characteristics). The lens is inserted into the anterior chamber with the leading haptic directed toward the opposite angle and centered over the pupil. A peripheral iridotomy is created with Vannas scissors followed by removal of the viscoelastic material using the irrigation aspiration device.

Posterior Chamber Lenses

YAG peripheral iridotomy (PI) is typically performed prior to the phakic lens implantation to avoid pressure elevation postoperatively. If not, surgical PI may be performed intraoperatively. The initial wound construction consists of a superior corneal or scleral tunnel incision and follows the same steps described for anterior chamber phakic IOLs previously described. Once the anterior chamber is filled with viscoelastic material, the phakic IOL haptics are carefully pushed into the retropupillary space. The lens is then centered over the pupil (Figure 15-2). Irrigation aspiration is then used to remove the viscoelastic material from the anterior segment of the eye. Clinical trials are currently being performed to determine the long-term stability and safety of these devices.

PRESBYOPIA CORRECTION

Presbyopia is a normal refractive stage that begins around the age of 40 characterized by loss of accommodation (near focus). Thickening of the lens prevents

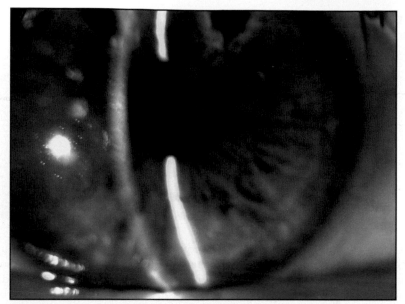

Figure 15-2. Vision posterior chamber phakic lens. (Courtesy of Tracy S. Swartz, OD, MS.)

changes in lenticular shape in response to relaxation and contraction of the zonular apparatus, leading to difficulties with near and intermediate vision tasks.[29]

Three structures in the eye can be targeted for the surgical correction of presbyopia: the crystalline lens, the cornea, and the sclera. The crystalline lens can be exchanged for various types of IOLs (monofocal, multifocal, and accommodative). The curvature of the cornea can be modified with the excimer laser (LASIK/PRK) in order to induce additional myopia in patients interested in monovision treatments. Procedures involving modification of the sclera can improve residual accommodation, but the mechanism of these specific treatments is still not well understood.

Intraocular Lenses

The crystalline lens can be exchanged for a monofocal IOL, a multifocal IOL, or an accommodating IOL. With implantation of a monofocal IOL, the nondominant eye is used for monovision with a refractive target known as unilateral myopization.[30]

Patients corrected with monofocal lenses are left with a single focal plane, which sometimes limits their ability to function. Multifocal and accommodative IOLs have been introduced as alternative methods to correct refractive errors in the presbyopic age group. The goal of using these lenses is to provide the patient with functional near and intermediate vision.

MULTIFOCAL IOLS

In multifocal IOLs (ReStor), a series of diffractive concentric apodized optical zones is engraved on the anterior surface of an Acrysof (Alcon Labs) IOL (Figure 15-3). Pupil size determines which optical zones are used by the patient's eye,

Figure 15-3. ReStor lens. (Courtesy of Tracy S. Swartz, OD, MS.)

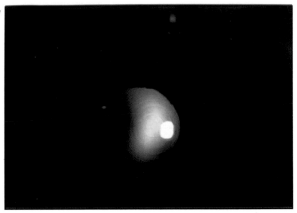

which are a function of the visual task required. For near tasks (miotic pupil), only the central zones are used; distance tasks utilize the more peripheral zones. The apodized optical zones provide different types of vision: near, intermediate, or distance.[31] Uncorrected corneal astigmatism may limit refractive outcomes with these types of IOLs. Multifocal lenses are placed in the capsular bag, using the same standard surgical techniques used for clear cornea phacoemulsification with posterior chamber IOLs.

Accommodative IOLs

Accommodating IOLs (Crystalens, AMO-Abbott, Abbott Park, IL) are placed in the capsular bag and, through a hinge mechanism, the lens is allowed to move back and forth to provide some degree of accommodation by changing the effective lens position.[31] Accommodative lenses are placed in the capsular bag, using the same standard surgical techniques used for clear cornea phacoemulsification with posterior chamber IOLs. Fibrosis of the capsular bag may limit the intended effect of these lenses.

Excimer Laser Corneal Procedures

Presbyopes may benefit from using the excimer laser to create a monovision ablation. In this technique the dominant eye is corrected for full distance vision and the nondominant eye is targeted for a myopic endpoint.[30] The degree of myopic correction for the nondominant eye is tailored according to the patient's age and visual needs. For patients in their mid-30s, a half monovision treatment (spherical equivalent of −0.75 D) is usually sufficient. In contrast, patients over the age of 40 should be offered a full monovision treatment with a planned post-operative spherical equivalent of −1.50 D. Conventional LASIK treatments are recommended for monovision eyes; depending on the preoperative refractive error, patients may require either a myopic or a hyperopic ablation to achieve the desired correction. Excimer laser ablations for monovision remain the preferred technique in our refractive surgery department,[30] where we have found a 92% satisfaction rate with this technique.[32]

The recent FDA approval of both multifocal and accommodative IOLs has shifted many refractive surgery practices away from excimer laser ablations for those patients who may already be in the presbyopic age range. Multifocal ablations have recently generated some interest. This technique uses the same surgical technique as LASIK, but the distance hyperopic correction is applied all over the 6-mm optical zone while the central 3-mm zone is made. There is a 1.5-mm circumferential transition zone. A 9.5-mm flap with a 4-mm hinge is created and excimer laser ablation is centered over the center of the pupil.[33]

BIOPTICS

Bioptics is the treatment of complex refractive errors with a combination of surgical techniques. It usually involves manipulation of 2 different structures of the eye, most commonly an IOL followed by corneal curvature modification. The concept of bioptics addresses the limitations of individual refractive procedures in correcting extremely high refractive errors. The goal of bioptics is to provide a suitable optical zone, a prolate cornea, and refractive predictability and stability. There is also the concept of reverse bioptics, which consists of corneal curvature modification prior to placement of an intraocular implant.[34]

Bioptics are indicated in patients with high refractive error and astigmatism, high refractive error with difficult refraction or IOL power calculation, moderate myopia with astigmatism and thin corneas, unexpected residual error after cataract surgery or phakic IOL implantation, and regression of refractive error after corneal surgery that cannot undergo further surgical treatment.

The most successful bioptics technique has been the combination of a phakic IOL with an excimer laser ablation for the treatment of high myopia.[34] In contrast, patients with high hyperopia rarely achieve correction with phakic IOLs because of their smaller anterior chambers. Several studies have evaluated the results of phakic IOL in different patient populations.[35] Presbyopic and myopic correction can be achieved with refractive lens exchange followed by a laser ablative procedure. This form of bioptics is rarely done in younger myopic patients because removing the natural lens causes loss of accommodation and there is also a higher risk of retinal detachment. Correcting hyperopia and presbyopia with refractive lens exchange is performed more often because of the limitations of the hyperopic treatment in individual procedures such as phakic IOL implantation and excimer laser ablation. Laser ablative procedures after cataract surgery are also common to correct miscalculated or unexpected residual refractive error. In cases of keratoconus and pellucid marginal degeneration, intracorneal ring segments may be used in combination with phakic or pseudophakic IOLs to correct irregular astigmatism and ametropia.

INCISIONAL PROCEDURES

Radial keratotomy (RK) was one of the first refractive procedures performed for the correction of low to moderate myopia.[36] Because of the potential complications (hyperopic shift) of RK and the improved safety and efficacy of excimer laser procedures, RK has fallen out of favor as the refractive procedure of choice. However, astigmatic keratotomy (AK), an incisional procedure similar to RK, is still used today to correct astigmatism in the setting of cataract surgery and PK.[37]

Radial Keratotomy

In RK, anywhere from 4 to 16 radial incisions are placed on the cornea to create a flattening effect. By utilizing peripheral cuts, the central optical zone of the cornea is flattened. The level of correction is based on the length and depth of incisions—higher levels of myopia are treated with longer and deeper incisions. Radial keratotomy can be performed in patients with low to moderate myopia. The surgeon uses a calibrated diamond knife to make a number of partial-thickness incisions (usually 8 or 16) in the peripheral cornea extending from the limbus to the paracentral cornea away from the visual axis. The incisions can be made from the periphery toward the center or from outside the central optical zone toward the limbus. Alternatively, the surgeon can make a shallow cut from the center outwards and retrace back to the center to deepen the incision. The central optical zone is ideally 7 mm to prevent postoperative complications such as glare, starburst, and halos; however, the degree of correction dictates the size of the incision and the remaining optical zone.[37]

Astigmatic Keratotomy

In AK, the incisions are positioned in the area of the greatest keratometric corneal astigmatism. AK employs the concept of coupling, whereby the incision in the steep meridian concurrently flattens the incised meridian and steepens the axis located 90 degrees away. Corneal sutures can be used to augment the steepening of the axis created by the corneal incision.

AK makes use of either paired transverse or arcuate incisions to relieve natural or surgically induced astigmatism. Transverse incisions ranging in size from 2 to 5 mm in length and arcuate incisions from 30 to 90 degrees produce a coupling ratio close to 1, which means that the amount of flattening in the most astigmatic axis equals the amount of steepening in the flattest axis.[38] As with RK, longer and deeper incisions can correct a greater degree of astigmatism than short or shallow incisions.

Incisional procedures are contraindicated in patients with ocular surface disease or with conditions known to interfere with normal wound healing as well as in biomechanically unstable corneas.

THERMAL PROCEDURES

Conductive keratoplasty (CK) is a refractive procedure that uses radiofrequency energy directed at the peripheral corneal stroma to shrink corneal collagen fibers, which results in central corneal steepening.[39] In 2002, the FDA approved the ViewPoint CK System for the correction of hyperopia and astigmatism. Collagen consists of a triple helix of polypeptide chains held together by covalent and hydrogen bonds. When heated to 65°C for approximately 1 minute, collagen will denature and shrink, producing a change in the refractive power of the cornea.[40] Because it does not involve incisions or tissue removal, this technique is considered a noninvasive method of refractive correction; therefore, postoperative complications such as dry eye, corneal haze, and central scarring commonly found in excimer laser procedures are not as common.

CK is indicated in patients with hyperopia between +0.75 D and +3.00 D as well as astigmatism less than 0.75 D and patients desiring presbyopic correction with monovision.[39]

In this procedure, the visual axis is marked followed by centration CK marker. Energy is delivered to the corneal stroma with a keratoplasty tip (Keratoplast;

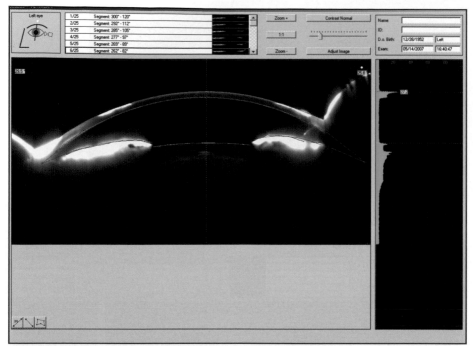

Figure 15-4. CK scars seen using Scheimpflug imaging. (Courtesy of Tracy S. Swartz, OD, MS.)

Refractec Inc, Irvine, CA) in a circle made of 8 spots around the optical zone (Figure 15-4). If a greater degree of correction is needed, more spots can be placed.

Laser thermokeratoplasty (LTK) also uses the concept of thermal energy direct-ed at the collagen fibrils of the corneal stroma to correct hyperopia and astigma-tism. LTK uses a laser to deliver the energy spots, instead of a keratoplasty tip as in CK.[41] Currently, the Sunrise Hyperion Noncontact Laser Thermokeratoplasty platform (Sunrise Technologies, Fremont, CA) is FDA-approved for the use of a holmium:YAG laser for the correction of 0.75 D to 3.50 D of spherical hyperopia. The continuous-wave diode laser thermokeratoplasty platform (Rodenstock; ProLaser Medical Systems Inc, Dusseldorf, Germany), still under investigation, uses a continuous-wave diode laser.[39] Long-term follow-up and data are needed to determine long-term refractive stability with these procedures.

INTRACORNEAL PROCEDURES

Intracorneal ring segments (ICRS) were designed as a reversible method to alter the curvature of the cornea and thus reduce refractive error.[42] Myopic cor-rections (flattening of the central cornea) are achieved by adding material to the periphery of the cornea. The thicker and smaller the segments, the higher the refractive correction. Implantation of ICRS is also useful in treating vision-threat-ening corneal disorders such as post-LASIK ectasia or keratoconus.[43]

There are 2 main types of ICRS: Intacs and Ferrara segments.[44] Intacs are the only FDA-approved ICRS (Figure 15-5). Intacs use a pair of semicircular PMMA segments with an arc length of 150 degrees and fixed external and internal diam-eters. The segments vary in thickness from 0.25 to 0.45 mm to correct myopia

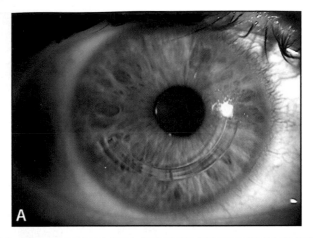

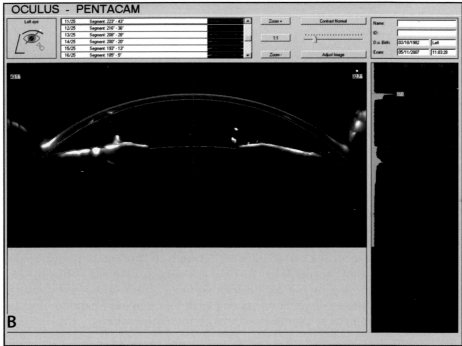

Figure 15-5. (A) Implantation of a single Intacs segment inferiorly. (Courtesy of Ming Wang, MD, PhD.) (B) Segment and femtosecond laser-created channel as viewed on Scheimpflug imaging. (Courtesy of Tracy S. Swartz, OD, MS.)

from −1.0 D to −4.0 D. Ferrara ring segments consist of 2 PMMA ring segments, each with an arc length of 160 degrees, but with varying diameters. The 6.0 mm segments are used to correct myopia up to −7.0 D and the 5.0 mm segments are used for higher degrees of myopia. The thickness of the segments ranges from 150 to 350 μm, depending on the amount of refractive correction needed.[44]

ICRS are indicated in patients with low myopia, astigmatism less than 1 D, and abnormal corneal topography (keratoconus) or patients with post-LASIK corneal ectasia. Patients with low myopia who desire a reversible method of refractive correction may also be offered ICRS. In addition, patients with mild to moderate levels of keratoconus or other keratectatic disorders can benefit from ICRS implantation if they have a clear central cornea (absence of scar of tissue), low spherical equivalents, and average keratometry readings less than 53.0 D.[45]

In order to insert ICRS, an initial incision is created with a diamond knife at 70% corneal thickness depth. A vacuum centering guide is used with a pocketing lever and a mechanical stromal spreader to create 2 intrastromal corneal tunnels with 180 degrees of arc clockwise and counterclockwise from the initial incision. The thickness of the ring segment to be implanted is based on the degree of refractive correction desired. The ICRS are soaked in topical antibiotic and are then slid into the tunnels with a Sinskey hook. The main incision is closed with a single 10-0 nylon suture (see Figure 15-4).

Alternatively, the surgeon can use a femtosecond laser to create the tunnels instead of the mechanical stromal spreader. The laser ensures a more accurate tunnel depth, width, and location, and the process is completed in 15 seconds.[45] Femtosecond corneal tunnels reduce corneal manipulation, avoid introduction of a foreign body or instrument into the corneal stroma, and therefore minimize the risk of infection and scar formation.

Asymmetric ISCRS segments can be used in cases of corneal ectasia post-LASIK or keratoconus. These segments may allow a better fit of soft or rigid contact lenses, thereby postponing penetrating or deep lamellar keratoplasty. This technique is most effective when the thinner segment is placed superiorly and the thicker segment inferiorly.[46]

PATIENT SCREENING AND FOLLOW-UP

Proper screening of patients seeking refractive surgery should include a review of the refractive history of the patient as well as a comprehensive ocular examination.

Review of the refractive history should include documentation of previous refractive errors obtained from medical records and old prescriptions (spectacles or contact lenses). Large refractive fluctuations (>1.0 D) or a history of recurrent changes in spectacles or contact lenses should raise a red flag. Refractive instability can have different etiologies, including dry eye conditions, biomechanically unstable corneas (keratoconus), or the development of cataracts. The patient should be carefully interrogated regarding previous refractive and intraocular procedures. Patients should also be asked about the use of contact lenses, including the duration of use, type of contact lens, history of contact lens-related complications (corneal ulcer or intolerance), and cleaning habits. Patients with fluctuating refractive errors should be counseled not to undergo surgery until their refractive error stabilizes.

Central corneal thickness (CCT) is of paramount importance in the proper selection of refractive surgery patients. CCT is used as a decision-making tool that assists the surgeon in the selection of the surgical technique. CCT is incorporated into the surgeon's algorithm, which also includes the magnitude of the refractive error, wavefront, and topographic information.

Traditionally, corneal pachymetry has been performed using contact techniques such as ultrasound corneal pachymetry. Pachymetry readings should be performed during the screening visits and immediately before and at the time of surgery. These ultrasound techniques are dependent on tissue hydration, and therefore measurement variations can occur. The goal of intraoperative pachymetry is to ensure that enough residual stromal bed thickness is present in order to safely perform the excimer laser ablation. Alternative techniques such as OCT[47] or Scheimpflug-based instruments (Pentacam)[48] have been used to create pachymetric maps of the cornea. In addition, elevation-based instruments can provide vital information on the posterior curvature of the cornea, which may allow quantification using the posterior float elevation map. These pachymetric maps allow the surgeon to ensure that a normal corneal thickness distribution exists, with a progressive thickening of the cornea from the center toward the periphery.

Pupil size determination should be routinely performed using either a millimeter ruler or an infrared pupillometer. The method used is not as important as the consistency of measurements, which should be performed by trained personnel under replicable lighting conditions. Pupil diameter should be assessed under scotopic (dim lights) and mesopic (light) conditions. Scotopic pupils will impact the amount of wavefront aberrations recorded as well as the patient's symptoms and refractive error.[5] In addition, the treated optical zone should be larger than the pupil size in order to reduce the induction of additional optical aberrations. In patients who complain of night driving difficulties, alpha-2 receptor antagonists (Alphagan, Allergan, Fullerton, CA), which promote pupil miosis, have been used with some success in selected cases.[49]

Computerized placido-based topography determines the keratometric power of the cornea. An axial map is created based on the curvature of the central 3 mm of the cornea to describe the total refractive power of the cornea.[48] The use of rigid gas-permeable or soft contact lenses induces corneal warpage, which may lead to the induction of topographic abnormalities.[50] If corneal warpage is suspected, contact lens use should be discontinued in order to allow the cornea to return to its baseline curvature.

As a general rule, topographic images showing abnormal inferior steepening, asymmetric warpage, or an abnormal inferior to superior ratio should raise a red flag. The presence of dry eye states may induce abnormalities in corneal topography, which may simulate abnormal corneal steepening. In patients with dry eye, topography should be performed after the instillation of a nonviscous artificial tear. If dry eye is suspected, optimization of the ocular surface should be performed and topographic and refractive assessment should be repeated at a later date.

Wavefront analysis is now an integral part of customized excimer laser ablations. Wavefront analysis allows objective determination of the patient's refractive state and quantification of the amount of higher order aberrations. More specifically, the presence of higher amounts of chromatic aberrations compared to the amount of corneal astigmatism should make the surgeon suspicious about the presence of a corneal ectatic disorder.[51] Wavefront information should be carefully analyzed, particularly in the presence of a dry eye states, which can interfere with these measurements. Customized laser ablations necessitate larger amounts of tissue ablation compared to conventional treatments and therefore should only be offered to those patients in whom sufficient corneal tissue is present in order to safely perform this surgery.

Patient follow-up is determined based on the type of procedure selected for the patient. LASIK patients are usually seen 1 day after surgery to ensure flap stability, followed by subsequent examinations at 1 week, 3 months, and 9 months. In our practice, we favor creation of LASIK flaps with a femtosecond laser and therefore our patients are asked to use a topical antibiotic drop 4 times a day and a topical steroid every hour for the first day, then 4 times a day for 1 week. The reason for the intense initial steroid therapy is based on the clinical observation that patients in whom LASIK flaps were created with earlier femtosecond laser models (15 and 30 mHZ) occasionally developed diffuse lamellar keratitis (DLK) at the edge of the flap. Advances with the current 60 kHZ femtosecond laser (Intralase, CA) have reduced the magnitude of this problem.

Patient follow-up after PRK is usually performed at 1 day; 1 week, when the bandage contact lens is removed; and then subsequent visits are schedule at 1, 3, and 9 months. Steroids are usually continued for longer periods of time for up to 1 month with a gradual taper in order to reduce the development of corneal haze after high myopic ablations. The patient's wound healing should be taken into consideration and no enhancements should be performed prior to 3 months, due to the refractive fluctuation that can occur during the early postoperative period.

Implantation of phakic IOLs is not recommended in patients with anterior segment pathology, corneal endothelial disorders or low cell counts, irregular astigmatism or refractive astigmatism greater than 1.5 D, corneal diameter less than 10 mm or greater than 14 mm, cataract, abnormal iris or damage to iris sphincter, ectopic pupil more than 2 mm from the center of the cornea, glaucoma, intraocular inflammation, corneal dystrophy or degeneration, history of retinal detachment or retinal changes, or ocular trauma that would affect the stability of the IOL. In order to be eligible for implantation of any type of IOL, patients must have an anterior chamber diameter between 11.6 and 13.0 mm, an anterior chamber depth of at least 3 mm, open iridocorneal angles, clear intraocular media, normal retinal exam, corneal curvature between 40 D and 47 D, no evidence of cataract or lens opacity, and endothelial cell count at least 1500 cells/mm^2. Phakic IOL patients are prescribed topical antibiotics and topical steroids to be used 4 times a day on the operated eye for 1 week. Patient visits are scheduled at 1 day, 1 week, 1 month, 6 months, and 1 year because the IOP needs careful monitoring.

Screening criteria and contraindications for patients desiring presbyLASIK are similar to those previously described for other excimer laser ablation techniques. This procedure is not FDA approved at this time.

MANAGEMENT OF COMPLICATIONS IN REFRACTIVE SURGERY

Excimer Laser Complications

Complications may occur intraoperatively or postoperatively and vary depending on the procedure. Dry eye is a common complication that should be ruled out prior to any refractive procedure for best results. Flap creation may cause disruption of the corneal nerve plexus which may exacerbate a pre-existing dry eye state (Figure 15-6). Patients seeking refractive surgery often suffer from some form of dry eye, which prevents them from wearing contact lenses comfortably.[52] Patients' complaints often include fluctuation in vision after periods of prolonged visual fixation, burning, and foreign-body sensation. Clinical findings include the presence of punctate epithelial erosions, unstable tear film with decreased tear breakup time and, in rare cases, reduction in tear production as evidenced by abnormal Schirmer's test. Optimization of the ocular surface should include

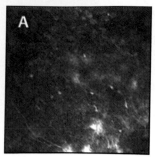
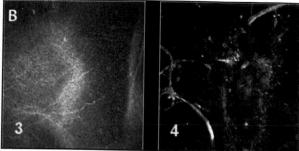

Figure 15-6. (A) Dry eye may result following keratorefractive procedure due to disruption of the corneal nerve plexus. At 3 months postoperatively, this LASIK patient showed reduced nerve axons. (B) Nerve tissue regenerates with time, often with improvement in dry eye symptoms following refractive surgery. (Courtesy of Heidelberg Engineering, Heidelberg, Germany.)

Figure 15-7. Truncated flap due to a jammed micro-keratome. (Courtesy of Tracy S. Swartz, OD, MS.)

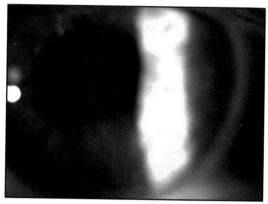

management of underlying blepharitis and frequent instillation of artificial tears. In patients in whom an inflammatory etiology is suspected to be the cause of the patient's dry eye symptoms, topical cyclosporine 0.05% has proven to improve refractive outcomes.[53] Punctal plugs should not be used in cases where an inflammatory ocular surface etiology is thought to be causing the patient's symptoms, because pooling of tears containing abnormal cytokines may further exacerbate damage to the ocular surface.

Flap Complications

LASIK flap-related complications can be divided into 2 groups: intraoperative and postoperative complications. Intraoperative complications such as truncated flaps (Figure 15-7), buttonholes (Figure 15-8), or torn (Figure 15-9) or free flaps are usually due to loss of suction during the microkeratome pass.[54] If a buttonhole is created or a flap cannot be lifted on the day of surgery, the procedure should be aborted and postponed. Once the cornea has undergone proper healing, the best option is to perform a PRK treatment months later to remove the abnormal LASIK flap. One-day postoperative visits ensure proper flap placement and identification of flap slippage, which increases the likelihood of epithelial ingrowth (Figures 15-10 and 15-11).

Epithelial defects may also occur during flap manipulation; these are easily managed with a soft contact lens and careful monitoring for the development of

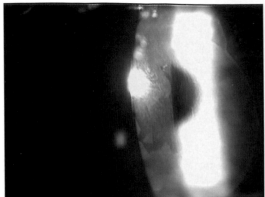

Figure 15-8. Button-hole flap. (Courtesy of Tracy S. Swartz, OD, MS.)

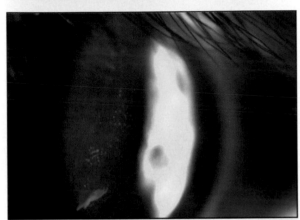

Figure 15-9. Torn flap with subsequent epithelial ingrowth. (Courtesy of Tracy S. Swartz, OD, MS.)

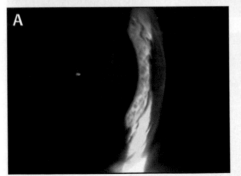

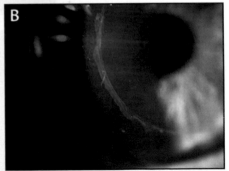

Figure 15-10. (A) Clean flap edge using a femtosecond laser. (B) Flap edge after a flap slip during sleep the night of surgery. (Courtesy of Ming Wang, MD, PhD.)

diffuse lamellar keratitis (DLK). Management options for DLK are based on the severity of the condition and can range from hourly topical steroid use to flap lift and irrigation under the flap with topical antibiotics.[55] DLK should be monitored frequently to prevent the development of a flap melt or irreversible scarring (Figures 15-12 and 15-13).

Complications associated with the femtosecond laser can occur in the presence of an inadequate tear meniscus, which can form between the suction ring and

Figure 15-11. Epithelial ingrowth following a flap-lift enhancement. (Courtesy of Tracy S. Swartz, OD, MS.)

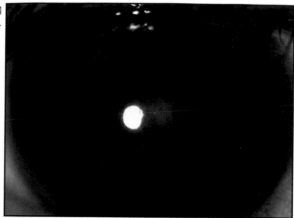

Figure 15-12. Grade 2 DLK noted 1 day postoperatively. (Courtesy of Tracy S. Swartz, OD, MS.)

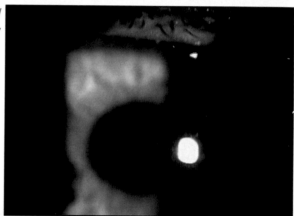

Figure 15-13. Toxic DLK tends to be severe, causing loss of best corrected vision and scarring. (Courtesy of Tracy S. Swartz, OD, MS.)

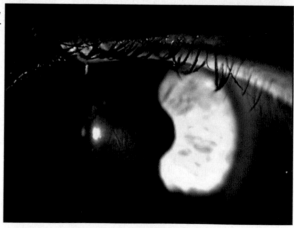

the peripheral cornea at the time of corneal applanation by the focusing lens. The ring should be carefully adjusted in order to eliminate the tear meniscus to ensure proper flap creation.

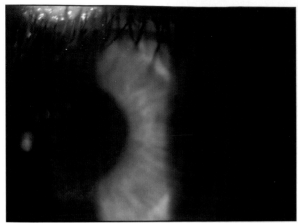

Figure 15-14. PRK haze. (Courtesy of Tracy S. Swartz, OD, MS.)

Haze After PRK

Haze formation after PRK is a serious complication associated with this procedure (Figure 15-14). Haze is thought to result from the accumulation of myofibroblast on the anterior corneal stroma and surface irregularities that create light scatter.[21] Clinically, haze is usually detected 1 to 3 months after surgery during slit-lamp examination and, in some cases, can become symptomatic. The development of haze tends to occur with excimer laser ablations greater than –6 D.[15] Current strategies for the prevention of haze after PRK include the use of MMC 0.002%; the duration of application varies from 30 seconds to up to 2 minutes.[18] The long-term effects of this preventative therapy have not been studied and caution is recommended when using this technique.

Aberropia

Aberropia is a term coined by Dr. Amar Agarwal from India in which patients with BCVA 20/20 vision in both eyes complain of difficulties with visual tasks despite normal topographies and minimal refractive errors.[56] Wavefront examination obtained on these patients usually reveals high amounts of higher-order aberrations such as coma or spherical aberration. Management of these patients is complicated and time-consuming, but very rewarding once the higher order aberrations are corrected.

Ectasia

Corneal ectasia can occur after both LASIK and PRK.[57] A large proportion of cases can occur in biomechanically unstable corneas with recognizable preoperative abnormalities in corneal topography, or insufficient residual stromal bed thickness after primary or enhancement procedures[12] (Figure 15-15). A small cohort of patients may also develop corneal ectasia without any recognizable risk factors.[25] Management of corneal ectasia can include lowering IOP[58] to reduce the strain on the cornea, gas permeable contact lenses, INTACS, and keratoplasty.[25] Collagen cross-linking has also been proposed for the management of postrefractive surgery ectasia as a method to reduce the keratometric progression of this condition.[25] Long-term prospective studies are needed to evaluate the long-term stability of this technique in this patient population.

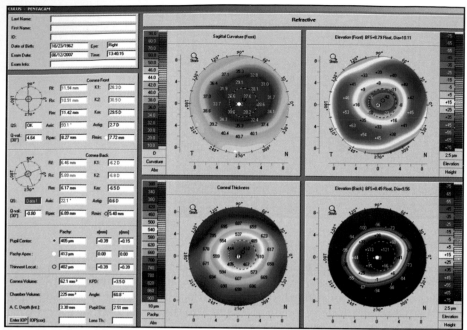

Figure 15-15. Ectasia following LASIK for a preoperative refraction of -11.00. (Courtesy of Tracy S. Swartz, OD, MS.)

Infections

Infectious keratitis after refractive surgery is an unusual but serious complication. Infection is more common among LASIK patients compared to PRK patients according to large populations studies.[59] The most common organisms are atypical mycobacteria, followed by both gram-positive and gram-negative organisms.[59] Fungal infections have also been reported. Management of infectious keratitis consists of lifting the LASIK flap and culturing the stromal bed and irrigating the stroma with antibiotic solutions. Patients should also be placed on a cycloplegic agent. Daily follow-ups are needed until the infection is thought to be under control.

Residual Refractive Errors

Residual refractive errors requiring an enhancement can occur in about 10% to 15% of patients according to our experience. Older age and the presence of preoperative dry eye have been associated with refractive regression after LASIK. In addition, poor epithelial wound healing may lead to surface irregularities.

Phakic IOL Complications

There are also a number of complications that may outweigh the benefits of phakic IOL implantation. Patients can experience corneal endothelial cell loss with the use of both anterior chamber and posterior chamber lenses.[60] Anterior subcapsular cataract formation/lens opacification can occur as a result of minor surgical trauma or uncontrolled intraocular inflammation (Figure 15-16). Lens opacifications can be managed with cataract surgery if they become visually sig-

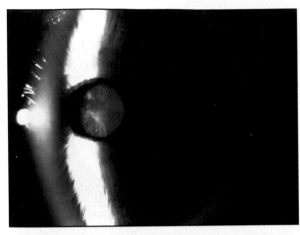

Figure 15-16. Anterior subscapular cataract following posterior chamber phakic lens implantation. (Courtesy of Tracy S. Swartz, OD, MS.)

nificant, but frequently lens opacification is often nonprogressive. Other potential complications include infection, decentration, glaucoma, and induction of higher order aberrations in patients with large pupils.[61] Careful surgical planning and execution can help decrease the incidence of these complications.

Incisional Procedures

Complications seen in RK patients include induced irregular astigmatism (Figure 15-17), hyperopic shifts,[36] decreased contrast sensitivity, and visual symptoms[62] such as glare, halo, and starburst. The induced aberrations may be partially corrected with an excimer laser surgery, although due to the biomechanical instability of these corneas results are not always predictable (Figure 15-18). In general, an overcorrection is initially desired, because these eyes tend to regress over time. Less common, but certainly possible complications, are microperforations, macroperforations, infection, and rupture of incisions from trauma.[63]

Intracorneal Ring Segments

Complications associated with these procedures include induced astigmatism, superficial wound site neovascularization, tunnel deposits and haze, induced hyperopia, undercorrection of refractive error, dry eye, epithelial defects, perforations, extension of the incision into the visual axis, shallow or uneven placement of the ICRS, infectious keratitis, sterile keratitis, chronic pain from contact between the corneal nerve and ICRS, decentration of the segments, stromal thinning, and corneal stromal edema around the incision and channel sites.[42-44]

Management of most of these complications is simple. Astigmatism and hyperopia can be managed by removing the superior segment, and undercorrection can be managed by implanting a superior segment (if only one segment was originally implanted).[45] If visual acuity is still unsatisfactory and contact lenses can be tolerated, the patient can be fitted with a contact lens. The use of the femtosecond laser to create the tunnels can reduce the incidence of incision-related and tunnel-related complications.[45] Complications such as infection, deposits, haze, misplacement, pain, decentration, stromal thinning, and edema can be managed by removing the segments, though extreme cases may require PK.[64] Awareness of risk factors for infection such as a history of diabetes, contact lens use, and trauma can also be preventative.

Figure 15-17. Irregular astigmatism following radial keratotomy. (Courtesy of Tracy S. Swartz, OD, MS.)

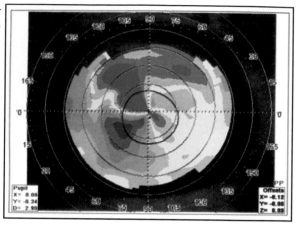

Figure 15-18. Conductive keratoplasty in patient who suffered a hyperopic shift following radial keratotomy. (Courtesy of Tracy S. Swartz, OD, MS.)

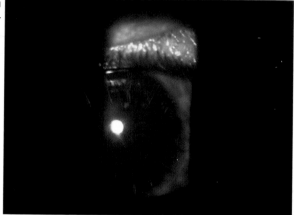

Thermal Procedures

There are few complications involved with CK and LTK, but the most common are surgically induced astigmatism[65] and regression.[39] Patients can experience regression of the refractive correction, so an initial overcorrection may lead to a more satisfactory long-term effect. Incidence of astigmatism decreases with more experienced surgeons, and it can be corrected with an enhancement procedure. Additionally, the residual refractive error can be corrected with an excimer laser procedure. Patients can also experience irregular astigmatism,[39] starburst, foreign-body sensation, and light sensitivity,[65] which eventually return to normal during the healing process.

NEWER TECHNOLOGIES: CORNEAL CROSS-LINKING

Corneal collagen cross-linking is a new non-FDA-approved therapeutic modality that has been used to halt the keratometric progression of ectasia in biomechanically unstable corneas. The procedure is performed under sterile conditions; after topical anesthetic application, the central 7-mm to 9-mm corneal epithelium is gently scrapped with a beaver blade. Riboflavin 0.1% solution is applied over the exposed corneal stromal 5 minutes prior to irradiation with

UV-A light. Treatment is initiated once the photosensitizer is thought to have sufficiently permeated the corneal stroma. UV-A light irradiation is administered using 2 independent UV diodes (370 nm wavelength) in order to obtain the desired irradiance of 3 mW/cm^2, which is monitored using a UV-A meter. The diodes are placed at a distance of 1 cm from the patient's cornea and the cornea is irradiated for 30 minutes; the riboflavin is administered every 5 minutes in order to ensure proper concentration and penetration of the photosensitizer into the corneal stroma. During the postoperative period, patients are treated with topical antibiotics until closure of the epithelial defect.

In clinical trials undertaken in Europe, keratometric progression of keratoconus has been shown to regress by a mean value of 2 D at a mean follow-up of 23 months after UV-A cross-linking.[66] The effect of collagen cross-linking on the corneal stroma keratocytes has been studied in both animal and human models. Animal models have demonstrated evidence of keratocyte apoptosis and necrosis, which have been shown to occur between 4 and 24 hours after collagen cross-linking.[67]

Confocal microscopy performed in human subjects after UV-A cross-linking has shown keratocyte rarefaction in the anterior and intermediate corneal stroma with associated edema. Keratocyte repopulation has been shown to approach baseline levels by 6 months after treatment.[68]

Further studies need to be conducted in order to assess the long-term effects of this treatment modality in terms of endothelial cell function and stromal clarity as well as keratometric progression of keratoconus. Applications of corneal collagen cross-linking include the manufacture of refractive inlays and onlays, which can potentially be modified with an excimer laser. In addition, there might be a role for collagen cross-linking in the management of corneal perforations as well as in stromal augmentation procedures.

CONCLUSION

The field of refractive surgery has undergone significant technological advances that have increased options for patients seeking surgical correction. Judicious scrutiny of the medical literature and attendance of advanced training courses are essential for the development of a safe refractive surgery practice.

REFERENCES

1. Available at: http://www.accessdata.fda.gov/scripts/cdrh/devicesatfda/index.cfm?start_search=11&Search_Term=LZS%20or%20LASIK&Approval_Date_From=&Approval_Date_To=&sort=approvaldatedesc&PAGENUM=10. Accessed July 25, 2007.

2. Maeda N. Wavefront technology in ophthalmology. *Curr Opin Ophthalmol.* 2001;12:294-299.

3. Chalita MR, Xu M, Krueger RR. Correlation of aberrations with visual symptoms using wavefront analysis in eyes after laser in situ keratomileusis. *J Refract Surg.* 2003;19(suppl):682-686.

4. Pallikaris IG, Kymionis GD, Panagopoulou SI, Siganos CS, Theodorakis MA, Pallikaris AI. Induced optical aberrations following formation of a laser in situ keratomileusis flap. *J Cataract Refract Surg.* 2002;28:1737-1741.

5. Krueger RR. The required technology for customized corneal ablation. *Ophthalmol Clin North Am.* 2004;17:vi, 143-159.

6. Roberts C. Biomechanics of the cornea and wavefront-guided laser refractive surgery. *J Refract Surg.* 2002;18(suppl):589-592.

7. Solomon KD, Holzer MP, Sandoval HP, et al. Refractive Surgery Survey 2001. *J Cataract Refract Surg.* 2002;28:346-355.

8. Stonecipher K, Ignacio TS, Stonecipher M. Advances in refractive surgery: microkeratome and femtosecond laser flap creation in relation to safety, efficacy, predictability, and biomechanical stability. *Curr Opin Ophthalmol.* 2006;17:368-372.

9. Sarayba MA, Ignacio TS, Binder PS, Tran DB. Comparative study of stromal bed quality by using mechanical, IntraLase femtosecond laser 15- and 30-kHz microkeratomes. *Cornea.* 2007;26:446-451.

10. Kezirian GM, Stonecipher KG. Comparison of the IntraLase femtosecond laser and mechanical keratomes for laser in situ keratomileusis. *J Cataract Refract Surg.* 2004;30:804-811.

11. Lifshitz T, Levy J, Klemperer I, Levinger S. Anterior chamber gas bubbles after corneal flap creation with a femtosecond laser. *J Cataract Refract Surg.* 2005;31:2227-2229.

12. Guirao A. Theoretical elastic response of the cornea to refractive surgery: risk factors for keratectasia. *J Refract Surg.* 2005;21:176-185.

13. Yee RW, Yee SB. Update on laser subepithelial keratectomy (LASEK). *Curr Opin Ophthalmol.* 2004;15:333-341.

14. Matsumoto JC, Chu YS. Epi-LASIK update: overview of techniques and patient management. *Int Ophthalmol Clin.* 2006;46:105-115.

15. Netto MV, Mohan RR, Ambrosio R Jr, Hutcheon AE, Zieske JD, Wilson SE. Wound healing in the cornea: a review of refractive surgery complications and new prospects for therapy. *Cornea.* 2005;24:509-522.

16. Siganos DS, Katsanevaki VJ, Pallikaris IG. Correlation of subepithelial haze and refractive regression 1 month after photorefractive keratectomy for myopia. *J Refract Surg.* 1999; 15:338-342.

17. Xu H, Liu S, Xia X, Huang P, Wang P, Wu X. Mitomycin C reduces haze formation in rabbits after excimer laser photorefractive keratectomy. *J Refract Surg.* 2001;17:342-349.

18. Netto MV, Mohan RR, Sinha S, Sharma A, Gupta PC, Wilson SE. Effect of prophylactic and therapeutic mitomycin C on corneal apoptosis, cellular proliferation, haze, and long-term keratocyte density in rabbits. *J Refract Surg.* 2006;22:562-574.

19. Rapuano CJ, Laibson PR. Excimer laser phototherapeutic keratectomy for anterior corneal pathology. *CLAO J.* 1994;20:253-257.

20. Muller LT, Candal EM, Epstein RJ, Dennis RF, Majmudar PA. Transepithelial phototherapeutic keratectomy/photorefractive keratectomy with adjunctive mitomycin-C for complicated LASIK flaps. *J Cataract Refract Surg.* 2005;31:291-296.

21. Netto MV, Mohan RR, Sinha S, Sharma A, Dupps W, Wilson SE. Stromal haze, myofibroblasts, and surface irregularity after PRK. *Exp Eye Res.* 2006;82:788-797.

22. Zhang M, Mai C, Nie S. Phototherapeutic keratectomy combined with photorefractive keratectomy for treatment of myopia with corneal scars. *J Tongji Med Univ.* 2000;20:347-348.

23. Dupps WJ Jr, Roberts C. Effect of acute biomechanical changes on corneal curvature after photokeratectomy. *J Refract Surg.* 2001;17:658-669.

24. Rapuano CJ. Excimer laser phototherapeutic keratectomy in eyes with anterior corneal dystrophies: short-term clinical outcomes with and without an antihyperopia treatment and poor effectiveness of ultrasound biomicroscopic evaluation. *Cornea.* 2005;24:20-31.

25. Klein SR, Epstein RJ, Randleman JB, Stulting RD. Corneal ectasia after laser in situ keratomileusis in patients without apparent preoperative risk factors. *Cornea.* 2006;25:388-403.

26. Albietz JM, Lenton LM, McLennan SG. Dry eye after LASIK: comparison of outcomes for Asian and Caucasian eyes. *Clin Exp Optom.* 2005;88:89-96.

27. Condon PI, O'Keefe M, Binder PS. Long-term results of laser in situ keratomileusis for high myopia: risk for ectasia. *J Cataract Refract Surg.* 2007;33:583-590.

28. Lovisolo CF, Reinstein DZ. Phakic intraocular lenses. *Surv Ophthalmol.* 2005;50:549-587.

29. Baikoff G, Matach G, Fontaine A, Ferraz C, Spera C. Correction of presbyopia with refractive multifocal phakic intraocular lenses. *J Cataract Refract Surg.* 2004;30:1454-1460.

30. Cox CA, Krueger RR. Monovision with laser vision correction. *Ophthalmol Clin North Am.* 2006;19:vi, 71-5.

31. Lane SS, Morris M, Nordan L, Packer M, Tarantino N, Wallace RB III. Multifocal intraocular lenses. *Ophthalmol Clin North Am.* 2006;19:vi, 89-105.

32. Miranda D, Krueger RR. Monovision laser in situ keratomileusis for pre-presbyopic and presbyopic patients. *J Refract Surg.* 2004;20:325-328.

33. Alio JL, Chaubard JJ, Caliz A, Sala E, Patel S. Correction of presbyopia by technovision central multifocal LASIK (presbyLASIK). *J Refract Surg.* 2006;22:453-460.

34. Leccisotti A. Bioptics: where do things stand? *Curr Opin Ophthalmol.* 2006;17:399-405.

35. Baikoff G, Bourgeon G, Jodai HJ, Fontaine A, Vieira Lellis F, Trinquet L. Pigment dispersion and Artisan implants: crystalline lens rise as a safety criterion [in French]. *J Fr Ophthalmol.* 2005;28:590-597.

36. McDonnell PJ. Refractive surgery. *Br J Ophthalmol.* 1999;83:1257-1260.

37. Choi DM, Thompson RW Jr, Price FW Jr. Incisional refractive surgery. *Curr Opin Ophthalmol.* 2002;13:237-241.

38. Raviv T, Epstein RJ. Astigmatism management. *Int Ophthalmol Clin.* 2000;40:183-198.

39. McDonald MB. Conductive keratoplasty: a radiofrequency-based technique for the correction of hyperopia. *Trans Am Ophthalmol Soc.* 2005;103:512-536.

40. Sporl E, Genth U, Schmalfuss K, Seiler T. Thermomechanical behavior of the cornea. *Ger J Ophthalmol.* 1996;5:322-327.

41. Brinkmann R, Radt B, Flamm C, Kampmeier J, Koop N, Birngruber R. Influence of temperature and time on thermally induced forces in corneal collagen and the effect on laser thermokeratoplasty. *J Cataract Refract Surg.* 2000;26:744-754.

42. Guell JL. Are intracorneal rings still useful in refractive surgery? *Curr Opin Ophthalmol.* 2005;16:260-265.

43. Kymionis GD, Tsiklis NS, Pallikaris AI, et al. Long-term follow-up of Intacs for post-LASIK corneal ectasia. *Ophthalmology.* 2006;113:1909-1917.

44. Ertan A, Colin J. Intracorneal rings for keratoconus and keratectasia. *J Cataract Refract Surg.* 2007;33:1303-1314.

45. Rabinowitz YS. Intacs for keratoconus. *Curr Opin Ophthalmol.* 2007;18:279-283.

46. Guell JL, Velasco F, Sanchez SI, Gris O, Garcia-Rojas M. Intracorneal ring segments after laser in situ keratomileusis. *J Refract Surg.* 2004;20:349-355.

47. Li Y, Netto MV, Shekhar R, Krueger RR, Huang D. A longitudinal study of LASIK flap and stromal thickness with high-speed optical coherence tomography. *Ophthalmology.* 2007;114:1124-1132.

48. Swartz T, Marten L, Wang M. Measuring the cornea: the latest developments in corneal topography. *Curr Opin Ophthalmol.* 2007;18:325-333.

49. Kesler A, Shemesh G, Rothkoff L, Lazar M. Effect of brimonidine tartrate 0.2% ophthalmic solution on pupil size. *J Cataract Refract Surg.* 2004;30:1707-1710.

50. Tsai PS, Dowidar A, Naseri A, McLeod SD. Predicting time to refractive stability after discontinuation of rigid contact lens wear before refractive surgery. *J Cataract Refract Surg.* 2004;30:2290-2294.

51. Alio JL, Shabayek MH. Corneal higher order aberrations: a method to grade keratoconus. *J Refract Surg.* 2006;22:539-545.

52. Gupta N, Naroo SA. Factors influencing patient choice of refractive surgery or contact lenses and choice of centre. *Contact Lens Anterior Eye.* 2006;29:17-23.

53. Roberts CW, Carniglia PE, Brazzo BG. Comparison of topical cyclosporine, punctal occlusion, and a combination for the treatment of dry eye. *Cornea.* 2007;26:805-809.

54. Gimbel HV, Penno EE, van Westenbrugge JA, Ferensowicz M, Furlong MT. Incidence and management of intraoperative and early postoperative complications in 1000 consecutive laser in situ keratomileusis cases. *Ophthalmology.* 1998;105:1839-1847.

55. Melki SA, Azar DT. LASIK complications: etiology, management, and prevention. *Surv Ophthalmol.* 2001;46:95-116.

56. Agarwal AAA, Agarwal S, Agarwal T. *Refractive Surgery: Worst Case Scenarios.* San Francisco, CA: ASCRS; 2006.

57. Dupps WJ Jr, Wilson SE. Biomechanics and wound healing in the cornea. *Exp Eye Res.* 2006;83:709-720.

58. Rabinowitz YS. Ectasia after laser in situ keratomileusis. *Curr Opin Ophthalmol.* 2006;17:421-426.

59. Solomon R, Donnenfeld ED, Azar DT, et al. Infectious keratitis after laser in situ keratomileusis: results of an ASCRS survey. *J Cataract Refract Surg.* 2003;29:2001-2006.

60. Lackner B, Pieh S, Schmidinger G, et al. Long-term results of implantation of phakic posterior chamber intraocular lenses. *J Cataract Refract Surg.* 2004;30:2269-2276.

61. Chandhrasri S, Knorz MC. Comparison of higher order aberrations and contrast sensitivity after LASIK, Verisyse phakic IOL, and Array multifocal IOL. *J Refract Surg.* 2006;22:231-236.

62. Holladay JT. Optical quality and refractive surgery. *Int Ophthalmol Clin.* 2003;43:119-136.

63. Artola A, Ayala MJ, Ruiz-Moreno JM, De La Hoz F, Alio JL. Rupture of radial keratotomy incisions by blunt trauma 6 years after combined photorefractive keratectomy/radial keratotomy. *J Refract Surg.* 2003;19:460-462.

64. Hofling-Lima AL, Branco BC, Romano AC, et al. Corneal infections after implantation of intracorneal ring segments. *Cornea.* 2004;23:547-549.

65. Du TT, Fan VC, Asbell PA. Conductive keratoplasty. *Curr Opin Ophthalmol.* 2007;18:334-337.

66. Wollensak G, Spoerl E, Seiler T. Riboflavin/ultraviolet-a-induced collagen crosslinking for the treatment of keratoconus. *Am J Ophthalmol.* 2003;135:620-627.

67. Wollensak G, Spoerl E, Wilsch M, Seiler T. Keratocyte apoptosis after corneal collagen cross-linking using riboflavin/UVA treatment. *Cornea.* 2004;23:43-49.

68. Mazzotta C, Balestrazzi A, Traversi C, et al. Treatment of progressive keratoconus by riboflavin-UVA-induced cross-linking of corneal collagen: ultrastructural analysis by Heidelberg Retinal Tomograph II in vivo confocal microscopy in humans. *Cornea.* 2007;26:390-397.

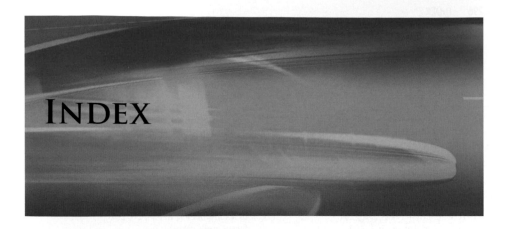

INDEX

aberropia, 287

abrasions, 14, 40, 191-192, 258

Acanthamoeba keratitis (AK), 19, 28, 29-30, 31, 32, 49, 226

accommodative intraocular lenses, 276

acid burns, 65, 197, 198

adhesins, 15

adhesives (glues), 128, 130, 193, 194, 259-261

AK (*Acanthamoeba* keratitis), 19, 28, 29-30, 31, 32, 49, 226

AK (astigmatic keratotomy), 239, 277, 278

AKC (atopic keratoconjunctivitis), 130, 132-133

ALK (anterior lamellar keratoplasty), 253-256

alkali burns, 65, 196, 197-198, 199

alkaptonuria, 144-145

AMG (amniotic membrane graft), 128, 137, 199, 214, 218, 259, 260, 262-263, 264-265

amino acid metabolism disorders, 144-145

amniotic membrane graft (AMG), 128, 137, 199, 214, 218, 259, 260, 262-263, 264-265

amyloidosis, 82-83, 87, 95-96, 145, 146, 147

anchoring plaques, 4

angle-supported lenses, 274

anterior lamellar keratoplasty (ALK), 253-256

anterior stromal puncture (ASP), 79, 257-258

aqueous tear deficiency

    diabetes, 148

    diagnosing, 64, 66, 67, 68, 69, 210, 211-212, 213

    dry eye classification, 202-203

    dry eye definitions, 201, 202

    neurotrophic keratopathy, 63, 66, 67

    non-Sjögren syndrome, 64, 202, 203, 205, 212

    nutrition, 8, 206

    Sjögren syndrome, 39, 40, 42-43, 64, 66, 202, 203, 204, 212

    systemic diseases, 123-124, 134, 136

arcus senilis, 93-94, 141, 142

argyrosis, 103

Artemis system, 229-231

artisan lenses, 274

ASP (anterior stromal puncture), 79, 257-258

astigmatic keratotomy (AK), 239, 277, 278

atopic keratoconjunctivitis (AKC), 130, 132-133

Avellino dystrophy, 81, 85, 146, 254

avulsions, 193

Axenfeld's anomaly and Axenfeld's syndrome, 153

bacterial keratitis, 13-22

    diagnosing, 15, 16, 17-19, 226

    inflammatory disorders, 14, 43, 44, 45-52, 132, 135

    management, 17, 18, 19-21, 30-33, 249

    ocular surface disorders, 14, 65

    postoperative risk for, 14, 15, 252, 288

    systemic diseases, 14, 127, 132, 135

    trauma, 14, 17, 191, 192

band keratopathy, 50, 87, 97-98, 130, 151, 152, 153, 261

basal cells, 2, 3-4, 10, 41, 70, 148, 226

Bell's phenomenon, 64, 68

Bietti crystalline corneoretinal dystrophy, 144

biomechanical property measurements, 239-240, 241

biopsy, 257

bioptics, 277

blunt trauma, 193

Bowen's disease, 166-167

Bowman's layer

    anatomy and physiology, 2, 5

    corneal dystrophies, 75, 79-80, 81, 85, 86, 88, 95, 97, 99, 100

    corneal ectatic disorders, 110

    diagnostic instrumentation, 231

    inflammatory disorders, 38

    metabolic disorders, 145, 151

    neoplasms, 163, 166, 168

    refractive surgery, 270, 271

    trauma, 191, 192

brawny edema, 16

bullous keratopathy, 4, 10, 14, 40, 70, 90, 91, 249, 250, 254, 263
burns, 65, 70, 196-200, 205, 249, 254, 261

cadaveric keratolimbal allograft (KLAL), 71-72
calcific band keratopathy, 50, 87, 97-98, 130, 151, 152, 153, 261
carbohydrate metabolism disorders, 4, 24, 65, 142, 143, 145-148, 155, 196, 205, 208, 209, 274, 289
catarrhal infiltrate or ulcers. *See* marginal keratitis
CCT (central corneal thickness), 281
CDB (corneal dystrophies of Bowman's layer), 79-80, 81
central cloudy dystrophy, 88, 95
central corneal thickness (CCT), 281
CH (corneal hysteresis), 240, 241
Chandler's syndrome, 101, 102
CHED (congenital hereditary endothelial dystrophy), 88, 92-93
chemical injuries, 65, 70, 196-200, 205, 249, 254, 261
chronic actinic keratopathy, 98-99
CHSD (congenital hereditary stromal dystrophy), 88
CIN (conjunctival and corneal intraepithelial neoplasia), 166-167
CK (conductive keratoplasty), 278-279, 290
CLAU (conjunctival limbal autograft), 71
climatic droplet keratopathy, 98-99
Coats' white ring, 100
Cogan microcystic dystrophy. *See* epithelial basement membrane dystrophy (EBMD)
Cogan-Reese syndrome. *See* iris nevus syndrome
Cogan's syndrome, 49, 53-54
collagen cross-linking, 116, 117, 118, 287, 290-291
compositional reflexes, 61-62, 63, 64, 68, 69
conductive keratoplasty (CK), 278-279, 290
confocal microscopy, 29-30, 112, 225-226, 227
congenital disorders, 49-50, 65, 88, 92-93, 152-154, 155, 205
congenital hereditary endothelial dystrophy (CHED), 88, 92-93
congenital hereditary stromal dystrophy (CHSD), 88
conjunctival and corneal intraepithelial neoplasia (CIN), 166-167
conjunctival flap, 199, 263
conjunctival limbal autograft (CLAU), 70-71
conjunctival melanoma, 103, 171-172
conjunctival nevus, 168
conjunctival squamous papilloma, 164, 165
connective tissue disorders, 40, 109, 148-150, 203, 208
copper deposition, 103, 130, 151-152, 153
cornea farinata, 89, 95
corneal arcus, 93-94, 141, 142
corneal chrysiasis, 103
corneal collagen cross-linking, 116, 117, 118, 287, 290-291
corneal dystrophies of Bowman's layer (CDB), 79-80, 81
corneal hyposthesia, 155
corneal hysteresis (CH), 240, 241

corneal resistance factor (CRF), 240, 241
crocodile shagreen, 88, 95
crystalline deposition, 85-87, 130, 141, 144, 150, 151
crystalline keratopathy, 252
cystinosis, 144

deep anterior lamellar keratoplasty (DALK), 7, 118-119, 254-256, 273
deep lamellar endothelial keratoplasty (DLEK), 91
defense mechanisms, 2, 5, 9, 13-14, 17, 21, 33, 38-39, 61-64, 66, 206
degenerative disorders, 89-91, 93-102
　　See also specific disorder
descemetoceles, 17, 18, 26, 262
Descemet's membrane
　　anatomy and physiology, 2, 7, 10
　　congenital disorders, 88, 154
　　corneal dystrophies, 7, 75, 88, 89, 90, 91, 94, 95, 103
　　corneal ectatic disorders, 111, 112, 118-119
　　inflammatory disorders, 50, 51
　　metabolic disorders, 130, 148, 152
　　microbial keratitis, 16, 17, 24
　　surgical procedures, 7, 51, 91, 118-119, 194, 195, 254, 255, 256-257
Descemet's stripping endothelial keratoplasty (DSEK), 7, 91, 256-257
Descemet's warts, 94
desmosomes, 2, 4
diabetes, 4, 24, 65, 147-148, 155, 205, 208, 209, 274, 289
DLEK (deep lamellar endothelial keratoplasty), 91
DLK (diffuse lamellar keratitis), 51, 283, 285, 286
dry eye, 201-223
　　classification, 202-206
　　diagnosing, 41, 64, 66, 67, 68, 69, 204, 208-213
　　diagnostic instrumentation, 64, 242, 244, 282
　　disorders/complications caused by, 14, 24, 39, 40, 41, 42-43, 99, 283-284, 288, 289
　　ocular surface defense, 61-64, 66, 206, 207
　　risk factors for, 203-207, 208, 209
　　　　diabetes, 65, 147, 148, 205, 208, 209
　　　　exposure keratopathy, 63-64, 66-68
　　　　inflammatory disorders, 41
　　　　neurotrophic keratopathy, 63, 64-66, 67, 68, 205
　　　　non-Sjögren syndrome, 64, 203, 205, 212
　　　　Sjögren's syndrome, 39, 40, 42-43, 64, 66, 203, 204, 212
　　　　surgical procedures, 41, 65, 206, 208, 249, 273, 281, 283-284
　　　　systemic diseases, 123-124, 127, 129, 134, 136, 137, 205, 206
　　　　trauma, 65, 110
　　treatment, 42-43, 66, 67, 68-69, 129, 214, 216-218, 264, 273, 278, 283-284
DSEK (Descemet's stripping endothelial keratoplasty), 7, 91, 256-257

EBMD (epithelial basement membrane dystrophy), 77-79, 258
ECM (extracellular matrix), 5-6, 15
ectasia, 109-122, 231, 238, 239, 243-244, 246, 271, 279, 280, 281, 282, 287-288, 290-291
edema, 9-10
Ehlers-Danlos syndrome (EDS), 148-149, 154
elevation maps, 233-236, 240, 242, 245-246, 282
endophthalmitis, 251, 252, 253, 256, 264, 266
endothelial rejection, 253
endothelium
    anatomy and physiology, 2, 7-8, 9-10
    congenital disorders, 153, 154
    corneal dystrophies, 7, 9, 10, 75, 84, 88, 89-93, 94, 101-102, 227, 228, 240, 249, 254
    corneal ectatic disorders, 112, 118-119
    diagnostic instrumentation, 8, 226-228, 229, 238
    inflammatory disorders, 49, 50, 51
    metabolic disorders, 146
    surgical procedures, 7, 91, 253, 254, 255, 256-257, 273, 283, 288
    trauma, 9, 193, 195
epidermolysis bullosa acquisita, 4
episcleritis, 53, 96, 124-125, 127, 128, 129, 136
epithelial basement membrane dystrophy (EBMD), 77-79, 258
epithelial-LASIK (epi-LASIK), 243, 246, 270, 271, 272
epithelium
    anatomy and physiology, 2-5, 8, 9, 10
    corneal dystrophies, 4, 75-79, 86, 87, 90, 93, 96, 98-100, 101, 102-103, 258
    corneal ectatic disorders, 110, 111
    diagnostic instrumentation, 226, 229, 230, 231, 238-239
    inflammatory disorders, 37-43, 45-47, 49, 51, 137
    metabolic disorders, 4, 97, 143, 144, 145, 146, 147-148, 149, 151
    microbial keratitis, 14, 15, 16, 17, 26-27, 29, 30, 31, 191
    neoplasms, 163, 164-168, 169-170, 171, 172, 174, 176-177
    ocular surface disorders, 61, 63, 66, 67-72, 132, 137, 166, 203, 206, 207, 211, 215-216
    surgical procedures
        pterygium excision, 266
        refractive corrections, 243, 246, 270, 271, 272, 273, 284-285, 286, 288, 289, 290-291
        superficial, 257-259, 261-263
        transplantations, 251-252, 253, 256
    systemic diseases, 125, 127, 128, 129, 131-132
    trauma, 14, 191, 192, 196, 197, 199
erythema multiforme major. See Stevens-Johnson syndrome (SJS)
erythema multiforme minor, 135
essential iris atrophy, 101, 102
evaporative dry eye, 61, 201, 202, 203-206, 210, 212, 213
excimer laser procedures, 269-273, 283-285
    See also specific technique
exposure keratopathy, 63-64, 66-68, 69
extracellular matrix (ECM), 5-6, 15

Fabry's disease, 142, 143
femtosecond lasers, 117, 270-271, 280, 281, 282-283, 285-286, 289
Ferry line, 102
fibrous histiocytoma, 174
filamentary keratitis, 39-43, 137
fish eye disease, 142
flap complications, 284-286
fleck dystrophy, 87-88
Fleischer ring, 102, 110, 111
fluorescein breakup time, 210
fluorescein prolifometry, 233-234
foreign bodies, 14, 100, 102, 103, 192-193, 198, 258
Fuchs' endothelial dystrophy, 7, 9, 10, 89-91, 227, 228, 240, 249, 254
fungal keratitis, 23-26
    diagnosing, 16, 19, 23, 24, 31-32, 226
    phlyctenulosis, 46, 47
    risk factors for, 23-24, 127, 192, 252, 288
    treatment, 23, 24-26, 263
furrow degeneration, 93

GAGs (glycosaminoglycans), 6, 84, 88, 145-147
gap junctions, 2, 4, 5
gelatinous drop-like dystrophy, 87, 147
generalized gangliosidosis, 142-143
ghost vessels, 50
glues, 128, 130, 193, 194, 259-261
glycocalyx, 5
glycosaminoglycans (GAGs), 6, 84, 88, 145-147
gold deposition, 103
gout, 97, 150, 151, 209
graft-versus-host disease, 14, 40, 137, 205
granular dystrophy, 80-82, 84, 85, 254, 258
gross anatomy, 1-2
guttae, 7

Hassall-Henle bodies, 94
hemidesmosomes, 2, 4
hereditary benign intraepithelial dyskeratosis (HBID), 165-166
herpes (simplex or zoster) virus
    corneal hyposthesia, 155
    inflammatory disorders, 38, 40, 46, 47, 49, 52, 100, 132, 135
    Kaposi's sarcoma, 173
    management, 26-27, 29, 30-32, 263
    neurotrophic keratopathy, 65
hormonal treatments, 218
Horner-Trantas dots, 131
HPV (human papillomavirus), 38, 164, 166
HSV. See herpes (simplex or zoster) virus
Hudson-Stahli line, 102
Hughes-Roper-Hall classification of chemical burns, 197
human fibrin-based glue, 260
human papillomavirus (HPV), 38, 164, 166
Hunter syndrome, 145, 147
hyaline degeneration, 98-99
hydrodynamic reflexes, 61-62, 63-64, 68, 205
hypercalcemia, 97, 130, 152, 153, 261
hyperlipoproteinemias, 86, 94, 141

hypolipoproteinemias, 141-142
hypopyon, 16, 17, 21, 24, 25, 30, 31
hyposthesia, 155
hysteresis, 240, 241

ICE (iridocorneal endothelial) syndrome, 91, 101-102, 256
ICRS (intracorneal ring segments), 116, 117-118, 239, 277, 279-281, 289
IK (interstitial keratitis), 48-54, 97, 99, 100, 147
immunoglobulin synthesis disorders, 148-150
immunologic diseases, 123-130, 133-137
    See also specific disease
immunomodulators, 218
incisional refractive surgery, 277-278, 289, 290
inflammatory disorders, 37-60
    degenerative, 96-98, 99-100, 261
    metabolic disorders, 145, 147, 150
    neoplasms, 164, 165-166, 168, 177
    ocular surface disorders, 65, 66-67
    systemic diseases, 125, 127, 128-129, 130-133, 134, 135-137
    See also specific disorder
"instantaneous curvature" maps, 232-233
integrated lacrimal functional unit, 206
interference, 236
interstitial keratitis (IK), 48-54, 97, 99, 100, 147
intracorneal ring segments (ICRS), 116, 117-118, 239, 277, 279-281, 289
intraocular lenses (IOLs), 150, 227, 231, 232, 237, 238, 273-276, 277, 283, 288-289
intraocular pressure measurements, 240
iridocorneal endothelial (ICE) syndrome, 91, 101-102, 256
iris cysts, 176-177
iris freckles, 175
iris masses and neoplasms, 175-178
iris melanocytoma, 176
iris melanoma, 177-178
iris nevus syndrome, 101, 102, 175
iris-claw lenses, 274
iron deposition, 100, 102, 110, 111

Kaposi's sarcoma, 49, 172-173
Kayser-Fleischer ring, 103, 152
keratoacanthoma, 165
keratoconjunctivitis, 39, 40, 45-48, 99, 130-133
    See also dry eye
keratoconus, 109-119
    connective tissue disorders, 109, 148-149, 150
    diagnosing, 110-111
    diagnostic instrumentation, 112-115, 229, 231, 236, 238, 240, 241, 242, 243, 246
    genetic factors, 91, 110
    iron deposition, 102, 110, 111
    management, 116-119, 249, 254, 277, 279, 280-281, 291
    postoperative ectasia, 109, 115, 116, 117
keratocytes, 5-6
keratoglobus, 111
keratoprosthesis, 134, 137, 199, 263-264
Khodadoust line, 253
KLAL (cadaveric keratolimbal allograft), 71-72

labrador keratopathy, 98-99
lacerations, 193-196, 198
lacrimal gland, functions of, 61, 62, 206, 207
lamellar keratoplasty, 249
    anterior techniques, 7, 118-119, 253-256, 273
    corneal dystrophies, 80, 82, 83, 85, 87, 91, 97, 99, 100
    corneal glue, 260
    mucolipidoses, 144
    neurotrophic keratopathy, 65
    posterior techniques, 7, 91, 256-257
LASEK (laser-assisted subepithelial keratomileusis), 39, 40, 270, 271, 272
laser thermokeratoplasty (LTK), 279, 290
LASIK (laser in situ keratomileusis)
    complications, 44, 65, 112, 115, 155, 208, 271, 273, 279, 280, 281, 283, 284, 287, 288
    diagnostic instrumentation, 112, 226, 228-229, 238, 239, 240, 243, 245, 246, 271
    indications for, 253, 275, 276
    iron deposition, 102
    patient follow-up, 282-283
    techniques, 270-271, 272
lattice dystrophy, 65, 82-83, 85, 96, 155, 254, 258
LCAT deficiency, 142
leishmaniasis, 49, 52-53
leprosy, 49, 51, 147, 155
limbal girdle of Vogt, 94
limbal guttering, 126, 127
limbal stem cell deficiency (LSCD), 69-72, 132, 137, 166, 264
limbal stem cell transplant (LSCT), 137, 199, 261-262
lipid keratopathy (or degeneration), 52, 100, 101
lipid metabolism disorders, 86, 94, 141-144
living-related conjunctival limbal allograft (lr-CLAL), 71, 72
"local" maps, 232-233
lr-CLAL (living-related conjunctival limbal allograft), 71, 72
LSCD (limbal stem cell deficiency), 69-72, 132, 137, 166, 264
LSCT (limbal stem cell transplant), 137, 199, 261-262
LTK (laser thermokeratoplasty), 279, 290
Lyme disease, 49, 52
lymphoid tumors, 173-174

mace, 197
macula occludens, 8
macular dystrophy, 65, 83-85, 254
map-dot-fingerprint dystrophy, 77-79, 258
Marfan syndrome, 149-150, 151, 154
marginal keratitis, 44-45, 96
marginal keratolysis. See Mooren's ulceration
Meesmann's dystrophy, 4, 75-77
megalocornea, 154
meibomian gland dysfunction (MGD), 14, 43, 45, 48, 133, 204, 208, 209, 210, 212, 213
meibomian gland, functions of, 61, 62
melanin deposition, 103
melanomas, 102, 169, 170, 171-172, 176, 177-178
Meretoja syndrome. See lattice dystrophy

mesodermal dysgenesis, 152-154
metabolic disorders, 65, 86, 93, 141-148, 150-152
MGD (meibomian gland dysfunction), 14, 43, 45, 48, 204, 208, 209, 210, 212, 213
microbial keratitis, definition of, 13
microcornea, 154
microplicae, 4
microvilli, 4, 8, 101
mineral metabolism disorders, 151-152, 153
mitogen-activated protein kinases, 207
monofocal intraocular lenses, 275
Mooren's ulceration, 70, 129-130
mucolipidoses, 143-144
mucopolysaccharides, 6, 143, 196
mucopolysaccharidoses, 142, 143, 145-147, 196
multifocal intraocular lenses, 275-276
multiple myeloma, 130
multiple sulfatase deficiency, 142, 143
Munson's sign, 110-111
mycotic keratitis. See fungal keratitis

necrotizing scleritis, 124, 125, 126, 127, 128-129, 266
nephropathic cystinosis, 144
neuroanatomic integration, 62, 64
neurotrophic keratopathy, 14, 24, 40, 63, 64-66, 67-68, 69, 205
non-Sjögren syndrome, 64, 203, 205, 212
nucleotide metabolism disorders, 150-151
nutrition, 8, 205-206, 208

OCP (ocular cicatricial pemphigoid), 14, 132, 133-135, 151, 205, 254, 261, 264
OCT (optical coherence tomography), 236-238
ocular chalcosis, 103
ocular cicatricial pemphigoid (OCP), 14, 132, 133-135, 151, 205, 254, 261, 264
ocular melanocytosis, 169
Ocular Response Analyzer, 239-240
onchocerciasis, 49, 53
optical coherence tomography (OCT), 236-238
osteogenesis imperfecta, 152

pachymetric maps, 228, 230, 234, 235, 236, 237, 238-239, 241, 271, 281-282
PAD (polymorphic amyloid degeneration), 95-96
PAM (primary acquired melanosis), 169-171
paracentral keratolysis, 126, 127, 128
parasitic keratitis
    diagnosing, 19, 28, 29-30, 31, 32, 226
    inflammatory disorders, 46, 47, 48, 49, 52-53
    Mooren's ulceration, 130
pellucid marginal corneal degeneration (PCMD), 109, 111, 112, 115-119, 231, 238, 240, 242, 243, 254, 277
penetrating keratoplasty (PK), 254
    chemical injuries, 199, 249
    corneal dystrophies, 80, 83, 85, 87, 88, 91, 92, 93, 97, 99, 100, 102
    corneal ectatic disorders, 116, 117, 118, 119
    inflammatory disorders, 39-40, 41, 48, 51, 52
    metabolic disorders, 143, 144

photorefractive keratectomy, 273
    postoperative complications, 39-40, 41, 52, 65, 67, 80, 85, 87, 93, 117, 118, 154, 155, 249, 251-253, 264, 289
    superficial corneal surgery, 263, 264
    systemic diseases, 128, 130, 134, 137
    techniques, 91, 249-251
peripheral ulcerative keratitis (PUK), 70, 96, 126, 127, 128, 129, 130
Peter's anomaly, 154
phakic intraocular lens, 227, 237, 238, 273-274, 275, 277, 283, 288-289
phlyctenular keratoconjunctivitis (PKC), 45-48
photorefractive keratectomy (PRK), 5
    diagnostic instrumentation, 239, 243, 246
    indications for, 39, 258-259, 272, 275, 284
    patient follow-up, 283
    postoperative complications of, 15, 39, 40, 65, 102, 115, 272, 273, 287, 288
    techniques, 272
phototherapeutic keratectomy (PTK), 79, 80, 82, 83, 85, 87, 98, 99, 100, 166, 273
pigmented corneal dystrophies, 102-103
pigmented neoplasms, 168-172
PK. See penetrating keratoplasty (PK)
PKC (phlyctenular keratoconjunctivitis), 45-48
placido imaging, 113, 231-233, 234, 236, 282
pleomorphism, 8, 50, 228
PLK (posterior lamellar keratoplasty), 7, 91, 256-257
polymegathism, 7, 228, 229
polymorphic amyloid degeneration (PAD), 95-96
porphyria, 150-151
posterior amorphous stromal dystrophy, 89
posterior blepharitis. See meibomian gland dysfunction (MGD)
posterior chamber lenses, 274
posterior embryotoxon, 153, 154
posterior keratoconus, 111
posterior lamellar keratoplasty (PLK), 7, 91, 256-257
posterior polymorphous dystrophy (PPMD), 91-92, 101
PPMD (posterior polymorphous dystrophy), 91-92, 101
pre-Descemet's dystrophy, 89
presbyopia, 231, 232, 273, 274-277, 278, 283
primary acquired melanosis (PAM), 169-171
PRK. See photorefractive keratectomy
progressive (essential) iris atrophy, 101, 102
protein metabolism disorders, 145
proteoglycans, 6, 9, 84
pterygium, 102, 254, 255, 259, 260, 262, 264-266
PTK (phototherapeutic keratectomy), 79, 80, 82, 83, 85, 87, 98, 99, 100, 166, 273
PUK (peripheral ulcerative keratitis), 70, 96, 126, 127, 128, 129, 130
punctate epithelial keratitis, 37-39, 43, 51, 67, 131, 132, 147-148, 197, 206
pupil size determination, 282

"Quad maps," 234, 235

racial melanosis, 168-169
radial keratotomy (RK), 65, 102, 244, 247, 277-278, 289, 290
recurrent corneal erosion (RCE), 4, 24, 40, 75, 76, 148, 191, 257-258
Reiger's anomaly and Reiger's syndrome, 153, 154
Reis-Bücklers dystrophy, 79-80, 155
residual refractive errors, 288, 290
resistance factor, 240, 241
rheumatoid arthritis, 40, 53-54, 97, 103, 123-128, 147
Rizutti's sign, 110
RK (radial keratotomy), 65, 102, 244, 247, 277-278, 289, 290
rosacea, 43-44, 46, 47

Salzmann's nodular degeneration, 50, 99-100, 102, 254, 255
Sanfilippo syndrome, 147
SBK (sub-Bowman's keratomileusis), 270
scanning slit, 234, 235
Scheimpflug imaging, 234-236, 237, 242
Schnyder's crystalline dystrophy, 85-87, 141
Schwalbe's line, 153
scleritis, 53, 124-125, 126, 127, 128, 151, 168, 266
scleromalacia perforans, 125, 126, 151
sclerosing keratitis, 126-127
sebaceous gland carcinoma, 174, 175
secondary Sjögren's syndrome, 123-124, 128, 129, 203
secretagogues, 218
sharp trauma, 193-196, 198
shield ulcers, 131, 133
siderosis, 102
silver deposition, 103
Sjögren syndrome, 39, 40, 42-43, 64, 66, 203, 204, 212, 254
    See also secondary Sjögren's syndrome
SJS (Stevens-Johnson syndrome), 14, 66, 70, 71, 135-137, 205, 261, 264
SK (superficial keratectomy), 79, 80, 82, 99, 100, 258-259
SLE (systemic lupus erythematosis), 39, 40, 128
slit scanning, 234, 235
SLK (superior limbic keratoconjunctivitis), 39, 40
specular microscopy, 226-228, 239
spheroidal degeneration, 98-99
sphingolipidoses, 142-143
SPK (superficial punctate keratitis), 37-39, 197
squamous cell carcinoma, 165, 167-168
squamous cells, 2, 3, 4-5
stellate wounds, 195
Stevens-Johnson syndrome (SJS), 14, 66, 70, 71, 135-137, 205, 261, 264
Stocker line, 102
striate melanokeratosis, 103
stroma
    anatomy and physiology, 2, 4, 5-7, 8-10
    congenital disorders, 49-50, 154
    corneal dystrophies, 75, 80-89, 90, 93, 95, 96, 99, 100, 102, 103, 141, 254, 258
    corneal ectatic disorders, 110, 111, 112, 115, 118-119

diagnostic instrumentation, 229, 230, 238, 240
inflammatory disorders, 37, 38, 39, 43, 45, 47, 48-54
limbal stem cell deficiency, 70
metabolic disorders, 141, 142, 144, 146, 148
microbial keratitis
    bacterial, 15, 16, 17, 18, 21, 252
    fungal, 25, 26
    parasitic, 30
    viral, 26-27, 29, 30, 38, 52
neoplasms, 163, 171, 177
surgical procedures, 6
    refractive corrections, 270-271, 282, 283, 287, 288, 289, 290-291
    superficial, 79, 257-258, 262-263
    transplants, 252, 254, 255, 256, 257
systemic diseases, 126, 127, 128, 130
thermal procedures, 278-279
trauma, 192, 193, 196, 197, 199
sub-Bowman's keratomileusis (SBK), 270
subepithelial neoplasia, 172-174
superficial corneal surgery, 257-264
    See also specific technique
superficial keratectomy (SK), 79, 80, 82, 99, 100, 258-259
superficial punctate keratitis (SPK), 37-39, 197
superior limbic keratoconjunctivitis (SLK), 39, 40
surface ablation techniques, 270, 272-273, 287, 288
    See also specific technique
swelling pressure, 9
symblepharon, 128, 135, 136, 137, 199, 200
syphilitic interstitial keratitis, 48-51
systemic diseases, 49, 123-137, 206
    See also specific disease
systemic interstitial keratitis, 49, 53-54
systemic lupus erythematosis (SLE), 39, 40, 128

tangential maps, 232-233, 234, 236
Tangier disease, 142
tear clearance, 13-14, 61, 62, 64, 68, 69
tear film
    anatomy and physiology, 4, 5, 8, 9
    composition, 41, 43, 61-62, 63, 64, 69, 134, 203, 205, 206-207, 212
    defense mechanisms, 13-14, 61-66
    dry eye definitions, 201, 202
    inflammatory disorders, 41, 43
    instability, 63, 64, 66, 206, 207, 210
    limbal stem cell deficiency, 69-70
    See also aqueous tear deficiency
tear film breakup time (TFBUT), 210, 211, 234
tear gas, 197
tear hyperosmolarity, 203, 205, 206-207, 212
Terrien's marginal degeneration, 96-97
TFBUT (tear film breakup time), 210, 211, 234
thermal procedures, 278-279, 290
Thiel-Behnke dystrophy, 79-80
Thygeson's superficial punctate keratitis (TSPK), 37-39, 43
tight junctions, 5, 8
tissue adhesives or glues, 128, 130, 193, 194, 259-261
tomography/topography, 234-238

topographic maps, 112-115, 229, 230, 231-236, 237, 241, 242, 243, 244, 245-246, 281-282
trauma, 191-200
  anatomy and physiology, 4, 9
  corneal dystrophies, 97, 100, 103
  corneal infections, 14, 17, 23-24, 191, 192
  diagnostic instrumentation, 242, 243
  inflammatory disorders, 39, 40, 41
  Mooren's ulceration, 130
  ocular surface disorders, 65, 110, 163, 165
  surgical procedures, 249, 254, 258, 259, 273, 283, 289
TSPK (Thygeson's superficial punctate keratitis), 37-39, 43
tuberculosis, 45-47, 48, 49, 51
tyrosinemia, 144

ultrasound measurement techniques, 228-231, 238-239, 271, 281-282

verisyse lenses, 274
vernal keratoconjunctivitis (VKC), 99, 130-133

very high-frequency (VHF) ultrasound eye scanner, 229-231
viral interstitial keratitis, 49, 52
viral keratitis
  corneal glue, 260
  corneal hyposthesia, 155
  inflammatory disorders, 38, 39, 40, 46, 47, 49, 52, 100, 130, 132, 135
  management, 26-27, 29, 30-33, 249, 263
  neoplasms, 164, 166, 172-173
  ocular surface disorders, 65
VKC (vernal keratoconjunctivitis), 99, 130-133
Vogt's striae, 110, 111

wavefront technology, 236, 269-270, 282
Wegener's granulomatosis (WG), 40, 53, 128-129
Wilson's disease, 103, 151-152, 153
wing cells, 2, 3, 4

zonula occludens, 5, 8
zoster virus. See herpes (simplex or zoster) virus

CURBSIDE
Consultation

The exciting and unique *Curbside Consultation Series* is designed to effectively provide ophthalmologists with practical, to the point, evidence-based answers to the questions most frequently asked during informal consultations between colleagues.

Each specialized book included in the *Curbside Consultation Series* offers quick access to current medical information with the ease and convenience of a conversation. Expert consultants who are recognized leaders in their fields provide their advice, preferences, and opinions to answer the tricky questions that require ophthalmologists to practice the "art" of medicine.

Written with a similar reader-friendly Q and A format and including images, diagrams, and references, each book in the *Curbside Consultation Series* will serve as a solid, go-to reference for practicing ophthalmologists and residents alike.

Series Editor: David F. Chang, MD

Curbside Consultation in Cataract Surgery:
49 Clinical Questions
David F. Chang, MD
288 pp., Soft Cover, 2007, ISBN 13 978-1-55642-799-2,
Order# 67999, **$79.95**

Curbside Consultation in Cornea and External Disease: 49 Clinical Questions
Francis W. Price Jr., MD
250 pp., Soft Cover, Due Early 2010,
ISBN 13 978-1-55642-931-6,
Order# 69316**, $79.95**

Curbside Consultation in Glaucoma:
49 Clinical Questions
Dale K. Heuer, MD
272 pp., Soft Cover, 2008, ISBN 13 978-1-55642-832-6,
Order# 68324, **$79.95**

Curbside Consultation in Neuro-Ophthalmology:
49 Clinical Questions
Andrew G. Lee, MD
240 pp., Soft Cover, 2009, ISBN 13 978-1-55642-840-1,
Order# 68401, **$79.95**

Curbside Consultation in Oculoplastics:
49 Clinical Questions
Robert C. Kersten, MD
250 pp., Soft Cover, Due Late 2010,
ISBN 13 978-1-55642-914-9,
Order# 69142, **$79.95**

Curbside Consultation of the Retina:
49 Clinical Questions
Sharon Fekrat, MD
240 pp., Soft Cover, 2010, ISBN 13 978-1-55642-885-2,
Order# 68852, **$79.95**

WWW.CURBSIDECONSULTATIONS.COM